The Coming of the Spirit of Pestilence

The Coming of the
Spirit of Pestilence

Introduced Infectious Diseases and Population Decline

among Northwest Coast Indians, 1774–1874

ROBERT BOYD

UBC PRESS

Vancouver and Toronto

UNIVERSITY OF WASHINGTON PRESS

Seattle and London

TO THE ANCESTORS

Published in the United States of America by the University of Washington Press,
P.O. Box 50096, Seattle, WA 98145-5096
Published simultaneously in Canada by UBC Press, 6344 Memorial Road,
Vancouver, British Columbia V6T 1Z2

Cataloging in Publication Data can be found at the back of the book.

The paper used in this publication is acid-free and recycled from 10 percent
post-consumer and at least 50 percent pre-consumer waste. It meets the
minimum requirements of American National Standard for Information
Sciences—Permanence of Paper for Printed Library Materials,
ANSI Z39.48-1984. ♻ ⊗

The Haida Indians, Native people of the Queen Charlotte Islands, associated the appearance of epidemic diseases with the "Pestilence spirit" or "spirit of the Pestilence," which arrived on large ships, like the first White men to visit their country. According to a Haida oral tradition that may recall the visit of explorer George Dixon in 1787, a dozen years after the first smallpox epidemic spread through the islands: "When . . . the first ship . . . came in sight they thought it was the spirit of the 'Pestilence,' and dancing on the shore, they waved their palms toward the newcomers to turn back. When the White people landed, they sent down to them their old men, who had only a few years to live anyway, expecting them to fall dead."

—Erna Gunther, *Indian Life on the Northwest Coast of North America*

Contents

Illustrations

TABLES

Preface

This book is a study of the introduction of infectious diseases among the Indians of the Northwest Coast culture area in the first century of contact (1774–1874) and of the effects of these new diseases on Native American population size, structure, interactions, and viability. The Pacific Northwest in 1774 was "virgin soil" for a long list of infectious diseases that had evolved in the Eastern Hemisphere. In the period covered in this volume, most diseases that could be maintained by Northwest Indian populations appeared in the area in epidemic form or became established in an endemic focus. Using all extant ethnohistorical data, chapters 2 through 7 reconstruct in detail six important epidemic episodes and establish a time frame for disease introduction on the Northwest Coast.

Previous researchers have maintained that the introduction of Old World diseases to the Americas after 1492 resulted in "the greatest demographic disaster in the history of the world" (Denevan 1976: 7). It has been difficult to test the hypothesis of disease-induced population decline in most parts of the Western Hemisphere. From the Northwest Coast, however, the relatively good quality of demographic data and late date of disease introduction provide a laboratory to test this theory. Chapters 8 and 9 examine all extant population estimates and censuses for two regions of the Native Northwest and assess the extent and nature of population decline in each.

The data demonstrate that disease was indeed the major cause of Indian depopulation in the Northwest. North of the forty-seventh parallel, the major cause of mortality was smallpox, which appeared in regularly spaced epidemic waves, whose timing was determined by chance introduction and the availability of a pool of non-immune susceptibles. In that portion of the southern coast where malaria appeared and became endemic, depopulation was more extensive. The introduction of the disease caused heavy mortality, which persisted particularly in later years among the young, accompanied by a decline in fertility.

Patterns such as these should have relevance in other areas where virulent Old World diseases were introduced to small-scale societies.

This book has been over 20 years in the making. It began, innocently enough, in autumn 1974 with a reading and conference class with Dr. Wayne Suttles, professor of anthropology at Portland State University, and evolved over the next 10 years into my doctoral dissertation, "The Introduction of Infectious Diseases among the Indians of the Pacific Northwest, 1774–1874" (University of Washington, 1985). The dissertation focused on three epidemics (smallpox in the 1770s, "fever and ague" in the 1830s, and smallpox in 1836–37) and population decline in three regions (North Coast, lower Columbia River valley, and the Plateau culture area). In 1993 the convergence of several events encouraged me to consider revising the dissertation in book form. Three new chapters were written, and a revised manuscript was submitted to the University of Washington Press in early 1995.

Earlier versions of several sections of the book have been published elsewhere. The first version of chapter 4 appeared as "Another Look at the 'Fever and Ague' of Western Oregon" in *Ethnohistory* 22(2) (1975). The greater part of chapters 2 and 6 were published as "Smallpox on the Northwest Coast: The First Epidemics" in *BC Studies* 101 and "The Pacific Northwest Coast Measles Epidemic of 1847–1848" in the *Oregon Historical Quarterly* 95(1), both in 1994. Data from the demographic chapters have been included in "Seasonal Population Movement on the Lower Columbia River: The Social and Ecological Context" (with Yvonne Hajda), *American Ethnologist* 14(2) (1987); "Population Decline from Two Epidemics on the Northwest Coast" in the Smithsonian Institution's *Disease and Demography in the Americas* (1992); and "Kalapuya Disease and Depopulation" in Mission Mill Museum's *What Price Eden? The Willamette Valley in Transition, 1812–1855* (1995). A summary article of my dissertation research, "Demographic History, 1774–1874" (commissioned in

1986), was printed in *Northwest Coast,* volume 7 of the Smithsonian's *Handbook of North American Indians* (1990); equivalent data from the Plateau culture area appear in *Plateau,* volume 14 of the *Handbook* (1998).

Travel grants from the University of Washington Department of Anthropology and the American Philosophical Society supported research at the Hudson's Bay Company Archives, the Royal British Columbia Archives, and the Bancroft Library. Research on the 1862 smallpox epidemic was made possible by a grant from the Toronto-based Hannah Institute for the History of Medicine.

Over the years, a number of people have helped in different ways in the writing of this book. Wayne Suttles initially kindled my interest in Northwest Coast Indian cultures, and it was under his tutelage that I discovered the wealth of information that may be found in the ethnohistorical record. The members of my Ph.D. committee, Eugene Hunn, Pamela Amoss, Donna Leonetti, Keith Murray, James Watson, and James Whorton, provided encouragement and advice over the five years during which the dissertation was researched and written. Other individuals who helped at various points along the way should be acknowledged and thanked here: Kenneth Ames, Jerome Cybulski, Henry Dobyns, Robert Galois, James Gibson, Yvonne Hajda, Roberta Hall, Michael Harkin, Susanne (Storie) Hilton, Dell Hymes, John Norris, Helen H. Norton, Robert Ruby, and the anonymous reviewers for the University of Washington Press. Thanks are also due to the staffs of the Regional Research Library of the Oregon Historical Society, the Northwest Collection at the University of Washington Library, and the Hudson's Bay Company Archives in Winnipeg; to Boris Gorodnitsky and Irina Gorodnitskaya, who translated Russian documents for chapter 5; to Dr. Ric Vrana of the Department of Geography at Portland State University, who drafted the maps; and to Pamela J. Bruton, Michael Duckworth, and Julidta Tarver of the University of Washington Press, who shepherded the manuscript through its final stages. I owe special debts to Dr. C. Dolores Gregory of the Portland Area Indian Health Service and to my family, whose steadfast emotional support during the difficult final years when this book was completed kept me going until I reached my goal. Any errors of interpretation in the final manuscript, of course, are mine alone.

The Coming of the Spirit of Pestilence

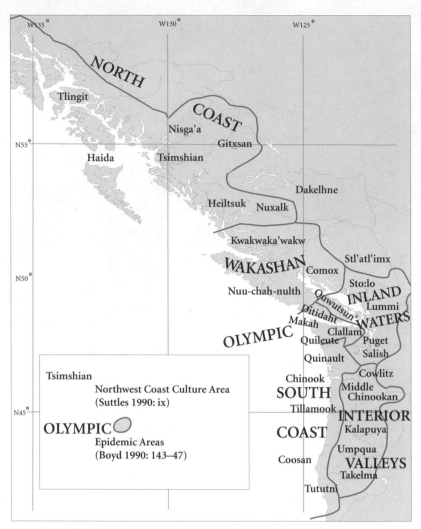

MAP 1. Northwest Coast Culture Area (with Epidemic Areas; see Chapter 10)

Introduction

The Northwest Coast is one of the best-known and most distinctive of all the Native American culture areas. It comprises all the Indian cultures of present-day Oregon and Washington west of the Cascade Mountains, British Columbia west of the Coast Range, and southeast Alaska. It includes such well-known peoples as the Tlingit, Haida, Kwakwaka'wakw (Kwakiutl), Nuu-chah-nulth (Nootka), Coast Salish (several groups), and Chinookans (map 1). Distinctive features of the culture area include a nonagricultural economy heavily reliant on aquatic foods, particularly salmon; an emphasis on woodworking using the ubiquitous western red cedar (plank houses, dugout canoes, and "bent-boxes"); political structures centering on family lines and local groups; guardian spirits, spirit quests, and winter ceremonies; and several distinctive subregional traits such as potlatching, totem poles, canoe burials, and the well-known "Northern art style" (Kroeber 1923; Drucker 1955).

In the late 1700s, when peoples of Euro-American descent began to visit the Northwest, they reported cultures that were vigorous, rich, diverse, and strong. After a century of Euro-American contact, however, these cultures were shattered: populations had plummeted, some groups had become extinct, and others were shadows of their former selves. From a precontact population conservatively estimated at over 180,000, only about 35,000 to 40,000 were left.

What happened to produce this change? It was not the result of wars or intentional destruction on the part of the newly arrived Euro-Americans, as some would have it. The change was brought about by the introduction of *microorganisms* that had evolved in the Eastern Hemisphere and were carried by the Euro-American immigrants, giving the newcomers a temporary biological advantage over the Native peoples of the Northwest Coast. The microorganisms caused diseases that had been unknown in this formerly isolated part of the world. And these diseases, in the Northwest as elsewhere in the Americas, caused the decimation of Native populations.

Until very recently, the role of disease introduction in Northwest history has been neither adequately studied nor fully understood.[1] As this book shows, Euro-American colonization of each subregion of the Northwest closely followed important epidemics among local Native Americans: the "fever and ague" in western Oregon after 1830, with Indian depopulation and a White majority by 1845; 1848 measles and 1853 smallpox in western Washington, with indigenous depopulation and a White majority by 1858; and 1862 smallpox and depopulation in Native coastal British Columbia and a White majority by the early 1880s.

Particularly since 1992, the five hundredth anniversary of Columbus's "discovery" of the Americas, the study of "disease transfer" has become important in the field of anthropology.[2] Disease transfer is an important element in the contact process between dissimilar peoples and cultures. It has had an important impact on world history, especially in explaining the expansion of Western culture. And it may be viewed as an example of biocultural evolution, where populations' abilities to adapt to new environments or environmental change determine whether they increase their numbers and prosper or suffer decline or extinction.

For several reasons, the Northwest Coast culture area, between the first Euro-American contact in 1774 and the last major epidemic in 1875, is an ideal laboratory for studying disease transfer.[3] First of all, many of the infectious

1. There is an encouraging trend to incorporate anthropological data and ideas on culture contact processes in studies of the history of western North America. See, e.g., White 1991: pt. 1.

2. For summaries of the latest research on the topic, see Verano and Ubelaker 1992; Dobyns 1993.

3. The only other region in the "New World" with documentation on disease introduction and depopulation equivalent in quality to the Northwest is Polynesia. For what is probably the most completely documented "disease and depopulation" study available, see McArthur 1967.

diseases brought to the Americas after 1492 appeared on the Northwest Coast during this period: smallpox and malaria were most important, though measles, tuberculosis, influenza, dysentery, and syphilis also had significant demographic impacts. The nature of the spread and the intensity of the effects of these diseases indicate that they were introduced to epidemiologically "virgin" populations. The Northwest Coast experience provides, in microcosm, an unusually graphic example of a process which has happened in many other parts of the world at much earlier times.

Second, given the relatively late date and the nature of the contact situation in the Northwest, the disease and depopulation experience is particularly well documented. Relatively good historical records allow reconstruction of processes of disease transfer and important epidemic episodes. Censuses of Native populations taken by the Hudson's Bay Company and early government officials allow reconstruction of depopulation trends. The data lend themselves well to the methods of the emerging fields of historical epidemiology and historical demography. Disease introduction and population decline in more accessible and densely populated regions of the aboriginal Americas occurred much closer to 1492, and most of the details of the phenomena have been lost.

This book tests the "disease and depopulation" hypothesis by establishing a chronology of disease introduction in the Northwest Coast (chapters 2–7), coordinating it with regional population histories, and ultimately demonstrating the effect of "new" diseases on the size, structure, interactions, and viability of historically known Northwest Indian populations (chapters 8–10). It illustrates how specific diseases or disease classes interact in different, patterned ways with small populations. And it provides a foundation for the generation of more-specific hypotheses about the interaction of new diseases and disease-caused population changes with technoenvironmental, social, ideological, and other relevant cultural subsystems in the Northwest Coast and, by extension, among other peoples and at earlier times.

Understanding the process of disease transfer is a first step in appreciating the humanity and richness of our indigenous forerunners in the Pacific Northwest. In the brief span of a century these peoples endured several consecutive plagues, many on a par with Europe's Black Death in terms of human suffering and cultural disruption. This experience needs to be recognized and acknowledged. Northwest Native peoples have preserved their cultural traditions to a remarkable extent, and anthropologists have chronicled what they could, but most of the rich, cumulated tradition can no longer be retrieved. Culturally, the loss of the Northwest Native Americans is ours as well.

This book is also about a phenomenon that continues today: the introduction of new diseases. Since 1875, the peoples of the Pacific Northwest, native and newcomer, have continued to experience and suffer from "new" diseases. Indian peoples have endured epidemics of tuberculosis and trachoma and (most recently) diabetes. Among immigrant Northwesterners, the 1918 influenza epidemic caused several thousand deaths. A polio epidemic arrived in the early fifties, and since the early 1980s, we have been dealing with a new plague, AIDS.[4]

What do we know about these new diseases? Where do they come from and why? How do they spread and how can we deal with them? What effects do they have on society? Specific answers, of course, will differ with each disease and will not be readily forthcoming. At present, our pool of knowledge on this entire phenomenon is much too shallow. But if we examine what happened with "new" diseases in the past, we can get some idea of where, why, and how they arose and how people dealt with them, and we can begin to appreciate their supreme importance for human history and the human condition.

4. On the latest "new" diseases to appear in contemporary society, see Garrett 1994.

1 / Historical Epidemiology

Background and Precedents

THE EPIDEMIOLOGICAL APPROACH TO HUMAN DISEASE

The epidemiological perspective on disease differs from the clinical perspective most people are used to. In clinical medicine human diseases are seen as being caused by particular varieties of "germs" that invade human hosts and cause an array of specific symptoms. The frame of reference is particularistic: the emphasis is on the individual host and a description of the disease entity as it manifests itself in symptoms that can be observed, treated, or cured in the individual. Epidemiology, in contrast, views disease from an "ecological" perspective (Burnet and White 1972: chap. 1) which emphasizes (1) the interaction between pathogen and human populations and (2) the relationships of both to the larger environment and cultural systems. Epidemiology is concerned with diseases as they are expressed, not in individuals, but in populations; it tries to isolate the determinants of diseases by studying disease distribution in space and time rather than pathogen or host characteristics.

How epidemiological studies work may be illustrated by an example. A classic study in the epidemiological literature is Dr. John Snow's 1855 paper "On the Mode of Communication of Cholera" (see Snow 1936), which examined a minor epidemic of cholera in a London neighborhood in August–September 1854. In the mid-1800s, the cause of cholera was unknown. Dr. Snow obtained a complete list of cholera deaths, with home addresses, from the General Register Office. He then plotted the addresses on a map. Geographically, the feature that most of the cases had in common was proximity to a single water source, the Broad Street Pump. Dr. Snow hypothesized that the disease was transmitted through this water. A friend examined the pump water under a microscope and noted the presence of "minute whitish flocculi" (now known to be the causal agent, the bacterium *Vibrio cholerae*). Snow also grouped the cases by time of death: 12 (2%) deaths occurred between 19 and 31 August; 344 (56%) were recorded in the first four days of September; and 168 (27%) occurred between 5 and 9 September, the day after the pump was closed. These two methods, mapping of cases and placement in a time line, are basic to epidemiological studies and are used in chapters 2 through 7 of this book.[1]

Another way of perceiving epidemiology is as a relationship between two different populations: host and parasite. Human beings serve as environments for a number of parasites, the vast majority of which are benign or even beneficial (Rosebury 1962). "Pathogens," however, are parasites that have adverse effects on their hosts, expressed in the form of debilitating diseases (Knight 1982: 2). Because parasites that kill their human hosts jeopardize their own existence, virulent diseases are sometimes seen as temporary stages in an evolutionary process ideally leading to a more balanced parasite-host relationship (Burnet and White 1972: 20). Parasite and host populations may "co-evolve" through time, though there are great differences in the tempo and kind of evolution. Parasites, with enormous numbers and short life spans, may evolve biologically at a rapid rate. Humans, with fewer numbers and longer

---

1. A major methodological difference between most epidemiological studies and the present study involves the data base. Instead of cases, the basic units in this book are documentary citations of disease: historical, ethnographic, and from the folk literature. Besides being a study on historical epidemiology, this book is also a species of ethnohistory, or the historical study of preliterate peoples. The historical sources, drawn from the writings of explorers, traders, missionaries, and early settlers, are evaluated according to the normal critical canons of historiography: who wrote it; where, when, and why was it written; is it reliable, a true statement of historical fact? Primary historical accounts provide the most valuable data on the disease experience, as they are grounded in space and time. Native accounts from the oral literature (tales and myths; Boas 1916: 565) have neither of these advantages and must be evaluated for what they are, as a form of literature and performance: incidents may be added or subtracted, diffuse from one culture to another, and otherwise be modified to satisfy the requirements of performance or the cultural message that is being transmitted (Hymes 1990). The oral literature may inform us of the presence of certain diseases; in some cases it may contain datable elements; but its major importance is to show the responses of Native peoples to diseases and the cultural constructions that they built around them.

life spans, change their genetic makeup relatively slowly; their usual response to changes in parasite populations is behavioral (or cultural), not biological.

STAGES IN HUMAN DISEASE HISTORY

Diseases are dynamic entities which evolve and spread and interact in different ways with different kinds of human societies. It is a small step beyond this observation to place human diseases in historical perspective and note their correspondence to different levels (or stages) of cultural development. Table 1, which incorporates the insights of several researchers on the evolution of human diseases, does just this and provides a broad framework that incorporates Northwest Coast disease history.

Until 1492, the human populations and human diseases of the Eastern and Western Hemispheres evolved in isolation from one another. Hunting and gathering societies in each hemisphere shared a pool of similar diseases, but as cultures evolved independently through village to urban stages, their disease pools diverged dramatically. For our purposes, the first four stages in table 1 are important. The Northwest Coast, before contact, was a variety of stage 1 (hunter-gatherers), with some characteristics of stage 2 (Neolithic villages). The most important diseases that were brought to the Northwest between 1775 and 1875 evolved in the Old World during stage 2 and stage 3 (urban civilization). And the actual process of disease introduction in the Northwest was but a very late chapter in stage 4 (interhemispheric exchange).

Stage 1: Hunter-Gatherer Diseases

Distinctive characteristics of hunter-gatherer populations include small group size, low population density, and a considerable degree of physical mobility. Hunter-gatherers are by definition nonagricultural, have few plant or animal domesticates, and do not practice wholesale modification of their environments. Because of their demographic characteristics, they cannot indefinitely support density-dependent diseases like smallpox, and their mobility protects them from excessive waste buildup and parasitic infection. The lack of agriculture usually implies broader-based, more healthy diets; the lack of domesticated animals means negligible exposure to their diseases; and relatively less environmental disturbance suggests less contact with disease

TABLE 1. Stages in the Relationships between Human Hosts and Parasites

Stage and Beginning Date	Demographic Characteristics	Health/Health Care System	Typical Diseases
1. Hunter-gatherers (ca. 40,000 B.P.)	Population stability (births = deaths) Small size of normally interacting unit General good health of population: diverse, balanced diet; exercise	Mobility promotes hygiene Limited modification of environment Transient contact with disease vectors and animal hosts	Chronic diseases maintained in individual (various *Treponema* species, *Mycobacterium leprae*, ringworm, *Herpes simplex*, and *H. zoster*) Transient vector-carried and zoonotic diseases Food poisoning
2. Neolithic villages (ca. 12,000 B.P. in Old World)	Population increase (fertility > mortality) Larger size of normally interacting group (villages of 500+) Decline in nutrition with transition from broad (wild) to narrow (domestic) food base	Sedentism creates hygiene (waste disposal) problems Significant modification of environment: tilling, deforestation, irrigation Closer contact with disease vectors and domesticated animals	Diseases related to poor hygiene: intestinal parasites, enteric viruses (dysentery) Deficiency diseases Vector-carried diseases favored by environmental modification: malaria, typhus, trypanosomiasis, schistosomiasis Chronic diseases of zoonotic origin (tuberculosis)

3. Urban civilization (ca. 5000 B.P. in Old World)	Urban areas: large, dense, continuous populations, economically dependent upon "Neolithic" (agricultural village) hinterland High fertility of villages compensates for high mortality of urban areas; differential migration	Significant class differences in hygiene and health care Widespread social interactions (intra- and extraregional) promote disease spread Intensified contact in agricultural areas with disease vectors and domesticated animal hosts	Density-dependent epidemic diseases arising from zoonotic hosts: smallpox, measles, influenza, colds (all respiratory); plague (vector); cholera (enteric) Continued importance of "Neolithic" diseases in agricultural hinterland
4. Interhemispheric exchange (500 B.P.)	Contact established between previously isolated populations: depopulation of New World; exponential increase of Old World populations	Conflict of previously isolated systems: health care, hygiene, sociocultural	Addition of Old World diseases to New World inventory: universalization of disease pools
5. Industrial and postindustrial world (ca. 150 B.P.)	Continued high fertility plus declining mortality throughout most of world; "demographic transition" to low mortality and fertility rates in most fully industrialized areas Advanced methods of contraception (birth control) in industrialized areas Increase in longevity	"Sanitary revolution" Vaccines and control of infectious diseases Health care sophistication Dietary shifts Environmental pollution	Environmental and occupational contaminants and diseases: cancers, "black lung," etc. Nutrition-related ailments: caries, diabetes, heart disease Changes in sexual habits: venereal herpes, AIDS Diseases of old age: Alzheimer's, osteoporosis, Parkinson's

SOURCES: See especially Cockburn 1959, 1963, 1967, 1971; as well as Polgar 1964; Fenner 1971; Armelagos and Dewey 1970; and Armelagos 1991. Characteristics of stage 5 have been summarized from Omran 1971; Rosen 1953; Corruccini and Kaul 1983.

vectors such as mosquitoes. Hunter-gatherers, it is often said, are healthy people. Relatively speaking (and in a precontact state), this is true.

But this does not mean that hunting-gathering peoples are disease free by any means. The ailments that they *do* have are quite consistent with the demographic and social characteristics of their stage. All hunter-gatherers have a high frequency of arthritis, indicative of physical stress. They are subject to internal parasites and food poisoning that result from incompletely prepared or contaminated food. And they harbor a class of chronic infections, which persist and remain infective in individuals for long periods of time.[2] Indigenous Northwest Coast ailments, as documented in the paleopathological record and oral literature, were typical of this stage, as well as including some afflictions that were more specific to the region. What is known about precontact Northwest Coast diseases is summarized in appendix 1 and tables 5 and 6 (see pp. 279–88).

Stage 2: Disease Patterns of Neolithic Villages

The Northwest Coast had some of the characteristics of the Neolithic stage: settled villages (for at least half of the year), as well as other (temporary) population concentrations; a greater continuity of settlement and generally larger populations than are usual for hunter-gatherers. Some hygiene and parasitic problems may have intensified due to population concentrations. Potential disease vectors—lice and anopheline mosquitoes—were present in the Northwest but carried few diseases before contact.

Agriculture and settled village life evolved independently in the two hemispheres, and it was during this stage that the disease histories of the two parts of the world began to diverge dramatically. The Old World (Eurasia and Africa) reached the Neolithic stage earlier and, because of its greater landmass and diversity of ecosystems disrupted by the changes associated with early agriculture, experienced a broader array of new diseases. The cutting of underbrush increased exposure to the mites and flies that carry the agents of scrub typhus and trypanosomiasis (sleeping sickness); irrigation increased human contact with the snails that harbor schistosomiasis; and most important of all,

2. These characteristics are summarized from Cleland 1928 and Basedow 1932 (Australian Aborigines); Polunin 1967, 1977 (Southeast Asian hunter-gatherers); Howell 1979 (South African !Kung); and Dunn 1968 and Service 1979 (general).

deforestation increased human contact with disease-carrying mosquitoes of the genera *Aëdes* (yellow fever) and *Anopheles* (malaria). Of these important "ecological" diseases, many did not transfer to the Americas; but when the organisms causing yellow fever and malaria came into contact with suitable American mosquito vectors, they caused epidemics and, in the case of malaria, significant population loss. The clinical and epidemiological characteristics of malaria, an important cause of Native American depopulation on the southern Northwest Coast, are summarized in appendix 2 (see pp. 289–93).

Stage 3: Disease Patterns of Urban Areas

Urban civilizations, of course, arose in both the Old World and in the Americas. But it was only in the Old World that the highly virulent, density-dependent "diseases of civilization" appeared. A major reason for this difference appears to relate to the presence in the Old World (and absence in the New) of domesticated animals which harbored the microbial ancestors of the "diseases of civilization." The smallpox virus, for instance, is similar to the virus that causes pox diseases in cattle; the measles virus is similar to that causing rinderpest and canine distemper; the influenza virus is similar to flu viruses of swine and poultry; and so on (Van Blerkom 1991; Fiennes 1978; Cockburn 1959, 1963, 1967, 1971).

Most of the "crowd diseases" affect only soft body parts, so we must turn to the written record to re-create their history. Smallpox first appears in Egyptian records in ca. 1200 B.C.; the first mentions of influenza, typhoid, dysentery, mumps, and diphtheria are by Hippocrates in 400 B.C. Measles was not recorded until A.D. 500 in Arabia, and then questionably. Other diseases have even later dates: cholera by 1517, whooping cough by 1519, and scarlet fever not until the 1600s, all in the Old World (Hare 1967).

The major crowd diseases smallpox, measles, influenza, and mumps are all viral and share the characteristics of rapid duration of infection plus immunity after recovery. In the late 1960s, epidemiologists studying measles endemicity and die-out in 19 island populations discovered an intriguing pattern: in populations above 300,000, measles was always present ("endemic"); in populations below that number, it died out, reappearing only when introduced from outside and disappearing again after an epidemic visitation (Black 1966). It was suggested that measles and other crowd diseases must therefore be evolutionary novelties, appearing after the rise of urban areas (Black 1966;

Cockburn 1959, 1963, 1967, 1971). This theory gains support from the relatively late documentation of most of these diseases in the historical record. A summary of the clinical and epidemiological characteristics of smallpox, the single most destructive introduced disease among Northwest Coast Native Americans, is presented in appendix 2.

With the crowd diseases present in densely populated areas, and "Neolithic" diseases persisting in the agricultural hinterlands in the Old World, an interesting dynamic took shape. Cities and rural villages existed in a symbiotic relationship—the one providing political control and networks; the other, food and a sustaining inflow of population. Historian William McNeill has pointed out that, periodically, the crowd diseases would break out of their urban settings and spread in epidemic form among the non-immune peripheral villages. McNeill suggests that this epidemiological effect was an important dynamic in the spread of major civilizations and demise of simpler cultures (1976, 1979).

Stage 4: Interhemispheric Exchange

After 1492, this pattern took on a whole new perspective. The urban civilizations of the Old World became donors of new diseases to a different set of "peripheral" peoples, those of the Americas. Although historian Alfred Crosby (1972) called this process the "Columbian Exchange," with respect to disease it was definitely lopsided. The most virulent Old World crowd diseases spread to the Americas, but the only significant ailments that moved in the other direction were syphilis and rheumatoid arthritis. Table 2 summarizes the latest thinking on interhemispheric disease exchange.

THE AMERICAN "PANDEMIC" OF THE 1520S

Shortly after interhemispheric contact was established, epidemics of new diseases appeared in both hemispheres: syphilis in Europe and influenza among the Indians of Hispaniola (Guerra 1988). The most important, however, was certainly the smallpox "pandemic" of the 1520s, which led to what geographer William Denevan has called "the greatest demographic disaster in the history of the world" (1976: 7). The pandemic began in 1519 in Santo Domingo, having been brought from Spain, probably by someone who was in the latency stage when the voyage began. Once introduced to the West Indies, smallpox

TABLE 2. Interhemispheric Exchange of Diseases

Native American Diseases[a]	Disease Imports
1. Salmonella and other food poisons	1. Smallpox
2. Fungal diseases: some tineas, blastomycosis, etc.	2. Malaria
	3. Viral influenza
3. Diseases caused by intestinal parasites: tapeworms, roundworms, pinworms	4. Yellow fever
	5. Measles
	6. Typhus
4. Streptococcus and staphylococcus	7. Bubonic plague
5. Shigellosis	8. Typhoid fever
6. Gastroenteritis	9. Cholera
7. Hepatitis	10. Pertussis
8. Encephalitis	11. Diphtheria
9. Viral pneumonia	12. Scarlatina
10. Tuberculosis	13. Chicken pox/shingles
11. Nonvenereal syphilis	14. Polio
12. Pinta	15. Amebiasis
13. Venereal syphilis	16. Trachoma
14. Rheumatoid arthritis	17. Hookworm and whipworm[b]
15. American trypanosomiasis	
16. American leishmaniasis	
17. Bartonellosis	

NOTE: Based on Newman 1976; Ramenofsky (in Kiple 1993: 322); Merbs 1992: 9. It should be noted that research on this subject is just beginning and that the reasons for assignation of some diseases to one list or the other are not always spelled out by the authors.

[a] Numbers 1–11 are found in both hemispheres; numbers 12–17 originated in the Americas. Rheumatoid arthritis and venereal syphilis are the only hypothesized American "gifts" to the Old World (Rothschild et al. 1988; Baker and Armelagos 1988).

[b] Definitely reported from a few precontact South American sites but questioned by archeoparasitologist Reinhard as indigenous to the Americas (1992: 241).

spread rapidly among an Indian population that was relatively dense and continuous and that had no acquired immunity or any knowledge of how to treat or control the disease. Cortez left the Indies for Mexico in 1519, and one of a party that followed to apprehend him came down with an active case of smallpox once they arrived on the Veracruz coast. According to Bernal Díaz del Castillo, "he infected the household in Cempoalla [a coastal city] where he was quartered; and it spread from one Indian to another, and they, being so numerous and eating and sleeping together, quickly infected the entire country." Until recently, historical accounts of the Mexican conquest have overlooked the fact that while Cortez and his small party of men were besieging Tenochtitlan, a smallpox epidemic was destroying the city's population. Details of the epidemic are recorded in the Florentine Codex and the Bernal Díaz del Castillo Chronicles. The disease spread, apparently (sources are sparse) south into Guatemala and Yucatan, preceding Alvarado's 1521 conquest of the Mayas, and over the Panamanian isthmus to the Andes, where a major epidemic cut down the population of the Incan Empire approximately eight years prior to the arrival of Pizarro (the above discussion has been summarized from Crosby 1972 and Ashburn 1947).

Dobyns (1966, 1983) hypothesizes that the pandemic of the 1520s spread the length and breadth of the hemisphere. As of 1996, however, the jury is still out on the true geographic extent of this calamitous visitation. It seems safest at this time to accept the conservative interpretation that smallpox spread throughout the Middle American and adjacent regions where maize agriculture supported a relatively dense and continuously distributed population. In the nonagricultural areas beyond, there is not yet enough evidence to say. The Pacific Northwest, however, may eventually supply an answer.

Archeologist Sarah Campbell (1989) has found evidence from the Northwest that she has interpreted as supporting Dobyns's hypothesis of a 1520s pandemic. A survey of a limited area of the middle Columbia uncovered significant reductions in the number and size of archeological components, structured features, and shell and bone residue, all coinciding in the early 1500s. This decline very likely represents a local population decrease, but Campbell acknowledges that other, nondisease explanations are possible. The hypothesis that this population decline was due to an epidemic is provocative and important but needs to be tested in comparable archeological regions in the Pacific Northwest before we can accept an early 1500s smallpox epidemic in the area, with all its implications for culture change, as fact.

MALARIA IN THE AMERICAS

The history of the introduction of malaria to the New World, unlike that of smallpox, is poorly known. But its effects were nearly as devastating. The malarial parasite seems not to have been native to the Americas. It must have been introduced during the colonial period to the three areas of the New World where heavy anopheline and human populations coexisted in pre-Columbian times, and where malaria has been prevalent up until the last century. In the early 1500s heavy mortality and depressed fertility from introduced malaria appear to have depopulated the Mesoamerican lowlands while leaving the arid central plateau relatively untouched (Friedlander 1970). Malaria was also endemic in the Mississippi Valley in the 1700s and 1800s, and it may have been a major factor in the population collapse of the Mississippian Mound Builders. When introduction occurred is not clear; malaria was certainly not present in 1539 when de Soto traversed the Southeast, but by 1680 at the latest, however, both *Plasmodium falciparum* and *vivax* were endemic in the Southeast (Rutman and Rutman 1976). Introduction of the virulent variety probably came with the intensification of the African slave trade in the early 1600s. Similarly, malaria may explain the depopulation of the Amazonian lowlands. The earliest Spanish explorers (e.g., Francisco de Orellana, 1542) reported dense populations; one century later, Spanish visitors found the land nearly abandoned (Ashburn 1947: 112–15). Because malaria was introduced in all these areas several centuries ago, the process was not well recorded and is only partially understood. The 1830s western Oregon experience with malaria introduction, as detailed in chapter 4, was probably similar in many respects and is much better recorded. The sources document the systemic upset that occurs on the cusp of change, when malaria was added to an already existing, more or less balanced cultural-ecological system. In this sense the western Oregon experience is an extremely important episode in the disease history of not only the Northwest but the rest of the world as well.

"VIRGIN-SOIL" EPIDEMICS

The smallpox epidemic of the 1520s, whatever its extent, was a classic example of a "virgin-soil" epidemic: a disease which spreads among a population that has never experienced it before. Virgin-soil populations generally lack immunity (acquired or inherited) to new diseases and have few or no cumulated cultural traditions (medicine, public health) to deal with them. There were several such epidemics in the early disease history of the Northwest Coast: 1770s smallpox (laying aside the possibility of a 1520s outbreak), 1830s malaria, 1838 influenza, 1844 dysentery, and 1848 measles (perhaps). One could also argue that for some peoples second outbreaks of a disease were also "virgin"—

in the sense that the population living at the time had never experienced the disease in question (though their ancestors did).

Virgin-soil epidemics are of great interest to epidemiologists and have been studied intensely.[3] They show clearly how a particular disease will spread through a given population when unimpeded by biological or cultural barriers. Virgin-soil epidemics also tend to have very high mortalities. In many cases, the human populations not only have not developed ways to deal with the disease but also have practices which tend to increase mortality beyond what would otherwise be expected. The following four social responses have just this effect.[4]

Flight and Subsequent Spread of the Epidemic

For the class of infectious viral diseases spread by droplet infection and with a latency period (such as smallpox and measles), flight was a particularly dangerous response. People generally flee to places where they have relatives and can be assured of refuge. In the case of the Amazonian Yanomamo in 1968, flight carried virgin-soil measles to the boundaries of the ethnolinguistic unit (Neel et al. 1970). Among the more mobile, mounted populations of the Great Plains in the early 1800s, flight facilitated the spread of epidemics over wide geographic areas (Ray 1976; Taylor 1977). On the Northwest Coast, given the various overlapping and interlocking social networks characteristic of the region, flight more likely produced a wavelike spread, but the availability of large dugout canoes created the potential (fulfilled in the 1862 smallpox epidemic) for rapid, long-range transmission.

Counterproductive Health Care

Most indigenous American health care systems were simply not equipped to deal with the new class of introduced contagious diseases (Newman 1976). Two treatments common on the Northwest Coast that not only were ineffective but actually increased mortality when used with the new diseases

---

3. See Crosby 1976, 1978 (historical populations); Neel et al. 1970 (the 1968 measles epidemic among the Amazonian Yanomamo); and Christiansen et al. 1952–53 (the 1951 measles epidemic among Greenland Inuit).

4. The basic discussion in this section is drawn from my 1985 dissertation, but see also McGrath 1991 for a similar classification.

were the practices of ingathering around an ill individual and the sweat-bath/cold-water treatment. The former was usual during curing sessions, which required an audience who kept time with drums during the shaman's singing and dancing. For precontact ailments, this practice was epidemiologically neutral and probably provided real psychological benefit; in the case of viral diseases spread by sneezing, it would facilitate transmission. Sweat bathing followed by immersion in cold water was a common treatment throughout aboriginal North America for lice, rheumatism, and other precontact ailments (Vogel 1970: 241–44). Numerous historical documents, however, state that the cold plunge, in particular, became deadly when used in association with the new class of febrile diseases. The cause of death is not known; fever associated with a cold plunge may cause shock (Taylor 1977) or induce death from pneumonia (Hodgson 1957).

Overload of Health Care Systems

Morbidity (number of people infected) in virgin-soil epidemics seems to be invariably high—in the Yanomamo and Greenland Inuit measles epidemics it approached 100%. Even in the worst conditions, of course, not everyone was sick simultaneously, because of the serial nature of most disease transmission. But the health care system would be severely taxed, and health care practitioners would not be able to treat all the sick. In some cases so many would be sick at once that very few people would be left to take care of the ill, and many that might recover with minimal care would die. Situations like this occurred during the plague epidemics of the Middle Ages and are recorded, for example, for the 1520 smallpox epidemic in Tenochtitlan (Sahagun 1975: 83) and for the New England Indians in 1634 (Crosby 1976: 296). Such conditions are likely for several Northwest Coast epidemics.

Cessation of Subsistence Activities
and Breakdown of the Social System

In the case of high-morbidity epidemics, normal subsistence activity may cease, and inadequate nourishment or even starvation may increase mortality among the ill. Smallpox epidemics among the Huron in the 1600s, according to the Jesuit Relations, had just this effect (Trigger 1976: chap. 8). The time of year, morbidity level, and duration of the epidemic are all important factors here. A lack of sufficient nourishment disproportionately affects the most vulnerable segments of the population: infants and the very old. During the Yanomamo measles epidemic, nursing ceased because many mothers were unable to provide milk, and many babies (nursing continued to three years) were unable to take the breast (Neel et al. 1970). On the Northwest Coast, epidemics that struck during the "lean season" of late winter/early spring would have been especially dangerous.

In severe cases of high morbidity and mortality among virgin-soil populations, all the above patterns may occur simultaneously and result in a general social breakdown.[5] Extreme situations like this, rarely noted in the surviving literature (e.g., Makah in 1853; see chapter 6), probably occurred among several Northwest Coast peoples during the high-morbidity/high-mortality smallpox epidemics of the 1770s and 1862 and during the "fever and ague" years of 1830 and 1831 on the lower Columbia.

5. The Mandan of the upper Missouri during the 1838 *Variola major* epidemic constitute the classic example. Here, due to the crowded conditions in the nucleated earth lodge villages, plus a susceptible population, transmission was very rapid and most were infected and came down with the disease at once. All normal social activity ceased, there were few to care for many who might otherwise have survived, and according to some sources, a general panic led many people to commit suicide rather than submit to the disease (Dollar 1977; Chardon 1932; Trimble 1988).

2 / The First Smallpox Epidemics
of the Historic Period

The first and by far the most devastating effect of Euro-American contact on Northwest Coast Indians was the introduction, in the late 1700s, of smallpox. Acting upon a virgin-soil population, the disease produced a high mortality, certainly in excess of the 30% average recorded for historic outbreaks (see appendix 2 for a summary of the clinical and epidemiological characteristic of smallpox) as well as an unknown degree of social and cultural disruption. This devastation, moreover, occurred during a shadowy period at the juncture of the protohistoric and historic eras, when no White eyewitnesses were on the scene to record its effects. Relatively little documentation on early smallpox has survived, and much of what has is duplicitous. The best way to reconstruct what actually happened during this crucial time is, following the tenets of historical epidemiology, to present all extant records, group them by geography and time period, and see what patterns emerge.

The possibility of smallpox penetration to the Northwest Coast before the beginning of the historic era cannot be ruled out on present evidence. Campbell's archeological case (1989) for Northwest participation in the hemispheric smallpox pandemic of the 1520s has been noted in chapter 1. Infectious diseases could have been introduced via shipwrecked oriental junks (Brooks 1876; Quimby 1985). Sporadic European contacts with potential for disease introduction include a possible wreck of a Manila galleon[1] in the 1500s (Cook 1973: 31–40) and the landings of Drake in 1579 and Chirikoff in 1741 at the south and north peripheries of the region, respectively. Direct contact with Europeans on the Northwest Coast did not begin until 1774, however, and it is from this time period that the first recorded references to smallpox in the region appear.

Following initial introduction, smallpox epidemics reappeared with some regularity on the Northwest Coast. The disease appears to have occurred among all Northwest Native peoples in the late 1700s; subsequent epidemics were more restricted in scope. In 1910, ethnologist James Mooney recorded four major epidemics in the Northwest, in 1781–82, 1836–37, 1852–53, and 1862 (1928: 13–14, 27, 30). My research has uncovered evidence for a fifth epidemic, in 1801–2, as well as a possible sixth outbreak in the winter of 1824–25. The periodicity of Northwest smallpox outbreaks is epidemiologically significant. The aboriginal populations of the Northwest Coast were never dense or continuous enough to support the uninterrupted presence of smallpox. The disease therefore appeared at intervals, dependent upon, first of all, introduction from outside the region and, second, the presence of a pool of non-immune susceptibles in the Indian population. Smallpox epidemics occurred roughly every generation (in the south, four epidemics were separated by gaps that averaged 26 years; in the north, there was a hiatus of about 60 years between the first and the second epidemic, and 26 years between the second and the third).

Evidence for the first epidemics comes from two classes of data: contemporary statements by Euro-American explorers and traders and remembered accounts, collected at a much later time and often mythologized, of Indian informants. References to smallpox in the early journals are, with few exceptions, limited to mentions of pockmarked individuals; no eyewitness accounts, by Whites, of actual epidemic visitations are known to exist.[2] Native remi-

---

1. Between 1565 and 1815, a Spanish trade galleon traveled annually between Acapulco and Manila, carrying American silver west along a route just north of the equator and silk, spices, and other Asian goods east with the Japanese Current at about 35° north latitude (north of Hawaii). See Schurz 1939.

2. In fact, considering the nature of Spanish and English contact in the 1770s, it would be surprising if we *did* have eyewitness accounts. The Spanish ships were never (at this time) in contact with the Indians for more than a month, usually much less, at any one time. Captain Cook was at Nootka exactly one month. Assuming the disease came on shipboard, and given the two-

niscences are valuable for their cultural and humanistic content but are difficult to date chronologically.

For early smallpox, therefore, the data base is often ambiguous and difficult to interpret. This is particularly so in reference to dating. The historical references I have found *tend* to cluster in three time frames (1770s, ca. 1800, 1824–25), but not exclusively so; the myth accounts, which exist outside chronological time, could relate to any or all early smallpox visitations. For these reasons I have chosen to include all smallpox references datable to ca. 1775–1825 in a single chapter, with the realization that future research may result in some shuffling of accounts and tightening of the sequence offered here.

SMALLPOX IN THE 1770S

Map 2 shows the distribution of smallpox references assignable to the decade of the 1770s. Map 3 shows known European landfalls (a possible source of smallpox) for the period from 1774 to 1779. The references cluster and may be discussed in three geographic regions: North Coast, Columbia River drainage, and Puget Sound/Strait of Georgia.

Historical Accounts

North Coast (Tlingit, Haida, Tsimshian, Kwukwaka̲'wakw). The first appearance of smallpox among the Tlingit is, relative to other groups, well recorded, with at least three citations in the historical literature. All were recorded from the Sitka area. The first comes from the journal of the English explorer Nathaniel Portlock, in 1787.

12 August 1787, Portlock's Harbor, 57°44′N
I expected to have seen a numerous tribe, and was quite surprised when I found that it consisted only of three men, three women, the same number of girls, two boys about twelve years old, and two infants. . . . I observed the oldest of the men to be very much marked with the small-pox, as was a girl who appeared to be about fourteen years

---

week latency period, sailors would have had to stay in one place for a considerable period of time to observe the epidemiological consequences of their visit. And throughout the decade of the seventies, Whites and Northwest Indians were in face-to-face contact for a total of less than four months. There was plenty of time between visits for an epidemic to spread and die out.

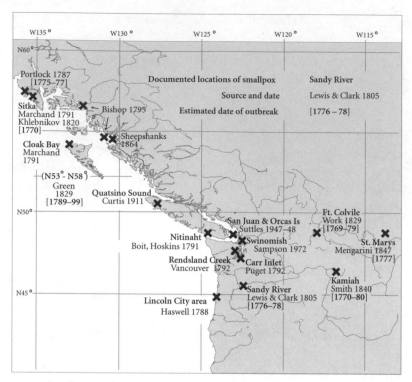

MAP 2. Smallpox in the Late 1700s

old. The old man endeavoured to describe the excessive torments he endured whilst he was afflicted with the disorder that had marked his face, and gave me to understand that it happened some years ago. This convinced me that they had had the smallpox among them at some distant period. He told me that the distemper carried off great numbers of the inhabitants, and that he himself had lost ten children by it; he had ten strokes tatooed on one of his arms, which I understood were marks for the number of children he had lost. I did not observe any of the children under ten or twelve years of age that were marked; therefore I have great reason to suppose that the disorder raged little more than that number of years ago [1775–1777]; and as the Spaniards were on this part of the coast in 1775, it is very probable that from them these poor wretches caught this fatal affliction. . . . A number of the Indians who visited us from the Eastward were marked with the small-pox, and one man who had lost an eye gave me to understand that he had lost it by that disorder; but none of the natives from the Westward had the least traces of it. I cannot account for this circumstance any other way than by supposing that the vessel from which these unfortunate people caught the infection, was in a harbor somewhere about Cape Edgecombe, and perhaps none of the natives further to the westward than this Sound had an oppor-

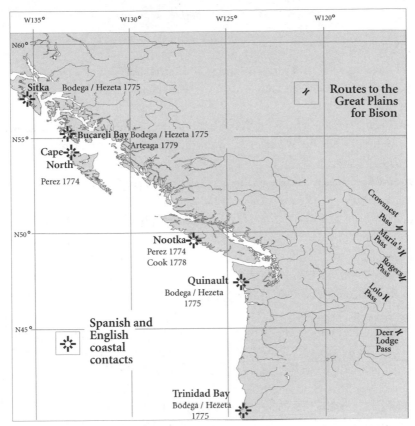

MAP 3. Extraregional Contacts in the 1770s: Spanish and English Coastal Contacts and Transmontane Routes to the Great Plains

tunity of having any intercourse with her, and by that means happily escaped the disorder. (Portlock 1789: 271–72)

Exactly four years after Portlock's observations, French explorer Étienne Marchand visited Sitka and similarly commented on the presence of pockmarked individuals:

It cannot be doubted that the small-pox has been introduced into the countries which border on Tchinkitanay Bay [Sitka Sound]; for several individuals of both sexes bear unequivocal marks of it; and they explained very clearly to Surgeon Roblet, who questioned them concerning the cause of these marks, that they proceeded from a disorder which made the face swell, and covered the body with virulent pustules that occasioned violent itchings; they even remarked that the French must be well acquainted with it, since some of them also bore the marks of it. In 1787, Captain

Portlock was witness of the ravages which it had made. . . . in the harbor to which he has given his name, and which is situated at no great distance to the north-west of Tchinkitanay towards the latitude of 57° 50′. (Fleurieu 1801: 1.328)

The third account from the Tlingit exists in three versions. That given below, from Kyrill Khlebnikov's 1820 report, is the oldest and assumed original.[3]

According to Saigakakh there was an epidemic of small pox there some 50 years ago, that is about 1770. He was a small child and barely remembers it, but he knows for a fact that there were only one or two persons left in each family. According to him it spread from Stakhin (Stikine) to Sitka, but did not go further north. The Kolosh [Tlingit] supposed that this illness was visited on them by the crow [sic: probably Raven, the local culture hero] as a punishment for the endless wars they waged among themselves. (Khlebnikov 1976: 29)

References for the Haida of the Queen Charlotte Islands and Tsimshian of the northern British Columbia mainland are sketchier but sufficient to indicate that smallpox was present among them as well. At Cloak Bay, Marchand noted "several" Haida with "the face deeply marked with the smallpox" (Fleurieu 1801: 1.438). A Tsimshian memory of the epidemic may be contained in a tale recorded in the 1860s, which recalled what happened when Whites first appeared in "a huge canoe." The newcomers shot a bird, rubbed two flints together to make fire, and boiled water in a metal pot over a fire. After each of these miraculous happenings, according to the tale, "the Indians all died," a probable reference to disease (Sheepshanks 1864: 42).

A very late account, which may refer to Haida, Tlingit, or both, comes from the 1829 journal of Anglican missionary Jonathan Green:

Some thirty or forty years since [1789–99], the small-pox made great ravages among them [coast natives between 53° and 58° N latitude]. This disease they call Tom Dyer, as some suppose from a sailor of this name who introduced it, though it is probable that it came across the continent. Many of their old men recollect, and they say, that it almost destroyed their country. (Green 1915: 39)

3. Two later versions were apparently copied from Khlebnikov with only minor variations (Romanov 1825: 27; Litke 1835: 217–18).

Green's estimated dates for initial smallpox (1789–99) are out of line with most other contemporary estimates, which range from 1769 to 1780. But his estimate may be correct, for a few North Coast references do indeed suggest a mid-1790s outbreak.[4]

The last datable North Coast record, collected from a Kwakwaka'wakw informant in the early 1900s by Edward Curtis, deals with the disappearance of the Hoyalas people of Quatsino Sound and their replacement by the Koskimo. Although Curtis's informant blames an epidemic for the dissolution of the Hoyalas, other accounts ascribe it to warfare, so the passage is not definitive proof of late-1700s smallpox in the area (Galois 1994: 361).

The Koskimo, who formerly lived at Kósŭŭ (on Cape Commerell) and later at Kwánëë (Deep Bay) came to their present location in the time of the great-great-grandfather of the informant Tsŭlniti, who was five years old when Fort Rupert was established in 1849.[5] . . . Quatsino Sound had been occupied by the populous Hoyalas. . . . An epidemic almost exterminated the Hoyalas, and the remnant scattered among the tribes to the south and on the eastern coast of Vancouver Island, wherever they had relatives by marriage. So great was the mortality in this epidemic that it was impossible for the survivors to bury the dead. They simply pulled the houses down over the bodies and left them. It was soon after the epidemic that the Koskimo moved into this region. (Curtis 1915: 306 n. 1)

4. From Charles Bishop's journal:

30 July 1795, Dundas Island (across Chatham Sound from Fort Simpson): "They are very numerous, and were much more so before the small Pox which raged here a few years since, and by Kowes Account, swept off two thirds of the People scarcely any that were affected Survived" (Bishop 1967: 83).

25 August 1795: "It seems the Small Pox is raging among them, and altho' Shakes is quite recovered, yet his Family are much affected by it and he has burried one of his Wives lately. His Eldest and favourite son is now ill of the terrible disease" (Bishop 1967: 91–92).

Although Dundas Island is in Tsimshian lands, Cow (Kowe) was the name of a line of chiefs associated with the Haida village at the entrance to Parry Passage (Gunther 1972: 124). Shakes was a name applied to a line of Stikine Tlingit chiefs. In 1795 a Russian fur-trading party at Yakutat Bay fled, "panic-stricken," when two Aleut hunters in the party contracted smallpox. De Laguna, ethnographer of the Yakutat Tlingit, associates this event with an outbreak that her informants said happened "before the Russians came, i.e., before they had established their post" (1972: 1.166–67).

5. If Tsŭlniti was born in 1844 and if we allow 20 years to the generation, his great-great-grandfather would have been born in 1764.

Franz Boas's large compendium of Kwakwaka'wakw oral *numaym* "quasi histories" contains several that deal with the Hoyalas/Koskimo. Version 1 of "Q!á'neqcᵉlakᵘ" states that "bad sickness comes from the north end of our world" (1935: 5); version 2 records a meeting with "the man with mouths on the body" (1935: 10). Elsewhere this person is described as "a man who now rolled around on the ground, now jumped into the water and went back ashore again. His body was covered all over with mouths which all laughed and shouted at the same time" (Boas 1975: 331). The "mouths" on the body most probably refer to smallpox sores. Jumping in the water was a way to deal with the fever; rolling around on the ground, with itching.

In 1885, a year before Boas's initial visit to the Kwakwaka'wakw, another visitor (George Dawson) hypothesized:

When the small-pox first ravaged the coast, after the coming of the whites, the Indians were not only much reduced in numbers, but became scattered, and new combinations were probably formed subsequently; while tribes and portions of tribes, once forming distinct village communities, drew together for mutual protection, when their numbers became small. (Dawson 1887: 4)

The long historical process of Kwakwaka'wakw village abandonment and consolidation is discussed in great detail in Robert Galois's *Kwakwaka'wakw Settlements* (1994).

The Columbia River Drainage (Flathead, Colville, Nez Perce, Chinookans, Tillamook). The Columbia River basin was opened to continuing Euro-American contact with the exploratory parties of Lewis and Clark and David Thompson in 1805–8. Four accounts written during the first half of the nineteenth century estimate dates for the initial appearance of smallpox. Three of these come from the Columbia Plateau, outside the Northwest Coast culture area. The most succinct is an 1829 report from Hudson's Bay Company's Fort Colvile, which notes: "Immense numbers of them were swept off by a dreadful visitation of the smallpox, that from the appearance of some individuals that bear marks of the disease, may have happened fifty or sixty years ago" (1769–79) (John Work, 1 April 1829, in Chance 1973: 120). More details of Plateau smallpox come from two documents from the 1840s. Derived independently by Presbyterian and Jesuit missionaries from Nez Perce and Flathead informants, they may refer to a single episode. Each says smallpox was acquired on a bison hunt: the Nez Perce account says among a joint party of Nez Perce and Flatheads; the Flathead version does not specify. The Nez Perce account says the disease was "the most virulent form of the smallpox." According to the Flathead: "The disease caused the growth of large red and black pustules over the entire body, particularly on the chest. Those developing red pustules died within a few days, but those who were plagued by black pustules died almost immediately." The Nez Perce version, dated 1840, estimated the event at "60 or perhaps 70 years ago" (1770–80); the Flathead version (from 1847) makes it "[a]bout seventy years ago" (1777).[6]

William Clark noted signs of the disease among both Upper Chinookans and Chinook proper in 1805–6:

3 April 1806, probably near the Sandy River
an old man who appeared of Some note among them and father to my guide brought forward a woman who was badly marked with the Small Pox and made Signs that they all died with the disorder which marked her face, and which She was very near dieing with when a Girl, from the age of this woman this Distructive disorder I judge must have been about 28 or 30 years past [1776–78], and about the time the Clatsops inform us that this disorder raged in their towns and distroyed their nation. (Lewis and Clark 1991: 65)[7]

A final reference from the lower Columbia region comes from the journal of the American vessel *Columbia,* one of the few ships to stop on the Oregon coast during the late 1700s. The journal noted "two or three of our visitors were much pitted with the small pox" near modern Lincoln City (Tillamook Salish area), on 10 August 1788 (Haswell in Howay 1941: 34).

---

6. Both passages are given in full in Boyd 1985: 79–80. The citations are from Asa Smith in Drury 1958: 136–37 (Nez Perce) and from Mengarini 1977: 193–94 (Flathead).

7. In what may be a reference to the effects of this outbreak, Robert Stuart, in a July 1812 visit to Chinookan villages on Sauvie Island near Portland, noted that the "Cathlanamencimens" (Lewis and Clark's Clannarminamow) were "once a very powerfull tribe, but now reduced by the small Pox to [about] 60 Men" (Stuart 1935: 32). (Sixty men implies a total population not far from Lewis and Clark's 1805 estimate of 280.) In 1968 the Oregon Archaeological Society (OAS) excavated Clannarminamow, site CO-9. Emory Strong noted that the site was much larger than indicated by Lewis and Clark's population estimate. The OAS findings seemed to offer an explanation for this discrepancy: "In the northernmost portion of the area at a depth of 121 centimeters human skeletal remains were encountered. . . . It soon became apparent that this was no ordinary burial, if indeed it was a burial at all. Nine skulls came to light all in odd positions, some resting on their sides, some on their faces and one even on the top of its head. The body bones were also in complete disarray as if they had been unceremoniously dumped there. This

Puget Sound and the Strait of Georgia (Southern and Central Coast Salish, Ditidaht). The journals of George Vancouver's 1792 exploration of Puget Sound and the Strait of Georgia contain several references to pockmarked Indians.

12 May 1792, Rendsland Creek, Hoods Canal (Twana territory)
[A]t the extremity of the inlet. . . . about sixty [people] . . . : one or two had visited us on the preceding Thursday morning [at Port Discovery]; particularly one man who had suffered very much from the small pox. This deplorable disease is not only common, but it is greatly to be apprehended is very fatal among them, as its indelible marks were seen on many; and several had lost the sight of one eye . . . owing most likely to the virulent effects of this baneful disorder. (Vancouver 1798: 1.241)

21 May 1792, Carr Inlet
[I]n the SW Corner of the Cove was a Small Village. . . . Two of the three in the Canoe had lost the Right Eye & were much pitted with the Small Pox, which Disorder in all probability is the Cause of that Defect. (Puget 1939: 198)[8]

In a summary statement on the Indians of Puget Sound and the Strait of Georgia, Peter Puget (1792) stated: "the Small pox most have had, and most terribly pitted they are; indeed many have lost their Eyes, & no Doubt it has raged with uncommon Inacteracy [*sic*] among them" (18 August 1792).[9]

The ethnohistorical records from this area are backed by several oral tra-

---

led us to believe that it may have been a secondary burial, the bones being buried in a common grave after body decomposition. This theory was later abandoned as skeletal remains were encountered throughout the entire excavation area at the same depth and all in the same complete disarray. Over 90 skulls in all were identified in the remaining course of excavation. Apparently at some point in the village's past history disaster struck, possibly in the form of some pestilence that had wiped out great numbers of the inhabitants. Later flooding of the site washed the bones into their present positions" (Jones 1972: 182). The archeologists' description makes a good case for epidemic depopulation. Assuming it is correct, association of the remains with the initial epidemic of smallpox, given Stuart's observation, seems most likely. But they could just as well have resulted from depopulation associated with a second visitation of smallpox in 1801–2, also noted by Lewis and Clark (see below, p. 40), or from the "fever and ague" epidemics of the 1830s (chapter 4).

8. On the Rendsland Creek account see also Menzies 1923: 29; on the Carr Inlet account see Vancouver 1798: 1.217 and Menzies 1923: 35.

9. Robert McKechnie (1972: 75) incorrectly identifies these Indians as Haida, because Puget penned the passage while in Queen Charlotte *Strait* (the Haida inhabit the Queen Charlotte *Islands*).

ditions, particularly from the lower Fraser and what are now Skagit, What-
com, and San Juan Counties of Washington State. Swinomish tribal historian
Martin Sampson recalled that "remains of the Swinomish who had lived . . .
before the first epidemic of smallpox" were found on the Whidbey Island
naval base and reinterred (1972: 27); the ancestors of the Nuwhaha were
"almost wiped out," though those on "upland lakes and prairies" were passed
over (25).

Wayne Suttles's Straits informants recalled that "two or three Lummi villages and one or two Samish villages were nearly wiped out by smallpox and
the survivors moved to mainland villages" (1954: 42). The Lummi myth "In
the Beginning" states that the "Taleqamec tribe" on San Juan Island was
"nearly exterminated . . . by a great plague." Survivors moved to Twolames
village (the source of the name "Lummi") at Sandy Point on Lopez Island
(Stern 1934: 107). In the late 1940s, Ruth Shelton (b. 1857) related to Suttles a
tradition passed on from her Samish forebears:

[T]he people of the village at Olga on Buck Bay, Orcas Island, mostly died of smallpox. . . . the original home of the Samish was on or near Mud Bay, Lopez Sound,
Lopez Island. After the smallpox came the survivors moved to the village on Guemes
Island across from Anacortes. Mrs. Shelton's great-grandmother or her great-great-
grandmother was a little girl when the smallpox came. . . . Allowing 20 years per generation, we might date her great-grandmother's childhood in the 1790s or her great-
great-grandmother's in the 1770s. (Suttles 1947–48)

Finally, historical records confirm that smallpox occurred on Vancouver
Island at the mouth of the Strait of Juan de Fuca, among the Nootkan Ditidaht.
On 28 June 1791, two crewmen of the *Columbia* noted its presence at Nitinaht
village.

abrest the Village of Nittenatt. . . . 'Twas evident that these Natives had been visited
by that scourge of mankind the Smallpox. The Spaniards as the natives say brought
it among them. (Boit in Howay 1941: 371)

Cassacan [a high-ranking noble] has also [besides venereal disease] had the small pox;
of which his face bears evident marks. Infamous Europeans, a scandal to the Christian
name; is it you who bring and leave in a country with people you deem savages the
most loathsome diseases? (Hoskins in Howay 1941: 196)

Correlation of Accounts

The ethnohistorical evidence presented so far reveals several patterns. The first concerns the geographical extent of the epidemic. All documented references appear on map 2. They clearly show that smallpox was widespread in the Pacific Northwest in the decade of the 1770s. The blank spaces on map 2 correspond in large part to peoples who were contacted late by Euro-Americans and for whom written documentation from the early period is consequently sparse. It is more than likely that smallpox occurred among most of these undocumented groups as well. Late-eighteenth-century conditions in the Northwest were favorable for a maximal spread of the disease. The epidemiological characteristics of smallpox, the flight reaction typical of virgin-soil populations, the relatively dense and continuous precontact populations, and the extensive social and economic networks characteristic of the aboriginal Pacific Northwest all suggest that smallpox, when first introduced, must have spread to the limits of settlement.

The evidence presented here can be taken to support an epidemic outbreak of smallpox that affected all of the peoples of the Pacific Northwest. As Henry Dobyns has suggested, the epidemic of the 1770s may simply be an extension of the pandemic known from other parts of western North America between 1779 and 1781. Smallpox in these years is documented from central Mexico, Baja California, the Pueblo southwest, and the Sioux and Blackfoot in the Great Plains. Geographically, an extension of the pandemic to include the Northwest is possible. But a major problem with this interpretation is that the dates do not match. Six of the above-cited Euro-American chroniclers[10] of the Pacific Northwest estimated, by the ages of pockmarked individuals or the ages of their informants, the year of the first smallpox outbreak. The range is from 1769 to 1780; the mean year is 1775. The coastal dates tend toward the earlier years of the decade; those of the interior favor the latter half of the range. There is also a possibility, of course, that the method of calculating is to blame—perhaps the chroniclers tended to overestimate the ages of their informants.

Origins

It is also possible that we are dealing with two or more regional outbreaks, each with its own history. The North Coast and Columbia River clusters, for

---

10. Jonathan Green's estimate (1789–99) is the exception.

instance, do not appear to share much more than rough contemporaneity. And the Central Coast cluster may also have a history of its own. The ethnohistorical sources mention two possible areas of origin for the initial outbreak of smallpox in the Northwest: from the Plains (for the Plateau cases) and from Spanish ships (for the coast). There is also evidence for a third route as well: from the Russian colony in Kamchatka to the Tlingit.

Kamchatka–Tlingit Route. In 1768, the Kamchatka Peninsula in eastern Siberia experienced a major smallpox epidemic. According to one observer, "5,368 persons were carried off" (Coxe 1780: 5). When Captain Cook's expedition stopped at Kamchatka in 1779, they "everywhere met with the Ruins of large Villages with no traces left of them but the Foundations of the Houses" (Samwell in Beaglehole 1967: 1252). The route of the disease is particularly interesting:

The small pox. . . . made its appearance in 1767 and 1768. It was brought into the country by a Russian vessel bound to the Eastern islands, for the purpose of hunting otters, foxes, and other animals. The person, who had in his blood the fatal germ, was a sailor from Okotsk, where he had taken remedies for the disorder, previous to his departure; but the recent marks of it were visible. Scarcely landed, he communicated this cruel malady to the poor Kamtschadales, which carried off three fourths of them. (de Lesseps 1790: 128)

The "Eastern islands" were the Kuriles, and probably the Aleutians as well, which were being visited by this time for furs.[11] The available literature on the Kamchatka epidemic does not name the "Russian vessel" that brought smallpox, but the timing suggests that it may have belonged to the "secret" surveying expedition of Petr Krenitsyn and Mikhail Levashov. Krenitsyn and Levashov left Okhotsk in October 1766 and, after an eight-day voyage, arrived at Kamchatka, where they remained for a year and a half, coincident with the Kamchatka epidemic. On 14 August 1768, after three weeks at sea, they arrived in the Aleutians. From a base on Unimak Island, exploring parties were sent as far west as 100 miles along the Alaska Peninsula. The expedition remained in the Aleutians for an entire year, during which time over

---

11. According to Alaska historian Raymond Fisher (1996: 18) "between 1756 and 1780 some forty-eight voyages were made" from Siberia to the Aleutians by Russian fur trappers in search of sea otter and fur seal pelts (my thanks to Pamela Amoss for locating this reference).

50 men were lost to "sickness" (mainly scurvy); the expedition returned to Kamchatka in August 1769. Of the voluminous records of this expedition, only a few short summaries have been published; the rest remain, untranslated and in manuscript, in the Russian Central State Archive of the Fleet (Glushankov 1973).

The link between the Kamchatka and Tlingit smallpox epidemics is weak, given the present state of knowledge. Aboriginal trade networks, however, existed between the Aleut, Chugach Eskimo, and northernmost Tlingit. The possible very early date of 1769 for Tlingit smallpox makes sense in terms of transmission from Kamchatka, but it does not agree with Portlock's observation that Tlingit from east of Sitka were pockmarked, while those from the west were not, or with Khlebnikov's assertion that the disease spread north from the Stikine River to Sitka.

Spanish Vessels. The most popular theory current among the (non-Spanish) Euro-American explorers of the Northwest Coast in the late 1700s was that smallpox had been introduced by Spanish explorers. Two of the accounts (Portlock among the Tlingit; Boit at Nitinaht) name the Spanish; a third (Green) suggests transmission from European ships, nationality not specified. Placing the blame on other nationalities for the introduction of baleful diseases and trade items (such as venereal disease, alcohol, and firearms) among the Indians was common practice at this time, however, so all such statements should be approached with caution. The timing of the first epidemic, nevertheless, implicates the Spanish. The six estimates for the date of the first Northwest outbreak fall between 1769 and 1780. European exploration of the coast began in 1774, with the Spanish Perez expedition. Two other Spanish voyages were undertaken in 1775 and 1779. The only other vessels on the coast in this time period belonged to the Cook expedition of 1778. Cook, however, stopped only at Resolution Cove in Nuu-chah-nulth territory, an area from which there is no record of smallpox at this time.

There are several problems with the Spanish origins theory, however. The first is the absence of any reference to smallpox in the Spanish records. Copies of nearly all the relevant logs are available at the Bancroft Library of the University of California. I have reviewed the most detailed of these and have failed to locate a single reference to any contagious disease which might be unambiguously interpreted as smallpox. Typical was the 1774 expedition, which suffered greatly from scurvy (see Beals 1989: 95, 114; de la Peña in Cutter 1969: 193), but no other disease is mentioned in that year's journals.

Second, although smallpox appeared in several epidemics in eighteenth-century Mexico, the source area for the Spanish ships, there were no outbreaks that coincided with the *exact* time of the Northwest Coast expeditions. There is no record of smallpox in Mexico in 1774 or 1776, and although there was an epidemic in 1779, it occurred in the autumn, whereas Arteaga's ships left the mainland in February (Cooper 1965). There was a smallpox outbreak in Baja California in 1781, but the disease did not take hold in upper California before 1838 (Valle 1973b). Given the size of central Mexico's population at this time, however, this point may be moot. The disease may have been endemic, with occasional rises in incidence that have been called "epidemics."

Finally, the duration of the sea voyage from Mexico to the Northwest was a potential barrier to transmission. The 1774 Perez expedition left San Blas (in Nayarit State) on 24 January, Monterey on 11 June, and arrived in the Queen Charlottes on 18 July (Beals 1989). The 1775 and 1779 sea voyages from San Blas (to Trinidad and Bucareli Bays, respectively) both lasted 11 weeks. Assuming one infected person at the beginning of the voyage, and given the normal progression of smallpox, after one month he would be either dead or recovered and no longer infectious. Sequential on-board infection might extend the danger period, but a minimum of 11 weeks remains a long time for even this eventuality.[12] Fomites, however, may have extended the window of opportunity for shipboard transmission.

Robert Fortuine (1989) suggests a 1774 introduction date for smallpox. But the source, a thirdhand summary of an English translation of the original Spanish journal, is suspect.[13] A reading of Don Francisco Mourelle's original Spanish "Navegacion" by Herbert Beals, translator of the Perez voyage manuscripts, has uncovered no mention of "marks of smallpox" (Beals, pers. comm., 1993). Warren Cook believes that smallpox originated with the 1779 Arteaga expedition and cites in support of his hypothesis an entry made at Bucareli Bay from Juan Francisco de la Bodega y Quadra's journal which refers to "an epidemic of unspecified nature" (1973: 81, 93).[14] Close analysis of the

---

12. On sea voyage barriers to disease transmission see Snow and Lanphear 1988.

13. Irving Rosse states that Mourelle "noticed the marks of small pox among the natives of Sitka Bay and Port Bucareli . . . in 1775" (1883: 25), thus leading to Fortuine's suggestion of "an introduction of the disease prior to that date" (1989: 228).

14. The relevant passage, from the 1912 translation by G. F. Barwick, follows.

20 May 1779, Bucareli Bay: "[T]he Commander found the greater part of his men seriously ill with an attack, which showed that just when we thought them most free they were in the great-

passage, however, suggests that the "unspecified epidemic" was probably scurvy, which was believed by the Spanish at that time to be contagious and spread by human contact.

This leaves the 1775 expedition of the *Santiago* (led by Bruno Hezeta) and *Sonora* (commanded by Juan Francisco de la Bodega y Quadra). Nathaniel Portlock believed that it was this voyage that brought smallpox to the coast; Warren Cook denies it (1973: 8), however, as there is no mention of small-pox in any of the 1775 journals. The 1775 journals, like those of the 1774 and 1779 Spanish voyages, are replete with references to scurvy. It is possible, as a few passages from the journals of Frays Miguel de la Campa Cos and Benito de la Sierra suggest, however, that there was a second disease on board the *Santiago*. On 22 July, off the Oregon coast, Campa Cos stated, "Those sick with scurvy and other illnesses continue to increase daily" (1964: 46). On 31 August, at Monterey, a special hospital was constructed for the sick, who included "thirty-six suffering from scurvy alone. There are others with various ailments, bringing the number up to fifty" (Campa Cos 1964: 59). On 2 November, off the southern California coast, "Don Juan Perez, the second captain, died of typhus, after an illness of nine days" (Sierra 1930: 238).

Of all the Spanish expeditions, the 1775 voyage is the most likely candidate for the introduction of smallpox to the coast. The date is correct (the mean year for the six estimates of the first outbreak), and the voyagers encountered Indians at four separate locations along the coast (Trinidad Bay, Quinault River, Bucareli Bay, and Sea Lion Cove). Two of the locations were in the territory of the Tlingit, who suffered from the epidemic; the Quinault

---

est danger; and seeing that several died suddenly in this way, he determined, on the advice of my surgeon Don Mariano Nuñez de Esquivel, to put ashore and make a shed for them on the beach; this D. Fernando Quiros caused to be erected very quickly, constructing it with the utmost convenience the place afforded, and, in the absence of D. Juan Garcéa, entrusting the superintendence to the said surgeon; and such was the care and watchfulness with which he looked after them, that although most of them were in the last stage, and the days at that season had proved very harsh, only two of them died, and he succeeded in a short time in rendering the rest of them sound and robust, and in stopping that epidemic, which was already feared as a plague on the 'Princesa'" (Bodega y Quadra 1779).

Confusion arises from the journal references to "contagion" and "epidemic," which would, of course, apply to smallpox but not to the most common sailors' ailment of the time, scurvy, which is a deficiency disease and not contagious. A later passage in Bodega y Quadra's journal, however, states: "the Commander thought it desirable to set sail . . . to Monterey, having regard also to the wretched condition his crew were in through scurvy, by which contagious disease he had lost eight men" (7 August 1779).

location is close to the Columbia River and Puget Sound, both foci of the initial outbreak; and Trinidad Bay (in the territory of the Yurok), though lacking in historical documentation, is 50 miles south of a village (the Point Saint George site, north of Crescent City) known, from archeological evidence, to have been abandoned about this time (according to oral tradition) because of an "epidemic" (Gould 1978: 135).

Great Plains Route. A third theory on the origins of the epidemic of the 1770s, popular with the trappers and traders of the North West Company and the Hudson's Bay Company in the early nineteenth century, was that smallpox spread from the Great Plains to the Plateau region and thence to the Pacific coast. The oral traditions collected from Nez Perce and Flathead in the later 1800s suggest this route, as we have seen. The fur company employees, however, were eyewitnesses to the smallpox epidemic in the Plains only; there were no Whites in the 1770s or 1780s in the Plateau. So the connection must have been made after the fact. The most explicit description of the Plains–Plateau diffusion route comes from North West Company employee Ross Cox, writing in 1811:

[T]he disease first proceeded from the banks of the Missouri. . . . travelled with destructive rapidity as far north as Athabasca and the shores of the Great Slave Lake, crossed the Rocky Mountains at the sources of the Missouri, and having fastened its deadly venom on the Snake Indians, spread its devastating course to the northward and westward, until its frightful progress was arrested by the Pacific Ocean. (Cox 1957: 169; see also Dunn 1845: 84–85)

For the northwest Plains, the assumed source of diffusion to the Plateau, there is an excellent account of the appearance of smallpox among the Blackfoot, given to North West Company explorer and geographer David Thompson by the Piegan informant Saukamappee in the winter of 1787–88. According to Saukamappee, at "the Stag River [probably the Red Deer River between Calgary and Edmonton] death came over us all, and swept [*sic*] more than half of us by the Smallpox, of which we knew nothing. . . . We caught it from the Snake Indians" (Thompson 1962: 245–46). The "Snake" in these accounts are assumed to be mounted Shoshonean Indians, who at this date ranged much farther north than their historic location in the upper Snake River drainage of Idaho. The Snake, in turn, would have contracted smallpox from sources to the south, ultimately from the Pueblos, where there was a documented outbreak in 1781. The disease would have been transmitted to Plateau peoples (Nez Perce and Flathead) from Snake and/or Blackfoot sources, in the Plains themselves, during the annual bison hunt.

It is notable that these extensive tribal contacts—Snake with Blackfoot, Plateau Indians with Plains Indians—were probably themselves the result of a recently adopted item in the culture of all the Indian groups involved, the horse. Francis Haines's historical research suggests, and local traditions support, a date of around 1730 for introduction of the horse to the Plateau, also from Shoshoneans to the south (Haines 1938). The annual Plains bison hunt of eastern Plateau peoples probably began after their adoption of horse culture.[15]

The major problem with the Plains origin theory is timing: all of the three estimated dates (1769–79, 1770–80, 1777) are earlier than the documented year of 1781 for the Plains; logically they should be later. The average of the three (1775), however, matches the hypothesized year for Spanish introduction on the coast.

One or Several Epidemics?

The above discussion represents the state of our knowledge on the origins of Pacific Northwest smallpox as of 1996. The data base is ambiguous and may be interpreted in several ways. There is still no final answer as to *when* smallpox first appeared, from *what area* and by which route it was introduced, or even if there was *one* regionwide epidemic or *several* localized ones.

Drawing on the primary sources, different researchers have suggested different solutions: for a Spanish introduction, medical historian Robert Fortuine (1989) favors the 1774 expedition; I (following Portlock) lean to 1775; historian Warren Cook (1973) favors 1779. For a Plains introduction, James Mooney (1928; following Ross Cox) favored 1781; geographer Cole Harris (1994, following Mooney) places it at 1782. My suggestion for a third route and date, from Kamchatka in 1769, was originally made in 1985 (pp. 86–87); it has not been considered further.

Before my 1985 dissertation, when I first raised the issue, no one had considered the likelihood of several localized epidemics. But in 1994, Harris, rely-

---

15. The dual factors of depletion of Plateau bison and increased mobility provided by horses were possible motivators for the Plains hunt (Anastasio 1972).

ing on the geographic discontinuities and clustering of the earliest accounts, held that multiple epidemics were a fact; in 1996 I presented the counterargument for a unitary epidemic, based largely on smallpox epidemiology and aboriginal Northwest social and demographic patterns. As of this writing, the issues have crystallized and positions have been taken. But definitive answers to all these questions remain elusive and are not apt to be forthcoming until new evidence is produced.

SMALLPOX IN THE FIRST DECADE OF THE 1800S

In the first decade of the 1800s, a generation after its initial appearance, smallpox reappeared on the Northwest Coast. As before, the epidemic proceeded unwitnessed and unrecorded by Euro-Americans.[16] Extant accounts consist largely of oral traditions collected from Indian informants well after the fact. The accounts come from four geographic areas: the Columbia Plateau, the lower Columbia River, southwest Washington, and the lower Fraser River. Unlike the initial visitation of smallpox, the early 1800s outbreak seems to have been limited in its extent to the central portion of the Northwest Coast. Origin in the Great Plains and transmission via interethnic contact seem certain.

Historical Accounts

Columbia Plateau. Michel Revais, ethnographer James Teit's mixed-blood Flathead informant, provided the most complete reconstruction of the epidemic's spread on the Plateau:[17]

"Smallpox came from the Crow. This was in the winter-time about 100 years ago [Revais was speaking in 1908 or 1909]. The people were in their winter camps. My grandmother

16. Unless a logbook or journal from one of the trading ships that visited the coast in 1801–2 is located and proves otherwise. Frederic Howay (1931: 135–40) gives the particulars on ships on the coast at this time; Lewis and Clark (1990: 155–56) name 13 shipmasters who traded on the Columbia in the 1805 season.

17. Revais was not a completely reliable informant, and Teit's historical reconstruction of tribal movements in the southern Plateau, based in part on his information, have since been shown to be incorrect (Murdock 1938). When dealing with Interior Salish, however, Revais was on more familiar ground, and the limited collateral information on smallpox in the Salish area supports his reconstruction.

was a little girl at the time, and living at Ntsuwê' ('little creek'), the first creek below
Dixon, Mont. The father of my father-in-law was a little boy and living at Kalispê'lEm,
eastern Washington. Both of them took the disease, but survived." The Flathead
suffered severely. . . . [they] are said to have been reduced to nearly half. . . . the disease . . . passed through the Flathead to the SEmtē'use, Pend d'Oreilles and Kalispel,
and on to the Spokan and Colvile, eventually dying out among the Salish tribes of the
Columbia river. (Teit 1930: 315, 316)

Other Plateau tribes who suffered from this epidemic included the Lakes,
Sanpoil, and Sinkiuse-Columbia. Teit's informants told him that the Okanagan, Nlaka'pamux, Secwepemc, and (to the south) "Shahaptian tribes" were
not affected (1930: 212, 315).

Confirmation of smallpox at this time among the Indians of the Colvile
District is found in the previously quoted passage from John Work's 1829
report, which went on to describe a "second ravage, but less destruction,"
that followed the initial outbreak by "about ten years" (1789–99). Similarly,
for the Nez Perce, missionary Asa Smith said: "The small pox again visited
this country soon after Lewis and Clark were here, perhaps two years after
[1808]; but it was a milder form, perhaps the varioloid & did not prove so
fatal. Many however died. The marks of this disease are now to be seen on
the faces of many of the old people" (6 February 1840, in Drury 1958: 137).

Lower Columbia. Although smallpox is not recorded among the Sahaptin
tribes of the middle Columbia at this time (Teit's informants, above, denied
it), its presence among the lower Columbia Chinookans is documented in
the Lewis and Clark journals. According to Meriwether Lewis:

7 February 1806
The smallpox has distroyed a great number of the natives in this quarter. It prevailed
about 4 years since among the Clatsops and distroy several hundred of them, four of
their chief fell victyms to it's ravages. those Clatsops are deposited in their canoes on
the bay a few miles below us. I think the later ravages of the small pox may well account
for the number of remains of vilages which we find deserted on the river and Sea coast
in this quarter. (Lewis and Clark 1990: 285)

The 1814 Biddle edition of the Lewis and Clark journals, which benefited from
ediorial additions by Clark himself, stated that "the Clatsops. . . . are represented as the remains of a much larger nation. . . . the survivors do not num-

ber more than fourteen houses and about two hundred souls" (Biddle 1814: 2.117).[18] The Lewis and Clark account is important: based on observations of an event which transpired only four years earlier, it is the most firmly grounded of all the early-1800s smallpox references. As such, it serves as a yardstick for all other accounts.

Southwest Washington. From the lower Columbia, smallpox spread along the coast to populated areas in the north. Twana informants from Hood's Canal, speaking in 1939–40, supplied the information on its route: "Disastrous epidemics, apparently of smallpox, struck the Twana in the time of informants' parents and grandparents (1800–1840). The most severe of these was early, perhaps about 1800, and came from the Lower Chehalis on Gray's Harbor via the Satsop; from the Twana it passed north to the Klallam and peoples of southern Vancouver Island" (Elmendorf 1960: 272).[19] Undated myths from this area may refer to a ca. 1800 epidemic (see above), as does the following Upper Chehalis historical tradition, of a vision associated with an epidemic:

Mrs. Mary Heck's grandfather.[20] . . . died when about eighteen years old, before married. Some kind of epidemic before whites came. Covered him with bark in house near Grand Mound. After ten days, his mother went out to weep. . . . Saw a man come round, it was her boy. He used to tell [his vision while "dead"]: he went to a place where having a big pow-wow. He was naked—no clothes—crack in wall in corner of house. People inside—dancing. He no sooner look than father spoke loud and said, "What do you want? No business, to come as you are where people are—naked! Go Way!" He came to found himself covered with bark. He sat down—ex—body—sores [*sic*]—brush it off. Saw maggots. Pretty well gone. Got up. Everyone gone. Recognized the place, went to river, washed body good and clean—went to place where family used to camp. Came to—ten days after. Says B[lucjay]. his Ta. [guardian spirit] brought him back. (Adamson 192–27)

Lower Fraser. Simon Fraser descended and ascended the river that bears his name in June and July 1808. On 24 June, at a Nlaka'pamux encampment

18. As noted earlier (n. 7), the depopulation of the Sauvie Island village of Clannarminamow recorded by Robert Stuart in 1812 may relate to this disease event.

19. As of this writing (1996), Elmendorf's Twana field notes are not available for examination, so it is an open question as to how he arrived at this reconstruction.

20. Mary Heck was "over 90" in 1926–27; her birthdate would have been 1836 or earlier; her grandfather was born perhaps ca. 1786 and reached the age of 18 in ca. 1804.

between Lytton and Spuzzum containing "upwards [of] five hundred souls," he wrote in his journal: "The small pox was in the camp, and several of the Natives were marked with it" (1960: 94). Fraser's wording is ambiguous: if smallpox was indeed *circulating* at the time, it would be contemporaneous with the outbreaks mentioned by Teit's informant and by Smith (above), which referred to smallpox in the Plateau culture area. Fraser's account could also be understood to refer only to pockmarked individuals, survivors of a previous outbreak. As an 1801–2 outbreak would have left more survivors than would one 30 years previous, the former interpretation is more likely. A date of 1801–2 is closest to the date that James Teit's lower Thompson (Nlaka'pamux) informants gave him for smallpox: "near the beginning of the century" (1900: 176).

Two oral traditions from Fraser River Salish informants appear to recall the visit of Simon Fraser and connect it with "sickness" and "pestilence." The most straightforward of these traditions is the Stl'atl'imx (Lillooet) legend "The Sun and the Moon." The story contains several episodes which are verified in Fraser's journal: the capsizing of a canoe that ran some rapids (21 June, downstream from Lytton; 1960: 91); an encounter with "enemy Indians" near the mouth of the river (2 July, pp. 104–8); the purchase and eating of dogs by some of the men (19 June, at Lytton, p. 87); and even, perhaps, the identification of Simon Fraser and his partner John Stuart with the "Sun and Moon" brothers (19 July, p. 87). The last part of the legend states: "The earth was all atremble during the travels of these four [Sun and Moon and their two sons]. Lots of people got sick. Some acted as if they were crazy, they danced, sang and had no time to eat until they were poor. This was not very long ago" (Elliott 1931: 176–77).

"Pestilence Was a Giant Called Stalacom," collected from Joe Splockton at Tsawwassen in the 1950s, less clearly refers to the 1808 voyage of Simon Fraser. In this tale, two Tsawwassen men went up the Fraser in a canoe, where they encountered the "giant" Stalacom. He rode back to Tsawwassen with them, but when the people became frightened and began to shoot at him, he fled back up the river. "[A]fter he had passed it wasn't long until along his path, wherever he had gone as he fled, all the people died. And Stalacom the giant, once he had done his work was never seen by the people again. And Tsawwassen, where many people had lived, was almost deserted for many years" (Appleby 1961: 47).

Tsawwassen depopulation is likely connected to the same disease event recalled by Wayne Suttles's informant Julius Charles (b. ca. 1865) and dated to before 1827:

[T]he shores of Boundary Bay and the drainages of the Serpentine, Nicomekl, and Campbell Rivers were once the territory of the "Snokomish," a tribe that spoke the Fraser River language [Halkomelem]. Most of them died of disease, probably small-pox. The rest married elsewhere. The Semiahmoo were intermarried with them and took over their territory. The Snokomish had a village on Blackie Spit, where Mr. Charles saw their "foundations." (Suttles 1947–48)

Julius Charles's recollections of smallpox at Birch Bay has a similar time frame.[21]

From the lower Fraser, the account of the Katzie shaman Old Pierre appears to mix mythology with datable events and may conflate two early smallpox outbreaks. The first part, clearly mythological, seems to recall a virgin-soil epidemic, with mortality at "three quarters," and is reproduced later in this chapter in the section on mythology. The second part (below) was dated by Sto:lo ethnographer Wilson Duff to the first decade of the 1800s (1952: 28).

My great-grandfather happened to be roaming in the mountains at this period, for his wife had recently given birth to twins, and according to custom, both parents and children had to remain in isolation for several months. The children were just begin-ning to walk when he returned to his village at the entrance to Pitt Lake, knowing nothing of the calamity that had overtaken its inhabitants. All his kinsmen and rela-tives lay dead inside their homes; only in one house did there survive a baby boy, who was vainly sucking at its mother's breast. They rescued the child, burned all the houses, together with the corpses that lay inside them, and built a new home for themselves several miles away. (Jenness 1955: 34)

Old Pierre's son, Simon, gave another version of the Pitt Lake calamity to Wayne Suttles in 1952, but with a significant addition: he gave the baby a name,

21. "When smallpox came to Birch Bay, they buried people in one house after another. Except for those who were away at the time, the only people who were saved were one family who used the wood of a little tree called *pcinełp* [probably Rocky Mountain juniper] for firewood. That killed the germs. They also put green cedar leaves in their mouths, as a man who bathes a corpse does. They buried the dead in back of the houses somewhere."

Słə́məxʷ.[22] Słə́məxʷ (rain) was a historical figure who was reputed to have "discovered gold somewhere above Pitt Lake" and who lived until (probably) "the 1880s." Given his age, it is likely that he was born after the second historical smallpox outbreak, not the first (Suttles, pers. comm., 5 November 1994).

Simon Pierre listed five villages above Katzie that "were wiped out, or nearly so, by smallpox before Fort Langley was founded" (in 1827). "These were *sna'-kʷaya* at Derby (the original site of Fort Langley, just downstream from the mouth of the Salmon River), *skʷɛ'ɛlic* on Bedford Channel north of the mouth of the Salmon River, *xʷə'wənaqʷ* at the mouth of the Whonock River, *sxayə'qs* at Ruskin at the mouth of the Stave River, and *xɛ'cəq'* at Hatzic" (Suttles 1955: 12).[23] The first decade of the 1800s is a possible date for the greater part of the "depopulation" of the village at Stanley Park (*ʔəẏálməxʷ*), from which "numerous skeletons" were uncovered during road construction, many of which were shipped off to the National Museum in Ottawa by ethnographer Charles Hill-Tout (1978: 2.53–54).

In fact, the "depopulation" of the Boundary Bay and lower Fraser villages may have been, not a single event, but a *process,* accentuated by several successive smallpox outbreaks, including all or some combination of the outbreaks recorded for the 1770s, 1800s, and 1820s. The Stanley Park village, which was not completely abandoned until 1887, exemplifies a second problem. Its last occupants were Squamish speakers. But it is an open question whether

---

22. "The tribe at Pitt Lake was wiped out by smallpox, all but one family. My great-grandfather saw a skunk swimming in the Pitt River, clubbed it, and took it home. He said it was supposed to keep off disease. He hung it in front of his house. Just then the smallpox came. His family was the only one that didn't get it. One morning there was no smoke coming from the other houses. They found a baby sucking its dead mother, and they raised him. This was Słə́məxʷ." Old Pierre (b. ca. 1861) was Simon Pierre's father and was about 20 years older than his son. Although both were certainly talking about the same historical event (smallpox depopulating Pitt Lake village), the fact that each referred to it in the time of "my great-grandfather" introduces a discrepancy. Perhaps "great-grandfather" should not be take literally (which places Duff's assumedly genealogical dating in question). Or perhaps Simon Pierre, further removed in time from the actual event, attributed it to the wrong ancestor. It is not possible to recheck the original sources—both informants, as well as the interviewers Duff and Jenness, are dead. Wayne Suttles, who collected the account from Simon Pierre in 1952, "can't account for why both OP and Simon said 'my great-grandfather'" (pers. comm., 5 November 1994). Such are the problems when dealing with oral (remembered) accounts.

23. In the Fraser delta ("opposite Tilbury Island") on 19 December 1824, Hudson's Bay trader John Work met a chief of "the Cahotitt [Kwantlen] tribe . . . marked with the small pox . . . a smart looking little man though pretty old" (1912: 222). Given the age of the chief, his pockmarks could easily be a heritage of the decade of either the 1800s or the 1770s.

it was Squamish speakers, Halkomelem speakers, or both who occupied the site a century earlier. It appears clear that the epidemic depopulation of the villages around the mouth of the Fraser was accompanied by shifts in ethnic territories (Suttles 1990b: 454–56; pers. comm., 5 November 1994), although at this late date, it is very difficult to sort out the particulars of the process.

A Heritage of Fear

The epidemic of the first decade of the 1800s left a heritage of confusion and fear, at least among the Chinook. In 1825 Dr. John Scouler said, "The Cheenooks to the present time speak of it with horror, & are exceedingly anxious to obtain that medicine which protects the whites, meaning vaccination" (1905: 204). Outsiders took advantage of this fear in two well-known instances. The first was the threat of smallpox used by the Cree berdache Kaúxuma-núpika to extort trade from the Indians; the second was the "disease in a bottle" threat used by Duncan McDougall of Fort Astor. Both occurred in summer 1811 on the Columbia River.

Representatives of the Pacific Fur Company, who had traveled on the ship *Tonquin* from New York, arrived at the mouth of the Columbia in April 1811. Here, on the south side a few miles east of Clatsop village and across the river from Chinook, they established Fort Astor. On 2 June, when the *Tonquin* set sail to Vancouver Island to trade for furs, 29 men were left at the fledgling post. They were soon joined by others.

On 15 June, in advance of the party of Canadian explorer David Thompson, nine Indians arrived from upstream, with a leader who spoke Cree (a language of the Canadian Shield). This Indian was the female berdache Kaúxuma-núpika (Schaeffer 1965: 197; called Kocomenepeca by Thompson), who (according to Thompson) considered herself a "prophetess" (1962: 367). Within a few days she was threatening the people at Chinook village with smallpox and, for her own safety, was taken under guard at the fort (Stuart 1935: 273). Thompson's party soon arrived, and in July they all returned upriver. Kaúxuma-núpika had apparently threatened people upstream on the Columbia with disease as well, for when the party arrived at The Cascades rapids, they had to reassure the Indians there that "the white men" had not "brought with them the Small Pox to destroy us" (1962: 367). Traditions of Kaúxuma-núpika's threats and prophecies survived for over a century among the Indians, and it has been suggested that they contributed to the rise of nativistic religions on the middle Columbia (Gibbs 1955–56: 305–6; Spier 1935: 25–29; Boyd 1996b: 175–77).

Left behind at Fort Astor, the Americans received (on 11 August) the ominous news of the massacre of the crew of the *Tonquin* by Nuu-chah-nulth Indians at Nootka Sound. Surrounded by potentially hostile Indians, Duncan McDougall, the fort head, took action. As retold by Washington Irving from now-lost Pacific Fur Company documents, McDougall assembled the principal Chinook and Clatsop men and said:

"The white men among you are few in number, it is true, but they are mighty in medicine. See here," continued he, drawing forth a small bottle and holding it before their eyes, "in this bottle I hold the small-pox, safely corked up; I have but to draw the cork, and let loose the pestilence, to sweep man, woman, and child from the face of the earth." The chiefs were struck with horror and alarm. (1964: 117)

McDougall's threat (according to Irving) was effective: the chiefs promised they would not harm his people. He even received a new name, "the Great Small-pox Chief." This incident, by itself, may appear insignificant. But in fact, the "disease in a bottle" threat was used more than once by Whites who wished to intimidate Indians and—like the prophecies of Kaúxuma-núpika—was adopted (in one form or another) by many Indian peoples as the explanation for the cause of new diseases (see chapter 4).

Epidemiology

Origins and Diffusion. Unlike the first smallpox epidemic, there does not seem to be any question about the origins of smallpox in the first decades of the 1800s. Michel Revais's account states explicitly that the disease "came from the Crow" and then proceeded in sequence, from east to west, among most of the interior Salish tribes of the Columbia Plateau. John Taylor's survey of epidemics in the northern Great Plains lists smallpox among the Crow, Shoshone, Arapaho, Cheyenne, Assiniboine, Sioux, and Chippewa in 1800–1803 (1977: 78–79). A separate maritime origin for the epidemic along the coast itself cannot be ruled out, but until documentary evidence surfaces to support such a claim, it seems best to consider the coastal and Plateau outbreaks as being directly related. The timing is right, and the geographic distribution,

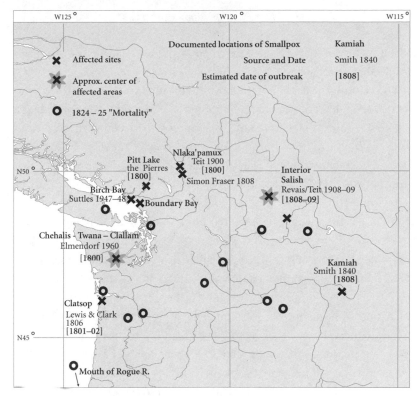

Documented locations of Smallpox

✖ Affected sites

✳ Approx. center of affected areas

⬤ 1824–25 "Mortality"

Source and Date

Estimated date of outbreak

Kamiah

Smith 1840

[1808]

Pitt Lake
the Pierres
[1800]

Nlaka'pamux
Teit 1900
[1800]
Simon Fraser 1808

Interior
Salish
Revais/Teit 1908–09
[1808–09]

N50°

Birch Bay
Suttles 1947–48 ✖✖ Boundary Bay

Chehalis – Twana – Clallam
Elmendorf 1960
[1800]

Kamiah
Smith 1840
[1808]

Clatsop ✖
Lewis & Clark
1806
[1801–02]

N45°

⬤ Mouth of Rogue R.

MAP 4. Smallpox in the Early 1800s

although not continuous, is close enough to be suggestive.[24] Map 4 shows documented locations of smallpox in the first decade of the 1800s.

Mortality. An important problem relating to smallpox in the first decade of the 1800s concerns the virulence of the smallpox strain and its effect on disease mortality. Taylor's data from the Plains suggest a "medium (10 to 25% of population)" mortality for this epidemic (1977: 78). John Work's Colvile report cites "less destruction" than the first epidemic, and Asa Smith's Nez Perce account speaks of "a milder form, perhaps the varioloid & did not prove

24. The possibility of successive outbreaks in the first decade of the 1800s must also be considered. Meriwether Lewis's date of 1801–2 for the Chinook appears to be firmly grounded and is close to the "about 1800" given by Elmendorf for the peoples of southwest Washington and the Olympic Peninsula and Duff for the Katzie account. But a literal reading of Revais on the Columbia Plateau peoples and Smith on the Nez Perce yields a date of 1808. Simon Fraser's ambiguous journal passage, seemingly backed up by two oral traditions, may also support 1808. Smallpox was *not* recorded in the Plains at this time, however.

so fatal." There is, indeed, great variation in strains of smallpox virus, from the fulminating form described so graphically in Mengarini's account of 1770s smallpox among the Flathead (see above), to the mild symptoms and low fatality rate (1% or less) of *Variola minor* (Smith's "varioloid") (see appendix 2). Symptoms, unfortunately, are not given in any of the accounts of early-1800s smallpox, so it is not possible to identify the strain of the disease on a clinical basis. Using mortality as a diagnostic, the evidence on the Northwest Coast is contradictory. Work's and Smith's descriptions indicate, relative to the first epidemic, fewer deaths, but the accounts for the coastal peoples suggest mortalities larger than would be expected from an outbreak of *Variola minor*.

What we may be witnessing, therefore, is not a difference in strain of smallpox influencing mortality but an epidemiological effect that did, indeed, produce a smaller proportion of fatalities in populations which had experienced an initial smallpox outbreak a generation earlier. Individuals who survive an initial bout with smallpox acquire a lifelong immunity to later attacks of the disease. In most (if not all) of the Indian populations of the Pacific Northwest in the first decade of the 1800s, therefore, there should have been a sizable proportion of immunes in that segment of the population over 20 or 30 years of age. Susceptibles to a second outbreak of smallpox would be concentrated in the segment of the population born since the first outbreak. Deaths in a second outbreak would indeed, other factors being held constant, form a smaller proportion of the total population. This epidemiological phenomenon may well explain the relative difference in fatalities between the two outbreaks reported by both Work and Smith.

Comparative Epidemiological Patterns. From an epidemiological perspective, other interesting patterns begin to emerge with smallpox in the first decade of the 1800s. Geographically, the second visitation appears to have occurred in a more restricted area than smallpox in the 1770s. The initial occurrence, of course, reduced the total population of the Pacific Northwest by a considerable amount. It also, undoubtedly, caused a change in the geographic distribution of the surviving populations. Some local groups were wiped out; others escaped with few fatalities. The accounts from the lower Columbia and Fraser River valleys, where denser populations must have made for more effective disease transmission, describe the depopulation and abandonment of village sites. A pattern of desertion of certain regions and regrouping and coalescence of survivors in more restricted areas (also reported from other parts of western North America as a result of epidemic depopulation and, for the coast, again in later years)[25] must have begun with the initial appearance of smallpox. The less continuous distribution of population over the land would create barriers to the transmission of epidemic diseases in subsequent years.

The timing of *later* smallpox epidemics was also affected by the phenomenon of immunity and susceptibility. In every case, a crucial factor in the ability of the disease to take hold and spread in classic epidemic form was the presence of a sufficiently large pool of susceptibles. For every epidemic following the virgin-soil episode in the 1770s, the pool of susceptibles was composed largely of individuals born since the preceding epidemic. There was a single generation gap between virgin-soil smallpox in the 1770s and the outbreak in the first decade of the 1800s on the Central Coast. Present evidence suggests a hiatus of over two generations (60 years) between smallpox in the 1770s and the epidemic of 1836–37 on the northern and southern coasts. Smallpox in the first decade of the 1800s was followed by a gap of either a single generation (the questionable 1824–25 "mortality") or two generations (the 1853 epidemic). One generation separated the 1836–37 North Coast epidemic from the 1862 epidemic.

THE 1824–25 "MORTALITY"

One of the unanticipated results of this research has been the discovery of scattered data that point to a significant epidemic mortality from an unknown disease (probably smallpox) throughout much of the southern coast and Columbia Plateau in 1824–25. The evidence is of three varieties: (1) ambiguous contemporary references to a "mortality," usually called "smallpox" when identified at all; (2) demographic data from the 1824–25 Fort George, 1827–29 Colvile, and 1829 Nez Percés censuses that suggest a major demographic disturbance in the region a few years previously; and (3) scattered recollections, from Indian informants of the late 1800s, of an epidemic in this time period.

Ethnohistorical and ethnographic sources from the coast which may refer to such an epidemic exist for Tututni, Tualatin Kalapuya, Chinookans, Quwutsun' (Cowichan), and Nuwhaha Puget Salish.[26] Different sources name different diseases. The Tualatin and Quwutsun' accounts say "small-

---

25. E.g., Cook 1976a; Ewers 1973: 109–12; Taylor 1977: 64–66; Krech 1978; this volume, chapter 8.

26. For the Tututni, see Parrish 1855: 499; quoted in chapter 5, this volume. For the Tualatin, see Frachtenberg 1914: 2. For the Chinookans, see Kennedy 1824–25; McKenzie 1825: 1 June; Scouler

pox" (as do others from the Plateau). Epidemiologically, sufficient time (one generation) had passed to allow a non-immune population large enough to support a third outbreak of smallpox. But it may have been the other spotted disease, measles, as suggested in the Tututni account and in a possibly garbled tradition recorded by Fort Vancouver physician Dr. Forbes Barclay in the 1840s: "The measles have been known to prevail in the Columbia in 1812 [*sic:* 1821?—the date of the arrival of the Hudson's Bay Company in the Northwest]—supposed to have been carried thither by the H. Bay Company from York factory where it prevailed at the same time" (in Larsell 1947: 90). Again, epidemiologically, the timing is correct: measles is documented from the Subarctic in 1819–23 (Krech 1981: 85) and from California in 1828 (Valle 1973a). But the Hudson's Bay records from the lower Columbia refer only to an ambiguous "mortality."

Three accounts mention the "mortality" in the family of Concomly, the chief of the Chinooks. Dr. Scouler's is most complete:

12 April 1824

Concomli or Madsu who is the greatest chief upon the river had lost two of his sons. While these two young men were sick Concomli had placed them under the care of a neighbouring chief who pretended to great skill in medicine, & cured diseases by singing over his patients. Under this method [of] cure both the young chiefs died, & the medicine chief was accused of procuring their death by enchantment. . . . To revenge this imaginary crime, the remaining son of Concomli had assassinated the medicine chief, & it was now expected that his friends, who are both numerous & powerful, would attempt to revenge his death. (1905: 165–66)

The two dead sons were "Chalakan & Choulits" (Kennedy 1824–25); the avenging son was Cassacas; and the shaman was "Tete Plume," who came from one of the "two Upper Villages at Cheenook" (McKenzie 1825: 1 June).

By late 1825 Concomly had lost "8 individuals of his family" to the "mortality," and the Chinooks had vacated a village at Point Ellis (Scouler 1905: 276–77). The Hudson's Bay people were concerned because the deaths had affected trade. At Chinook village, "this casualty . . . tended to slacken the exertions of the surviving part of the family for a considerable time, who instead

---

1905: 276–77. For the Quwutsun', see Scouler 1905: 203; *Daily British Colonist,* 19 December 1862. For the Nuwhaha, see Sampson 1972: 25.

of collecting furs, were occupied in going round the villages in the vicinity howling like wolves and begging property to sooth their sordid [*sic*] for the loss of their near relatives" (Kennedy 1824–25).

Two Quwutsun' accounts that name smallpox date to this time period. Off Point Roberts in August 1825, Dr. Scouler met the "Cowitchen chief, Chapea . . . [who] had in his retinue an Indian deeply marked with small-pox" (1905: 203). This passage, by itself, could refer to an earlier outbreak. More specific, however, is the following, from a 19 December article in the *Daily British Colonist* (Victoria) newspaper, written just after the major smallpox epidemic of 1862 (chapter 7).

The old people of the [Quwutsun'] tribe relate that some thirty or forty years ago [1822–32] there was a similar state of affairs to the present—that the weather was very foggy—*hiyou smoke*—and that there was an unusually plentiful catch of salmon, but that the Indians did not live to benefit, by the abundance, the smallpox having cut them off in great numbers; they were consequently in great fear that a like calamity may now befall them.

Several of the Fraser River traditions given earlier of village abandonment "before the founding of Fort Langley [1827]" may incorporate memories of an 1824–25 disease visitation. The only mainland Salishan account that specifically dates to a third- or fourth-decade epidemic, however, is Swinomish historian Martin Sampson's tradition for the Nuwhaha (northernmost Puget Salish):

[T]he last scourge in the 1830s [*sic*] reached every village, leaving only about 200 out of over 1,000 people. Only one out of a village on Jarman Prairie was saved, a baby girl. A visiting uncle found her in her dead mother's arms, moved her to the north side of the Prairie, and left her in a shelter. He then went back to the houses on the bank of the Samish river, and after making sure that no others were alive, set the torch to all of the buildings. Checking the houses on Friday Creek and finding all of the inhabitants dead, he also burned this village. There, as a further sanitary measure, he took off all his clothing and tossed his garments on the flames.[27] (Sampson 1972: 25)

27. The sole surviving orphan theme recalls the earlier Pitt River account and may be a borrowed element. But the geographic details and chronological timing support the depopulation as a purely local, late event.

The only definitely dated Plateau record is from the Cayuse (27 March 1825): "The returns have fallen off this Season about 300 Skins; this seems to have arisen from a Mortality that took place in the course of the Winter among the Cai-uses which prevented them from hunting" (Simpson 1968: 127). All the other Plateau accounts are based on recollections of ethnographic informants consulted by James Teit and Andrew Splawn in the late 1800s. Teit gives 1825 as the date for a smallpox epidemic among the Columbia Salish (1928: 97) and 1831–32 for the Coeur d'Alene and Okanagan (1930: 3, 40, 212); Splawn makes it 1836 for Columbia River peoples.[28] Splawn's Sahaptin informants said that smallpox frightened the Yakamas, who "fled to the mountains . . . so terror-stricken that they left their sick to die along the trail. . . . more than half the Indians died along the Columbia from its mouth to Kettle Falls" (1944: 426, 393).

Additional evidence from three contemporary censuses or semicensuses of Columbia drainage peoples taken by Hudson's Bay officials suggest that Splawn's description of geographic extent is correct. The Fort George (Astoria) estimate of 1824–25 (Kennedy 1824–25) gives winter populations of some Chinookan villages slightly lower than those expected from the 1805 Lewis and Clark estimate, which may reflect some deaths from the "mortality" reported in contemporary lower Columbia sources. The 1829 Fort Nez Percés estimate also has total numbers slightly under that of Lewis and Clark. The 1827 Fort Colvile census has a distinctive pattern of low percentages of children among downstream, riverside populations, consistent with a hypothesis of an epidemic disease which attacked especially children, transmitted between continuously distributed winter (1824–25) villages. Given the contemporary epidemiological and demographic environment of the Plateau, a mild strain of smallpox or measles could easily produce such a pattern. I interpret this evidence as a minor epidemic, probably of smallpox, along (at least) the banks of the Columbia River in the winter of 1824–25.

28. Teit's 1831–32 is not defensible ethnohistorically: smallpox is unmentioned in contemporary documents. Splawn's 1836 appears to have been estimated from the probable date of the adolescent vision quest of his informant, We-i-pah, plus awareness of the 1836–37 smallpox epidemic on the North and South Coasts (chapter 5). Since We-i-pah was "an old man when the first settler came to this valley in 1861" (Splawn 1944: 426), however, 1836 is almost certainly too late. And again, contemporary ethnohistorical sources are mute on smallpox at this time on the Plateau. For these reasons I am assuming that both Teit's and Splawn's accounts refer to an earlier time, likely 1824–25.

MYTHOLOGICAL ACCOUNTS OF EPIDEMICS AND DEPOPULATION

Northwest Coast myth accounts by their very nature are set outside linear time and are not easily dated. But myths may include internal evidence for early epidemic visitations or depopulation of villages by epidemic disease, though it may be disguised or included incidentally in the narrative. And there are sometimes clues that help narrow down the time frame during which such disease events and/or mortalities may have occurred. Such clues, from genealogy, datable events, and archeology, when present, are noted in what follows.

The relevant myth accounts lend themselves to organization by theme, and each major theme seems to be limited to a specific geographic region. The themes, in other words, may be interpreted as local culturally specific explanations of catastrophes that were both new and devastating to the Indian peoples. Northwest Indians attempted to explain such events through mythology, in a framework that was meaningful to them in their own cultures. Given varying disease histories (beyond the initial virgin-soil experience) and varying cultural traditions, themes fall naturally into four regional clusters: North Coast, lower Fraser, Washington coast, and lower Columbia.

North Coast (Tlingit, Haida, Tsimshian, Heiltsuk)

North Coast myths that may recall early smallpox epidemics and resultant depopulation were not collected until the first decade of the 1900s, well over a century after the initial virgin-soil experience, 60 years after the second epidemic, and 40 years after the last. Two themes (the "magic plume" and depredations of a sea monster) concern village depopulation; although disease is mentioned incidentally, other natural catastrophes (volcanism, tsunamis) were probably more important. But a third group of stories, which concern the "Pestilence spirit," clearly recall epidemic visitations.

The oral traditions of the Haida people contain several myths which involve the spirit translated as "Pestilence." The collecting ethnographer, John Swanton, stated that "in recent years" the spirit was "particularly associated with smallpox" (1905b: 303 n. 16). But Pestilence stories certainly predate the 1862 smallpox epidemic that Swanton knew; Erna Gunther (1972: 121) cites one that she thought was a recollection of the 1787 visit of explorer George Dixon. And the associations of "Pestilence" with large boats and some variation on "sparks" or "flashing eyes" that cause people to drop dead (certainly guns) suggest that belief in the spirit came with the first Euro-American vessels during the late 1700s. "Big-Tail," related by John Moody at Skidegate in 1900 or 1901, states it best:

Pestilence came [into a house]. His canoe was like a white man's vessel. Sparks flew out of it. They [the sparks] went through the house. For that reason the supernatural beings [invited to a feast] were afraid. The things that come out of it are what cause sickness. The supernatural beings feared they would strike them. . . . when he [the nephew of Supernatural-being-at-whose-voice-the-ravens-sit-on-the sea] untied a little something against the roof of the house, which was like a hollow tube closed with knots at both ends, Pestilence's canoe was quickly turned about.[29] (Swanton 1905b: 299)

The Yakutat Tlingit believed that epidemics came in "disease boats." According to ethnographer Frederica de Laguna:

Epidemics were believed to be the work of spirits that came in boats, sometimes paddling in canoes, or riding in a sailing ship or even in a steamboat. They were invisible to any eyes but those of the shaman. In the boat were all those who had previously died of the disease, and in this way they traveled to the Land of the Dead, "way back," where go the souls of those who died nonviolent deaths. Some persons received such disease spirits as their yek [guardian spirit], and so became shamans. A shaman could see the "boat of sickness," containing all those who had died of the disease. As people died they entered the boat, and when the epidemic had run its course in one locality, the boat would sail away, perhaps to go to another. (1972: 2.710)[30]

Lower Fraser

Among the lower Fraser peoples there are several variations on a myth that has the world experiencing several disasters, ending with a smallpox epidemic that preceded the coming of the Whites. Some Christian influence is apparent in these stories, perhaps diffused to the coast with a Christianized form

---

29. A second Pestilence tale from the Haida is "Story of the Shaman, G.a'ndox's-Father" (Swanton 1905b: 311–15); a Tsimshian example is "The Princess Who Rejected Her Cousin" (Boas 1916: 185–92).

30. An example of a Tlingit "disease boat" tale is "How Qałax̱aetł Became a Shaman" (de Laguna 1972: 2.713).

of the Plateau Prophet Dance in the early 1800s (Suttles 1957) and/or influenced by the chronologies transmitted through pictures shown in the Catholic Ladder, a teaching device first used in the area by Catholic missionaries in the 1840s. Two sets of these myths, each including a short and a long version, for Squamish, Chilliwack, and Katzie, from four different informants, are given below.

In 1888, Franz Boas recorded a Squamish creation tale from the Squamish chief, Joseph. Qa'is, the Sun (who also figures in Old Pierre's chronology; see below), created the earth but destroyed it four times in succession when the "people became evil." The first time the people were turned to stone; the second time a fire "burnt the earth completely"; the third time there was a flood (complete with a large boat and mountain); and the fourth time "Qa'is sent the smallpox and one winter with deep snow to the people as punishment for their wickedness" (1975: 92).

Charles Hill-Tout's lengthier Squamish version, collected from an "aged informant" in the 1890s, links the smallpox visitation with a different natural disaster:

[A] dreadful misfortune befell them. . . . One salmon season the fish were found to be covered with running sores and blotches, which rendered them unfit for food. But as the people depended very largely upon these salmon for their winter's food supply, they were obliged to catch and cure them as best they could, and store them away for food. They put off eating them till no other food was available, and then began a terrible time of sickness and distress. A dreadful skin disease, loathsome to look upon, broke out upon all alike. None were spared. Men, women, and children sickened, took the disease and died in agony by hundreds, so that when the spring arrived and fresh food was procurable, there was scarcely a person left of all their numbers to get it. Camp after camp, village after village, was left desolate. The remains of which, said the old man, in answer to my queries on this, are found today in the old camp sites or midden-heaps over which the forest has been growing for so many generations. Little by little the remnant left by the disease grew into a nation once more, and when the first white men sailed up the Squamish in their big boats, the tribe was strong and numerous again. (Hill-Tout 1978: 2.22)

The Katzie shaman Old Pierre, noted earlier, related a chronology that has the people drowning and dispersing in a great flood, then starving in a long snowstorm before the third disaster, "a great sickness":

After many generations, the people again multiplied until for the third time the smoke of their fires floated over the valley like a dense fog. The news reached them from the east that a great sickness was travelling over the land, a sickness that no medicine could cure, and no person escape. Terrified, they held council with one another and decided to send their wives, with half the children, to their parents' homes, so that every adult might die in the place where he or she was raised. Then the wind carried the smallpox sickness among them. Some crawled away into the woods to die; many died in their houses. Altogether about three-quarters of the Indians perished. (Jenness 1955: 34)[31]

The version collected from the Chilliwack informant Albert Louie in 1965 retains the flood, drops the snowstorm, and identifies the disease as smallpox, which killed "oh, half the Indians" (Wells 1987: 160).

Middle Fraser

Though technically the middle Fraser (Stl'atl'imx and Nlaka'pamux) peoples are members of the Plateau culture area and therefore outside the scope of this volume, two myths should be mentioned here, both because they suggest a coastal origin for a deadly disease and because they share with the lower Fraser accounts a theme of a few survivors who became ancestors to people alive today. Both were collected by James Teit around the turn of the century. The Nlaka'pamux (Thompson) story, "The Origin of the Spuzzum People," is most complete:

A father and son . . . hunting. . . . came upon a village of strange people. . . . their languages were mutually unintelligible. They must have belonged to the coast tribes [the man and his son buy a copper hammer]. On reaching home, they showed their won-

---

31. In 1985, following Wilson Duff, I assigned Old Pierre's Katzie account and the variant from the Squamish to "around 1800," though I expressed some doubts about the dating (Duff 1952: 28; Boyd 1985: 111). In 1994, however, geographer Cole Harris lumped these two accounts with all others from the lower Fraser and assigned them to the first epidemic. On rereading all relevant records, I now think that *both* researchers are probably correct. Old Pierre's description of the Pitt Lake village depopulation, quoted earlier, was the one part of his entire narrative that was associated with a specific ancestor, and which Duff dated, apparently genealogically, to 1800. But the earlier, mythologized portion, given above, appears to describe a virgin-soil disease event. Old Pierre's narrative, in other words, may conflate memories of two disease events, a phenomenon common in remembered oral traditions when the events are similar and closely spaced (Vansina 1985: 175).

derful purchase to their friends; and the people of all the houses, including the x̣ax̣a'
people [pit-dwellers], flocked to see it. After all had examined it, they repaired to their
respective houses, and went to sleep; but none of those who had looked at or had
touched the copper hammer awoke again. They all died that night. . . . two young men
away training in the mountains. . . . on their return home . . . to one of the houses on
the south side of the creek . . . they found all the people dead. They entered the other
house, and found all the people dead there also; then they crossed the creek to the
house of the x̣ax̣a', but found them dead likewise. Then they repaired to the remaining house, where the people were also dead excepting an old woman and her two young
granddaughters, who were the only people who had not gone to see the wonderful
copper hammer. . . . the girls married the two men, and they had numerous children,
from whom it is said most of the Spuzzum people are descended. (Teit 1912a: 275–76)

The related Stl'atl'imx (Lillooet) story, "The Poor Man; or, the Origin of
Copper," sets the action at Green Lake (headwaters of the upper Lillooet),
where "all died" from "some disease . . . except an old woman and her grand-
son." The two found a copper (a coastal wealth item) and became rich, the
boy married and had sons, and "the Green Lake people became very numerous again" (Teit 1912b: 343–44).

Coastal Washington

A small body of myths from the area between the mouth of the Columbia
and Port Townsend on the Olympic Peninsula seem to recall an early epidemic. A Chinook myth, "The Transformers," and a Humptulips (Lower
Chehalis) myth, "Musp' and Kəmo'ʟ," share a theme of a woman who laughs
and the people of a village all fall dead. The Chinook version was collected
from a "woman born about 1830" (Curtis 1911: 116–23); the Humptulips story,
from informant Lucy Heck, 70 years old in 1926, and dated by her to a time
frame preceding about 1830.[32] Both tales mention, in their second sections,
selective deaths of children, a phenomenon which might be interpreted as
indicating two successive epidemics and acquired immunity. The Humptulips
story bears quotation (in part):

32. The informant recalled that the story was told to her by her stepfather at her marriage
(reconstructed date, ca. 1876) and dated to a period over two generations earlier (to before 1836,
calculating 20 years per generation; or before 1826, calculating 25 years per generation).

Chief Woodpecker lived on the present site of Humptulip city. The village was composed of twelve large houses. . . . Sʟʟ'o'cən. . . . a pretty young girl . . . from a place above Humptulip City. . . . was getting ready to laugh with Bluejay. . . . By the time she had finished laughing, everyone in the house, including Bluejay, had fallen dead. Their tongues lolled out and their eyes fairly bulged from their heads. Then she went to another house and cried, "I am going to laugh with Bluejay! Ha ha, ho." Every last person in the house dropped dead. She went to another. . . . And again all the people dropped dead on the spot. She went from one house to another and every occupant died. . . . every person in the village was dead. . . . she set out for her own village ten miles further up the river. (Adamson 1934: 329–30)

In part 2, Sʟʟ'o'cən has two sons, who travel back to Humptulips and find the eleven houses full of skeletons. They burn the remains and set out on a journey during which they visit five prairies in succession and at each kill and cut open the stomach of a cannibal; children emerge and are rejuvenated. "'What shall we do to increase the population here? There are so few people left.' . . . little rolls of dirt became people" (Adamson 1934: 338).

Lower Columbia

From the lower Columbia and Oregon coast there are two myths of note. The most dramatic of these is certainly "The Sun's Myth," collected from the Chinook informant Charles Cultee by Franz Boas in 1891. The story tells of a man who travels to a distant place 10 months to the east where he stays in the lodge of a woman, admires "that thing shining all over" (the sun) hanging from the roof, and is given it as a present when homesickness causes him to leave.

As versified by Dell Hymes, the myth builds dramatically. On his return home, the man with the sun visits four villages of his father's brothers, and for reasons that are not explicitly stated, the inhabitants of each village die. Finally he reaches his father's village.

> Again he would go.
> Now his too, his town,
>   he would be near his town.
> In vain he would try to stand, that one,
>   see, something would pull his feet.

His reason would become nothing,
 he would do it to his town,
  crush, crush, crush, crush;
 all his town he would destroy
  and he would destroy his relatives.
He would recover:
 his town (is) nothing,
  the dead fill the ground.
He would become
 "Qa! qa! qa! qa!,"
  he would cry out.
In vain he would try to bathe;
 in vain he would try to shake off what he wears,
  and his flesh would be pulled.
Sometimes he would roll about on rocks;
 he would think,
  perhaps it will break apart;
  he would abandon hope.
Now again he would cry out,
 and he wept.
   (Hymes, pers. comm., 24 January 1994)[33]

Hymes originally thought this story recalled the devastating "fever and ague" epidemics of the 1830s (chapter 4); he is now inclined to think it refers instead to the first smallpox epidemic, the one that "raged in the towns" of the Clatsops and "distroyed their nation," to use William Clark's language. "It fits the culture-internal explanation of what had happened seamlessly— something brought on the culture from within, breaking the implicit compact with the powers of the world" (Hymes, pers. comm., 24 January 1994). The vagueness of the myth lends itself to different interpretations, but (as in the case of the Kwakwa̱ka̱'wakw man with "mouths" all over his body) there are clues, both symptomatic and epidemiological, that point to smallpox. "In vain" the man tries "to shake off what he wears, and his flesh" is "pulled"; he tries to bathe; he rolls around on the rocks to rid himself of that which causes death. Despite the absence of references to sores, these words are suggestive

33. This is an excerpt from Hymes's latest revision. For the complete myth, see Hymes 1975.

of the itching pain and fever associated with (especially) confluent smallpox. Epidemiologically, deaths and total mortality follow his stay in each of the five villages, also suggestive of smallpox. And the loss of reason, abandonment of hope, and grief are all typical of survivors of a devastating epidemic. This story, related by a lineal descendant of survivors of the first epidemics, is probably the most dramatic of any of the Northwest Coast oral traditions recalling epidemics.[34]

34. The Alsea myth "The Five Thunderers" may be related to the Chinookan "Sun's Myth." Collected in 1900 from one of the last speakers of Alsea, it tells of five brothers who "travel all over the world in a canoe." They visit five villages; in each something is "killing all the people." Although the "agents" of death in each case are nondisease and precontact (a bur, cannibal women, fleas, starvation, and calico salmon) (Frachtenberg 1920: 91–109), epidemiologically this myth could recall a virulent contagious disease like smallpox. And (though this is admittedly speculative) some of the "agents" *may* refer, symbolically, to smallpox symptoms (e.g., flea = itching, calico salmon = pockmark) (Dell Hymes, pers. comm.).

3 / Diseases Caused by Treponemata and Mycobacteria

Precontact and Postcontact Forms

INTRODUCTION: THE PRECONTACT EVIDENCE

The two major chronic diseases of the Northwest Coast during the early contact period, syphilis and tuberculosis, are caused by microbes that belong to two widespread genera of disease-causing organisms: *Treponema* and *Mycobacterium*. *Treponema* is a spirochete genus that includes *T. pallidum*, the germ that produces (in subspecific forms) venereal syphilis and nonvenereal bejel and yaws; a second treponemal species causes the indigenous American skin disease pinta. *Mycobacterium* includes species that cause tuberculosis (*M. tuberculosis*) and leprosy (*M. leprae*; see appendix 3); many of the remaining fifty-odd mycobacterial species cause tuberculosis-like symptoms in humans.

Although varieties of both mycobacteria and treponemata existed in both hemispheres before contact, until very recently the pre-Columbian distribution of syphilis and tuberculosis remained a mystery. Since 1988, there has been a rapid increase in paleopathological evidence on the origins of syphilis. Baker and Armelagos (1988) have shown that there are a great number of syphilitic bones in the pre-Columbian Americas and virtually none in the pre-1492 Old World. The work of Rothschild and Rothschild (1996) has revealed a concentration of syphilitic bones in the midlatitude agricultural zone of the Americas versus nonsyphilitic (yaws and pinta) treponemal bones in outlying areas.[1]

---

1. For the native American treponematoses, "bone enlargement resulting from proliferative periostitis," occurring particularly in "bones that have minimal overlying soft tissue," such

Similarly, since 1973, when physical anthropologists reported the existence of acid-fast tubercular bacilli in a Peruvian mummy dated to A.D. 700, paleopathological evidence for pre-Columbian American tuberculosis has been increasing. It now appears that tuberculosis and/or allied mycobacterial diseases were present in all of the more densely populated regions of the Americas.[2]

Although both syphilis and tuberculosis were apparently native to other parts of the Americas, there is currently no paleopathological evidence for either disease in the Northwest Coast culture area. Indigenous syphilis was found as far west as New Mexico (Rothschild and Rothschild 1996: 558). Precontact tuberculosis or an allied mycobacterial disease existed as close as North Dakota and Arizona (Buikstra and Williams 1991: 162). Present evidence, therefore, implies that both diseases were introduced to the Northwest after contact by Europeans. And the reaction of Northwest Indian populations to syphilis and tuberculosis suggests that they were (for the most part) "virgin soil" for both diseases.

But the real picture is not one of simple introduction—there may have been diseases caused by other mycobacteria and treponemata in the Northwest before contact. Since 1990, we have known that a form of treponematosis (probably yaws) was indigenous to the Northwest. In that year physical anthropologist Jerome Cybulski reported five skeletal remains from two coastal British Columbia sites dated at 325 and 1490 B.C. with probable treponemal lesions (Cybulski 1990: 57; 1994: 81). Given the geographic extent of indigenous American tuberculosis and the population density of the Pacific coast, a Northwest tuberculosis or tuberculosis-like mycobacterial disease is possible.

Although paleopathological evidence for a precontact treponemal relative of syphilis appears sound, ethnohistorical evidence for such a disease is slim. There is a good chance that some of the many passages in the oral literature

---

as "the calvarium and tibia," is diagnostic (Ortner, Tuross, and Stix 1992: 343). Yaws produces a high frequency of surface periostitis on hands and feet, especially in subadults; syphilis is low frequency, with many examples of the distinctive "sabershins," largely in adults (Rothschild and Rothschild 1996).

2. For the Peruvian mummy, see Allison, Mendoza, and Pezzia 1973. In 1981, using the diagnostic of "resorptive" bone lesions in three or fewer lower thoracic and upper lumbar vertebrae, paleopathologist Jane Buikstra and colleagues identified a "tuberculosis-like pathology" in large regions of agricultural native America, in particular the North American Midwest. Although some researchers suggested that these remains may have been the product of nontubercular mycobacteria (Clark et al. 1987), the case for pre-Columbian American tuberculosis was sealed

which refer to scabs and sores in fact refer to treponemal disease. Although a definitive description is highly unlikely, the best possibilities are those that mention symptoms shared by all nonvenereal treponematoses, namely, lesions in children, focused on the hands and feet. Two variants of a Nisga'a tradition, for instance, describe a slave girl with scabs on "Her hands, her feet" (Boas 1902: 189–90) or "her legs and arms" (Barbeau and Beynon 1987: 1.201), which are likened to an "abalone shell" or "abalone pearl," reminiscent of the lesions of pinta. And two historic accounts, both from 1786 at Nootka, are also *suggestive* of nonvenereal treponematoses:

6 July 1786

Mr Mackay had already gained the affections of [Maquinna's] Family by the Cure of the Chief's Child, who was much indisposed with scabby hands and legs; this seemed indeed to be the prevailing complaint among all their Children. (Strange 1929: 22)

25 July 1786

[W]e saw no diseases among this People that did not proceed from nastiness [i.e., filth], or such as are incident to old Age. Their most common disorder is the itch, which with them appears to be of two kinds: the common kind ["itch" is the colloquial term for scabies, but pediculosis is more likely here], and one of a more inveterate nature, which greatly annoys their Childrens' Feet. They appeared ignorant of any remedies for these complaints, and received thankfully our assistance. (Walker 1982: 79)

INTRODUCED VENEREAL DISEASES

Despite the presence of an indigenous form of treponemal disease, there is no doubt that venereal treponematosis (syphilis) and its venereal companion gonorrhea were introduced to the Northwest Coast by the earliest maritime explorers and fur traders. The diseases may have come with the Spanish explorations of 1774 and 1775, but there is no documentary evidence to support this possibility.[3]

---

in 1994 with the recovery of *M. tuberculosis* DNA from a 1,000-year-old Peruvian mummy (Salo et al. 1994).

3. Venereal disease *was* recorded among the crew of the 1779 Spanish expedition to the Northwest Coast, particularly among those who were natives of San Blas in Mexico (Martinez 1915: 23–24, 59, 64).

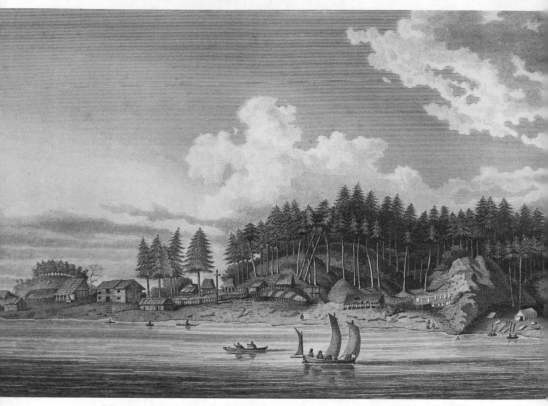

FIG. 1. The Spanish settlement at Friendly Cove, Nootka Sound, was the earliest year-round White settlement on the Northwest Coast and an early focus of venereal disease and pulmonary tuberculosis. This drawing, made in 1792, is from vol. 1 of George Vancouver's *Voyage of Discovery*, between pp. 388 and 389. (Courtesy of the Oregon Historical Society, Portland, negative no. OrHi 96960.)

For the Cook expedition of 1778, however, there is abundant evidence for venereal introduction, both gonorrhea and syphilis. The sailors of the Cook expedition appear to have been the venereal equivalent of Typhoid Mary: they have been implicated in the introduction of venereal diseases to New Zealand, Tonga, Tahiti, and Hawaii in addition to the Nuu-chah-nulth peoples of Nootka Sound (fig. 1).[4] Ship surgeon David Samwell's 1786 broadside "Observations respecting the Introduction of the Venereal Disease into the Sandwich Islands" shows that the spread of the disease was a topic of discussion (and, one might assume, guilt) in Cook's time as well.

4. All of this evidence is examined in Watt 1979.

Stage 1: Traders and Prostitution

Cook's sailors set a pattern which would be repeated and shortly institution-alized during the maritime fur-trading period (1778 on) of Northwest Coast history (Gibson 1988; Cole and Darling 1990). Samwell describes how it began:

6 April 1778

[W]e had seen none of their young Women tho' we had often given the men to under-stand how agreeable their Company would be to us & how profitable to themselves, in consequence of which they about this time brought two or three Girls to the Ships . . . exceedingly dirty . . . removed with Soap & warm water. . . . they were prevailed upon to sleep on board the Ships, or rather forced to it by their Fathers or other Relations who brought them on board. . . . Their Fathers . . . made the Bargain & received the price of Prostitution of their Daughters, which was commonly a Pewter plate well scoured for one Night. When they found this was a profitable Trade they brought more young women to the Ships. . . . [Thus] they found means at last to disburthen our young Gentry of their Kitchen furniture, many of us leaving this Harbour not being able to muster a plate to eat our Salt beef from. (Samwell in Beaglehole 1967: 1095)

Samwell thought these women were the "daughters" of the men they met, but he was wrong. After two more weeks of contact, William Ellis had figured out who they were:

22 April 1778

It was a prevailing opinion, that the women brought on this occasion were not of their own tribe, but belonging to some other which they had overcome in battle. What led us to suppose so, was the different treatment which was observed between these and those who were not exposed in this manner. The former were mute, did not dare to look up, appeared quite dejected, and were totally under the command of those who brought them; the latter on the contrary were as full of conversation as the men, behaved with ease, and (comparatively speaking) evidently were under no kind of controul. (Ellis 1782: 1.216–17)

These women were slaves. The Northwest Coast institution of slavery was practiced throughout most of the region from southeast Alaska to the central Oregon coast. Slaves were indeed generally captured in warfare with alien (nonrelated) peoples and tended to be women and children, as men were hastily dispatched. They were valued for their labor and prestige and were lodged in the houses of their owners, who tended to be highborn people of economic means (Donald 1996). Slave owners were often traders as well and knew how to conduct a transaction to their own benefit. They were quick to see that they could use their slaves in a new way to bring wealth into their hands. The Northwest Coast institution of (female) slavery dovetailed nicely with the demographic and mercantile characteristics of the maritime new-comers: these were, after all, crews which were exclusively male, mostly young, and separated by thousands of miles and several months from their coun-trywomen on what was essentially a speculative, capitalist endeavor. The sit-uation was ripe for the spread of venereal disease. Similar statements from Nuu-chah-nulth peoples on the use of slaves as prostitutes are found in traders' journals from the 1780s and 1790s.[5]

What happened at Nootka was repeated at other coastal landfalls. The ear-liest reference of its sort from the Queen Charlottes notes that Haida men were "jealous of their women" but "not only permitted but even persuaded" some of them "to accept the invitations of our people" (Lauder 1789: 111).[6] When Alejandro Malaspina visited the Tlingit of Port Mulgrave (Yakutat Bay) in June 1791, he noted: "From the first they indicated that their women were at our disposal" (1934, entry of 27 June 1791). The Spaniards assumed these sirens were slaves.

5. E.g., Alexander Walker in 1786 (1982: 87); Jacinto Caamaño in 1790 (1790: 157); Dionisio Alcala Galiano in 1792 (1991: 184); José Mozino in 1792 (1970: 43); and John Jewitt in 1803–5 (1975: 39). But when members of Vancouver's 1792 expedition approached upper-class women, they were rebuffed. Edward Bell said Makah women would "burst into tears" and "hide themselves in the bottom of their canoes" (1792, entry of 11 May). Peter Puget said, "Those of the Inferior Class easily gave themselves up to Prostitution, three or four Common Looking Glasses or other trifling articles would always purchase their favors.... A young girl belonging [related?] to Clussanimulth named Tlakcaw . . . contrived by Excellent management and distribution of her Smiles to receive innumerable presents from her admirers, but without granting her favors to anyone" (1793, entry of 15 May).

The members of Vancouver's expedition appear to have propositioned Indian women at every opportunity. Sometimes they were successful, as at Chinook (20 May 1792, Boit in Howay 1941: 399), Quinault (December 1792, Vancouver 1798: 2.84), and Skagit (2 June 1792, Vancouver 1798: 2.286); sometimes not, as among Straits Salish (July 1792, Manby) and Twana (3 August 1792, Puget). The different responses probably related to whether the contacted people had any previous experience with sailors and whom the sailors met—free women or slaves.

6. By the early 1790s, references from Cloak Bay and Queen Charlotte Sound stated: "The men and the old women who offered young girls as articles of trade, took great care to point out that they did not wear the American ornament [labret, or lip plug] which had appeared to dis-

Stage 2: Primary Syphilis

The eventual outcome of these sexual encounters was venereal disease. Initial cases were reported within 10–13 years after the first mention of sale of sexual services to sailors among contacted peoples, to wit, on the southwest coast of Vancouver Island:

June 1791, village Nittenat
Cassacan we found troubled with the venereal to a great degree. . . . on questioning . . . he says sometime since a vessel came to this place; to the Captain of which he sold a female prisoner or slave girl for several sheets of copper: on the vessels going away, the girl was sent ashore; he afterwards cohabited with the girl, who shortly after died; caught the fatal disease and communicated it to his wife; who, he says, has it equally as bad as himself: thus this most banefull disorder will e'er long prove fatal to this pair, and possibly spread throughout the village; making the most dreadful destruction: we dressed Cassacan, but he would not permit us to, his wife; and gave him several medicines; which he received most thankfully. (Hoskins in Howay 1941: 196)

On a return visit six months later Cassacan "still retains the loathsome disease" (258); he also had pockmarks, which indicated he had survived an attack of smallpox (see chapter 2).

The earliest reference to venereal disease among the Haida was in 1799, at Cloak Bay, site of the Comte de Fleurieu's 1791 description of prostitution:

20 March 1799, Tatance [Dadens]
Altatsee . . . carried me to see his brother who was sick at the next house. He had the Venereal and had been in the same situation I found him in for six months they told me; they being utterly ignorant of the nature of the disease, and what it arose from, and were very thankful when I told them we would send him something from the Ship that would cure him. (Sturgis 1978: 56)[7]

---

please strangers, and that in their lip there was no incision. The countenance of these young victims was decent, their look timid; and they announced, by their embarrassment, that it was without their consent that an offer was made of their persons" (Fleurieu 1801: 1.443). "The young women were well featured. We had them on board at from ten to twenty years of age. Their fathers would instruct them how to behave while our men had to do with them" (Bartlett 1925: 298).

7. Two days later, Sturgis's journal referred to "the old woman" and "her numerous seraglio, with which she accomodates [*sic*] all vessels that stop here" (1978: 60).

The oldest, possible reference to venereal disease among the Tlingit is from 25 April 1803 (Banner in Ramsay 1976: 160).

For the Chinook the earliest record is from November 1805, in the Lewis and Clark journals:

18 November 1805

[O]ne woman in a desperate situation, covered with Sores Scabs & ulsers no doubt the effects of venereal disorder which Several of this nation which I have Seen appears to have. (Clark in Lewis and Clark 1990: 65)

21 November 1805

The women have more privalages than is Common amongst Indians—Pocks & Venerial is Common amongst them. I Saw one man & one woman who appeared to be all in Scabs, & Several men with the venereal. (Lewis in Lewis and Clark 1990: 74)

Passages from the next two months relate that the Americans were approached by "[a]n old woman & wife to a Cheif [Delashelwit: p. 416] of the Chinooks" and "her 6 young Squars I believe for the purpose of gratifying the passions of the men of our party" (Clark) (1990: 75), and "Cusalah . . . the young Clot Sop Chief . . . in a Canoe with his young brother & 2 Squars . . . he offered a woman to each of us" (Clark) (1990: 136).[8] Members of Lewis and Clark's party came down with the "Louis veneri" and were treated by Lewis with topical applications of mercury. The commander later gave an indication of the prevalence of venereal disease among Native men:

[T]his disorder . . . is witnessed in but few individuals, at least the males who are always sufficiently exposed to the observations or inspection of the physician in my whole rout down this river I did not see more than two or three with the gonnaerea and about double that number with the pox. (1990: 239–40)

For the quarter century following Lewis and Clark, the only extant references to venereal diseases among Indians come from the lower Columbia,

---

8. The high-ranking Chinookans were obviously old pros at this activity by 1805 and may have been drawing from a stable of female slaves. Clark noted that one of the slaves of Delashelwit's wife had a tattoo on her left arm which read "J. Bowmon"; as early as 1796 a slave belonging to Chief Shelathwell had a child by a "Mr. Williams" of a 1792 (Gray or Vancouver?) expedition (Bishop 1967: 267).

although we can be sure that the other established foci—at Nootka Sound, Cloak Bay, and Sitka—remained active and that the infections were spread to adjacent peoples. The themes already established about venereal disease in the Northwest continue through the 1810s and 1820s. Wherever Euro-American males established a presence, syphilis and gonorrhea followed.

Fort Astor (after 1814, Fort George) was established on the south bank of the mouth of the Columbia in 1811. The recently published, unexpurgated journal of Alexander Henry (1992), who was stationed at the fort in 1814, preserves some interesting statistics on venereal prevalence among Whites. A roster dated 4 April showed 50 employees, 9 of whom (18%) were "Confined to their Room with the venereal disease, and a man to attend upon them." An additional 7 (14%) were "Able men . . . more or less affected with the venereal," making a grand total of 16, or 32%, of the total workforce at the fort who had active cases (1992: 711).[9] Earlier in the journal Henry stated that he feared "at least half" would come down with the disease (679); later this was amended to "few or none are exempt from it" (718), a remarkably high prevalence. The hospitalized cases were treated to "a course of Mercury" (718); most of these eventually submitted to "corrosive sublimate" (719). These were gruesome treatments; Henry held that the men were "stupidly blind to their own welfare" (718). But things did not change with the arrival of the British on 23 April; later in the year Ross Cox described the (apocryphal?) treatment of a gentleman (perhaps Duncan McDougall, the fort head) who was thrust into a freshly slaughtered horse's paunch by a Clatsop shaman (Cox 1957: 236–37).[10]

9. It is interesting that Henry's list shows none of the 10 Hawaiians as infected, yet earlier he stated that Hawaii was a source of the venereal; nor are any of the 6 gentlemen listed, though on 10 May he stated that 3 of them "took each . . . a woman," and on the twelfth "Mr. J[acques]. C[artier]. discharged his lady she being far gone, with the venereal, so much so that he is already attacked by two pimples" (1992: 741).

10. Cox also described the Indian side of the traffic in bodies: "Numbers of the women reside during certain periods of the year in small huts about the fort from which it is difficult to keep the men. They generally retire with the fall of the leaf to their respective villages, and during the winter months seldom visit Fort George. But on the arrival of the spring and autumn brigades from the interior they pour in from all parts and beseige our *voyageurs* much after the manner which their frail sisters at Portsmouth adopt when attacking the crews of a newly arrived India fleet. Mothers participate with their daughters in the proceeds arising from prostitution. . . . husbands share with their wives the wages of infamy. [Cox probably did not realize that most of these women were slaves.] Disease is the natural consequence of this state of general demoralization, and numbers of the unfortunate beings suffer dreadfully from the effects of their promiscuous intercourse" (1957: 166–67).

Ten years later, just before the transfer of the newly arrived Hudson's Bay Company's headquarters from Fort George to Fort Vancouver, George Simpson said:

Nine Whites out of Ten who have been resident at Fort George have undergone a course of Mercury. . . . Several of the Flat Head Women at the Establishment keep Female Slaves and it was the practice to allow them be let out among the newly arrived Servants for the purpose of prostitution; indeed the Princess of Wales (Mr. [Archibald] McKenzie's [the post head] Woman) carried on this shameful traffick to a greater extent than any other having 8 or 10 female Slaves, it is now however broke off altho with some difficulty . . . it deprived them ["all the Women in the Fort"] of a very important source of Revenue. These wretched Slaves often change proprieters two or three times in the course of a Season . . . they are brought to a premature end by Disease when they are left prey to the Dogs & Crows. (1968: 99, 101)

Two more issues should be addressed here. First, the situation at Fort George was extreme. There is absolutely no doubt that the problem of venereal disease in the general vicinity of fur-trading establishments was quite real, judging by the continual reference in later Hudson's Bay Company fort journals to individuals suffering from cases of venereal disease or "pox" and unable to work or undergoing treatment with mercury. But neither are there any statistics which indicate the degree of venereal prevalence recorded by Alexander Henry. It is possible that the Hudson's Bay people were simply more circumspect about the issues, but it also seems likely that preventive measures such as that mentioned by Simpson had some effect, as did the unstated Company policy of encouraging common-law unions between male employees and Indian women. The problem at the forts was really not that much different from what occurred around other all-male establishments on the Western frontier, such as mining camps. And it really did not start to improve until settlement brought Euro-American women to the frontier and the former market "dried up." The situation that encouraged the spread of venereal diseases in the early-contact-period Northwest was quite clearly driven by two factors—demography and economics. When those two factors changed and Indians gained regular access to physicians and Western medicines, venereal disease became less of a problem among them.

A second point which needs to be made and which underlines this hypothesis is that, away from the forts, where there were few single Euro-American males and no economic motive to support prostitution, the practice was virtually nonexistent and so was venereal disease. Those explorers and trappers who knew and visited Native peoples on the coast and in the interior consistently pointed out the difference between these two regions in the prevalence of prostitution and venereal disease.[11] Ross Cox, referring to Sahaptins, said, "Prostitution is unknown among them; and I believe no inducement would tempt them to commit a breach of chastity" (1957: 87). Among all of the historical documents from the Plateau culture area before reservations were established in the late 1850s, there are virtually no references to Indians with venereal diseases.[12] On the coast itself, away from the main avenues of commerce and contacts with outsiders, Native peoples remained free of venereal disease. In 1841, when Sir George Simpson visited the Kwakwaka'wakw of McNeill's Harbor, he remarked that "these people have comparatively few diseases among them. They have kept pretty free of syphilis by having had little or no intercourse with foreign seamen, for sailing vessels never attempted, as a matter of business, the channel between Vancouver's Island and the mainland" (1847: 1.114).

Wherever coastal peoples had regular contacts with outsiders (regardless of nationality) during the 1830s and 1840s, prostitution and venereal disease took hold.[13] Dr. Romanowsky, Russian-American Company physician at Sitka in the 1840s, dated the rise in syphilis at Sitka to 1822, when Tlingit were allowed

11. For example, on 21 March 1806 Patrick Gass, a member of the Lewis and Clark expedition, wrote that among the Clatsop, Chinook, Cathlamet, Tillamook, and Chehalis, "women are much inclined to venery, and like those on the Missouri are sold to prostitution at an easy rate.... To the honour of the Flatheads [Nez Perce], who live on the west side of the Rocky Mountains, and extend some distance down the Columbia, we must mention them as an exception; as they do not exhibit those loose feelings of carnal desire, nor appear addicted to the common customs of prostitution; and they are the only nation on the whole route where any thing like chastity is regarded" (1958: 229–30).

12. A good part of this difference was cultural: Plateau peoples rarely owned slaves (Donald 1996); they were more "democratic," with fewer internal social divisions, and less driven by a desire for wealth and prestige than were the "mercantilistic" peoples of the coast. But the rest was historic: less severe depopulation from epidemic disease and less sociocultural disruption, more adoption of elements of Christianity into vigorous nativistic religions, and (distant from the competitive American versus British fur-trading practices of the coast) a more congenial relationship with the Hudson's Bay people of the interior posts.

13. On the Queen Charlottes, in May 1829, "I learned from him [Chief Kowe] today, that all the young women of the tribe visit ships for the purpose of gain by prostitution" (Green 1915: 68). Most of these ships were American. In 1841, at the Hudson's Bay Company's Fort Simpson, established among the Tsimshian in 1833, "Syphilis, I was sorry to observe, was very prevalent"

"to settle on the northwest side of the Fortress walls." Soon he noted, "A part of the native women, who live in the woods during the whole year, indulge in orgies of lovemaking [*sic*] with the Europeans employed in Novoarchangelsk [Sitka]." In 1842 and several years afterward many of these women were forcibly brought to the settlement's hospital, where the doctor treated their syphilis, and a decline in the annual number of cases in Sitka followed (Romanowsky and Frankenhauser 1962: 36). But Romanowsky believed that the disease was spreading nevertheless among the Tlingit population of the Alexander Archipelago:

As they maintain continuous intercourse with other natives of the same tribe living at remarkable distances, they may contract not only the Syphilis from them, but transplant it upon others as well . . . the Toens or Elders who possess slaves . . . can sell them and send them from one place to the other into slavery; this transplantation of often infected persons, also helps in spreading this disease. (Romanowsky and Frankenhauser 1962: 36)

Romanowsky also gave a clinical description of syphilis among the Tlingit and described how it differed from that among the Russians:

According to my observations, the Syphilis of the local Americans differs by its outward form as well as by its characteristics altogether from the one occurring in Europe. The following are the common forms of this disease under which they appear here: 1) Blennorrhea of the urethra with men and of the vagina with women. 2) Ulcers (Ulcers syphilitics). Most frequent are primary ulcers which in spite of their remarkable spreading area, have often a smooth, flat and clean surface, rarely covered with a puslike layer. The edges are not rough or elevated and are by themselves not penetrating into

---

(Simpson 1847: 1.123). And at the Russian establishment at Sitka, ca. 1832, in a passage reminiscent of the situation at Fort George: "In addition to these dealings [wage labor], the Kolosh [Tlingit] have found another profit which they consider necessary for their manner of living. Many of them bring their slaves and young girls and invite the Russians to use them. The owner takes everything that the girl receives. And this new branch of their industry also brings them every possession the promyshlenniks [Russian employees] have. Officials of the [Russian-American] Company are involved in these relations, as well as many visitors who have come to the colonies aboard ships from Europe. . . . They spread disease everywhere to a great degree" (Khlebnikov 1976: 71).

the depth. With one word, they have the appearance of a simple ulcer and they yield easily to the normal treatment. Therefore our form of Syphilis may be called a degenerated or Pseudosyphilis: pure syphilitic ulcers occur very seldom. The secondary stage occurs in the form of Buboes which also occur rarely. This disease causes only milder phenomena with natives. Very often they drag this malady around for years without suffering from secondary phenomena in spite of their disorderliness and uncleanliness. . . . From the quality of the syphilitic toxin which affects the natives only slightly, one could draw the conclusion, that it is not contagious at all, however we see a quite contrary result with Europeans, who are not only catching the Syphilis from having an unclean intercourse with a native, but who are exposed also to all the secondary phenomena occurring in Europe. (Romanowsky and Frankenhauser 1962: 36)

This passage, by a physician who had examined and treated both Indian and White syphilitics over several years, strongly makes a point that was noted incidentally in early writings: in general, the outward symptoms of syphilis were more severe in Whites; Indians often tolerated less severe symptoms for a very long time. Two other examples support this. The first is from the lower Columbia in 1806: "from the uce of certain simples together with their diet, they support this disorder with but little inconvenience for many years" (Lewis in Lewis and Clark 1990: 240).[14] The second refers to the Northwest Coast as a whole, in 1841:

[N]one of these tribes is free from the ravages of syphilis. This affliction, indigenous without doubt to America, seems to be constitutional, even among peoples who have never come in contact with the white races. Yet this scourge appears to be far less serious in this land than in Europe. Despite the hideous sores this causes, the natives continue about their work; and although they have no method to bring about a cure, yet they appear to live to a ripe old age. (Duflot de Mofras 1937: 2.173)

What these accounts mean is not easy to determine. Although it is possible that some of these passages confuse syphilis with other skin diseases, it could be that we are dealing with two different forms of treponemal disease, native and introduced, interacting with one another. There is some cross-

14. On Chinookans, see also Stuart 1935: 10; Henry 1992: 703; and Ross 1849: 98.

immunity between forms of treponemal diseases. People who have syphilis are immune to yaws (Watt 1979: 152), and yaws (if one has had a chronic case since childhood) may protect from syphilis. This phenomenon has been noted in Polynesia, where it has been hypothesized that in areas where yaws was prevalent (e.g., Tahiti) there was some resistance to sailor-introduced syphilis, while in areas where yaws was less common (e.g., Hawaii), the population had little native immunity to introduced syphilis and suffered accordingly (Pirie 1972; Smith 1975). Something similar might have taken place on the Northwest Coast.

Although some sources above suggest that many Northwest Indians tolerated syphilis at low levels for long periods of time, others document cases where introduced venereal disease had direful effects. In early 1814 Alexander Henry recorded that the Astorians had to prod the Clatsop "Calpoh's family to come and remove the body of their deceased Slave Girl, and bury it. . . . The Body was in amost wretched state in the last Stage of Venereal, black and Swollen" (Henry 1992: 670). Under the cross-immunity theory, those Indians who had experienced a bout of childhood indigenous treponematosis would tolerate introduced venereal syphilis; those who had not had the childhood disease would have no immunity to adult venereal syphilis and suffer from its worst effects.

Stage 3: Venereal Sterility

The effects of venereal disease might also be carried on to the next generation, that is, to children conceived by or born to women with a chronic case. As it took roughly 10–15 years between first contact and the first notice of venereal disease among Indians, it took another generation before observers started noticing the effects on the birth rate. As early as 1792 the Spanish anticipated such a result at Nootka, based on what they had seen in the Baja California missions.[15] But by the time a decline might have been noted (ca. 1816), Nootka was off the main trade routes and there is a paucity of documentation (al-

15. According to José Mozino: "The *taises* ["chiefs" or high-ranking men] themselves prostitute these [lower-ranking] women, especially to foreigners, in order to take advantage of the profit earned from this business. . . . This wantonness has surely been sad for those small settlements, which are gradually weakened by the ravages of venereal disease; within a few years it can ruin them so that the entire race will perish. . . . These, sterilized by this pernicious contagion, ought to fear the unfortunate fate of the people of Baja California, of whose race there

though midcentury discussions of Nuu-chah-nulth depopulation rank syphilitic sterility as an important factor; see Sproat 1868: chap. 27).

The process *is* documented on the lower Columbia. In 1839, the Hudson's Bay representative at Chinook maintained: "The indians are very fast dying off [Mr. Birnie] says seven-eights have disappeared owing to venereal disease chiefly" (Hinds 1839). This is an overstatement, as the bulk of the decline was due to mortality from "fever and ague" (see chapter 4). But as far as decline in the birth rate was concerned, Birnie noted that "syphilis is so common that it must prove a great source of sterility." A year and a half after Birnie's observation, the first missionary to the Chinook and Clatsop stated: "They are very few in number, and their number is continually decreasing" (Frost 1934: 359).

But two children are now living out of ten or twelve that were born, to our knowledge, among the Indians of our neighbourhood, since last November. . . . I saw several of those that died natural deaths, which were perfect masses of putrefaction before they expired, in consequence of disease which they had inherited from their parents. (Lee and Frost 1844: 314)

Both chronic gonorrhea and syphilis can produce sterility, miscarriages, and stillbirths, as well as congenital syphilis, with its own suite of symptoms, in infants (Arnold, Odom, and James 1990: 422). In 1845, the missionary to these people reported to his superior the following:

26 February 1845
This day I had an interview with J. L. Parish, a local preacher from Clatsop. . . . From his account of the Clatsop and Cheenooks Indians, they are passing away like the dew; there are but four children under one year old in both tribes. He thinks less than ten under six years old and over one. There are perhaps in the Clatsop tribe, 100; Cheenook, 300, including young and old. (Gary 1923: 275)

---

scarcely remains one or two, the rest consumed by the raging syphilis, which the sailors of our ships have spread among them" (1970: 43–44).

For a contemporary (ca. 1770) account of the effect of syphilis in Baja California, see Cook 1935. There have been several studies of disease and depopulation in the California missions (both Alta and Baja); all assign a preeminent role to syphilis as a cause of decline of Indian birth rates (which, coupled with high death rates from epidemic disease, caused rapid depopulation). The lengthiest discussion of syphilis is in Cook 1937. See also Jackson 1983, 1994.

In 1848, the measles epidemic and, in 1853, smallpox (chapter 6) claimed even more children. And in the absence of any effective medical treatment for venereal diseases, the birth rate remained low.

The negotiators of the unratified western Oregon treaties of 1851 made a special request to the commissioner of Indian Affairs for "erecting one or more Hospitals for the reception and treatment of diseased Indians, a number of whom are labouring under chronic or constitutional venereal, contracted in their intercourse with the whites" (Gaines, Skinner, and Allen 1851). In 1853 George Gibbs said the Chinook and Cowlitz were "diseased beyond remedy, syphilis being with them hereditary as well as acquired" (1855: 455). But nothing was destined to be done for the remnants of the western Oregon peoples until they were gathered together on the polyglot reservations at Grand Ronde and Siletz in 1855–56. The medical records from Grand Ronde show very high rates of gonorrhea, with 210 cases (out of a total population of ca. 1,900) being treated in October 1856 alone. Gonorrhea, amenable to medication, declined to 35 cases by October 1857. Syphilis, with many fewer cases, was more deadly and without penicillin could not be cured. There were 18 cases treated in both October 1856 and October 1857 (monthly numbers ranged from 8 to 24), and between August 1856 and April 1858 (four months uncounted), there were 14 deaths directly attributable to the disease, or about 1 per month. As Anson Henry, the reservation doctor, noted in his October 1856 report, this disease could only be conquered by a change in behavior (Henry 1856–58).

Similar, though less severe, situations occurred on other reservations in western Oregon and western Washington. But a full examination of them takes us past the early contact, "epidemic" period in the United States and beyond the scope of this book. The early contact period extended somewhat longer in British Columbia: reservations were established around Victoria in the 1850s but not on the northern coast until the 1880s (Kew 1990: 159–60). Regular access to physicians and a check on the spread of venereal diseases in British Columbia therefore occurred later than in the States.

From the late 1850s throughout the 1860s, the focus for the spread of venereal (and other) diseases to the Native peoples of coastal British Columbia was the "Northerners' Encampment" on the outskirts of Victoria (see also chapter 7). Here North Coast Indians congregated in large numbers for commerce—which unfortunately included prostitution—with the Whites. Speaking in 1863, the medical officer of H.M.S. *Beaver* stated:

The open practice of habitual Prostitution is not considered a disgrace, but as a highly legitimate and very lucrative calling, nor does the Indian warrior consider it as in any way derogatory to his manhood to subsist on the earnings of his squaws at this shameful trade. Every spring a large fleet of Canoes comes down to Victoria, from Queen Charlotte Island, bringing a number of young girls with them: during the summer time these girls assemble on the roadsides a little way out of Victoria, and there engage in Prostitution, returning in the autumn to their northern home with their earnings. Can it be then a matter of wonder that Syphilis is very prevalent, and that every new generation will show with greater force the ravages caused by this disease? (*Beaver* 1863)

At the Northerners' Encampment free women participated in the trade. It was yet another way for North Coast people, recently enriched by the fur trade, to plow more money into even more elaborate potlatching (Wayne Suttles, pers. comm., 5 November 1994) and thereby raise their social standing. The long-distance, annual migration of the "Northerners" facilitated the spread of venereal disease into areas not yet settled by Whites. Haidas from the Queen Charlottes, Tsimshians, Stikine Tlingits, and Kwakwaka'wakw were present in the Northerners' Encampment; venereal disease was introduced to many of their home communities with the canoes returning from Victoria.

Peoples in the vicinity of Victoria who did not frequent the Northerners' Encampment remained relatively untouched by venereal disease. In his three years on the Makah reservation (1861–64?) James Swan saw "but three cases . . . of syphilitic bubo. One was a squaw, who had contracted the disease in Victoria; the other two, men of the tribe to whom on her return she had imparted it" (1870: 79). In 1864, Robert Brown of the Vancouver Island Exploring Expedition said: "In Cowichan & Nanaimo there is little or no prostitution. . . . Little or none along the West Coast except at Alberni where there was a saw Mill. . . . Even yet amongst tribes where whites have little visited is there a strict respect for the virtue of their women."

By the late 1860s second-generation cases of syphilis were being reported on the British Columbia coast, and the cycle that had begun in the south was repeating itself in the north:

There is undoubted testimony of old Hudson Bay Company officials who first came to the Coast about 55 years ago that then both Syphilis and Scrofula were uncommon among the Indian races and now venereal in its various forms and Scrofula are at present the blight and curse of the whole native race. . . . The primary form of the disease most commonly observed is of a sloughing of phagedonic form accompanied by suppurating buboes, the indurated sore I have very rarely seen and the constitutional symptoms rarely manifest themselves by the skin. . . . Syphilis now prevails extensively both in its acute and congenital forms affecting the whole mass of the Indian population diminishing their power of procreation, arresting fertility and in cases where conception has taken place, being either followed by abortion or children notably deficient in virility and vitality few of whom live to maturity. . . . Syphilis invariably falls most severely on that race which previously had been least subject to it such has been observed when the disease was first introduced into the Sandwich Islands spreading with a rapidity and by a contagion different both in degree and kind to what is found [in] civilized (Syphilized?) countries. (Comrie 1869)

As is often the case with historical accounts dealing with disease and death on the Northwest Coast, this passage is both sensationalistic and overstated. But the pattern of introduction and change that it describes is undoubtedly real and was familiar to the Euro-American colonists.

TUBERCULOSIS

Stage 1: Consumption

Although some form of mycobacterial disease may have been present before contact, there is no doubt that classic tuberculosis was introduced to the Northwest Coast at a very early date. Two members (and possibly more) of Cook's third voyage died of "consumption" (Watt 1979: 149), the colloquial English term for pulmonary tuberculosis, then epidemic in Europe. Cook's ships remained at Nootka Sound for a month in spring 1788; other maritime traders visited coastal locations intermittently from 1774 on. The Spanish established a post at Nootka Sound that was occupied continuously from 1790 to 1795, the first instance of sustained contact between a Euro-American population and a Native Northwest Coast people. Tuberculosis in a Northwest Indian was first documented in May 1793, at Nootka: "We were visited by Harrase & his Son, the latter could speak & understand English better than any other Native in the Sound, but we were sorry now to perceive him much emaciated with a pulmonary consumption attended with great debility, frequently short cough & purulent expectoration" (Menzies 1793).

Tuberculosis is communicated via droplet infection—in a sneeze or cough or through spitting. The bacilli usually lodge in the lungs, where an initial lesion is formed; they may later spread to other locations via the lymph nodes (Benenson 1995: 488; Clark et al. 1987: 49). Children are most apt to develop an active case following initial infection, but usually the disease remains dormant for a while and reappears later in life, especially when the patient has been weakened by malnutrition or other diseases. In comparison with other droplet-borne infections, tuberculosis does not spread easily. Close physical contact and poor hygiene aid in its transmission. Native Northwest Coast housing, which encouraged such close contact (especially during winter, when both nutrition and hygiene were compromised), certainly had some effect.

Following the initial report of consumption in an Indian in 1793, there is no mention of the disease in any historic records for over 30 years. A Clackamas recollection suggests (by its placement of tuberculosis in a series of introduced diseases) that tuberculosis took hold in western Oregon in the 1820s:

Soon after the myth (white) people had come to this land, they brought with them all sorts of illnesses. . . . At first they merely announced it, they said that a disease is coming. A person will cough, forthwith his breath will be shortened (and he will not be able to breath as well as usual), and then he will die (of tuberculosis).

Some one man was seated there when they announced (predicted this). He stood up, he said (in jest), "Oh I am coughing right now. ʔhuʔ ʔhuʔ ʔhuʔ ʔhuʔʔ" he did. He said, "The cough has gotten me now!" They told him, "Do not speak like that! The sickness that is coming is bad." "Humph," he replied to them. I do not know how long after, and then they (the Indians in Western Oregon) got to coughing. The very first one was he who had laughed at it. The cough got him, he died forthwith. Children would be running about, they would start to cough, they would run, and soon after while they were still running they would drop right there, they would die. She said, many of them died (like that), or more slowly. The cough (tuberculosis) killed them. (Jacobs 1958–59: 2.545–46)

After 1793, the next historical reports of tuberculosis come from the Willamette Mission school, established for Indian orphans in 1835. Several deaths from consumption, most among local Kalapuyans, were recorded there in the 1830s (Carey 1922; Bailey 1986: 101, 166). The earliest, a 14-year-old boy of the "Silelah" (probably the Siuslaw village *čá·lila*) tribe, who died of "bleeding at the lungs" on 19 August 1835, was recorded with some detail in the teacher's diary:

19 August 1835

died Kenotish one of the Indian lads who came to live with us last April, his disease was pulmonary consumption which seized upon him soon after coming here—his sufferings have been very great which he has born with exemplary patience his remains were decently interred this evening with appropriate exercises in a rural spot selected for a burying place not far from the Mission house.

Kenotish's brother, after examining the body and grieving, "meditated revenge" on two of the missionaries, but "prevented by another Indian . . . they killed seven [Yamhill Kalapuyan] indians" instead (Shepard 1834–35).

This passage contains the first recorded example of probable revenge killings following the death of a Northwest Indian from an introduced disease. The year after Kenotish's death, the second recorded Indian death from consumption, of the Chinookan chief Cassino's son, near the Hudson's Bay Company's Fort Vancouver, was also followed by an attempt at a revenge killing. The subject in this case was the boy's stepmother, who fled from an angry Cassino and found refuge among her people at the mouth of the Columbia (Parker 1838: 256; Kane 1971: 92). And following the first recorded Indian deaths (of the chief's son and nephew) from consumption at the newly established Fort Nisqually, Dr. William Tolmie, who had given them cough medicine, was frightened by rumors that another nephew wanted to assassinate him. Instead, "an Indian sorceror and trader" was slain (1885: 33).

Consumption apparently became prevalent along the Oregon coast about this time, and the Indians had an explanation for it. According to ethnographer George Gibbs:

The Indians state that within the last twenty years a great many all along the coast have died of the Doctor's sickness. This account of the disease is that a medicine man or woman, wishing to destroy an individual, has dealings with the evil spirit (with his particular demon), in secret and goes through certain forms of incantations in secret. Immediately a disease insect with a very hard shell and a number of legs punctuates [*sic*] into the vitals of the victim, feeding on the tissues & increasing in size. Meanwhile the sufferer loses all appetite for food, coughs, becomes very much emaciated, and finally dies. There is no fever, no eruption, & not much pain. What the disease really is has not been ascertained but Dr Milhau surmises from the prevalence of scrofula that it is consumption. (1857)

The idea of penetration by a disease-causing organism or object as the cause of tuberculosis is consistent with Native beliefs, as verified by a Coos tradition:

Shamans and tuberculosis
A strong shaman, when a person was continually spitting (from consumption) . . . said . . . "It is like *gu" me'* worm that is eating on him there inside him. That is what is making him cough." . . . Then indeed he worked on the person . . . and when he took it out, they all saw it (the worm). Indeed then the sick person got well. (Jacobs 1939: 93)

Perhaps the Indians associated this new wasting disease with an older one, caused by native intestinal parasites such as the tapeworm or roundworm (see appendix 1).

Dr. Milhau also told Gibbs that, on the Oregon coast as elsewhere, shamans who were unsuccessful in treating tuberculosis were killed:

14 November 1856
The death of an Indian with this disease (tuberculosis) throws the whole village into a state of excitement and the Indians proceed immediately to kill off all the suspected doctors and make indiscriminate slaughter of all suspected persons until the disease disappears, so that between the disease and the means to prevent it a large number have been buried. (Cited in Beckham 1986: 31)

Consumption was also prevalent among Tlingit Indians near Sitka by the 1840s (Romanowsky and Frankenhauser 1962: 63–64). Sitka had been occupied by Russians since 1799. Statistics from three years show that Indians died from consumption more often than Whites, and women (who also tended to be Indian) died more frequently than men. Between 1845 and 1846 there were 51 deaths, 10 of which were from consumption; in 1846–47, there were 26 deaths, 6 by consumption; and in 1847–48, there were 35 deaths, 10 by consumption. The doctors theorized that fewer Russians died because they had been exposed to, and survived, the disease in childhood (in Russia); Tlingits had no such resistance.

Stage 2: Scrofula

Consumption, or tuberculosis of the lungs, is the variety currently most familiar to Euro-Americans. But a second form, scrofula, which affects the lymph glands, had become prevalent in the Northwest by the mid–nineteenth century.[16] In 1852 a French traveler stated that the Chinook "[m]ore than any other are lymphatic and prey to scrofulous illnesses" (Saint-Amant 1854: 382), and in 1855 Dr. Israel Moses gave a more detailed diagnosis from Chinook village: "Many are absolutely deformed by the enlargement of the cervical glands, frequently suppurating, discharging, and forming frightful cicatrices" (1855: 38). A recent medical description of "scrofuloderma" is "reddish granulations, edematous, exudative, and crusted" located over the cervical lymph nodes (Arnold, Odom, and James 1990: 381).

With the establishment of reservations, scrofula was noted with great regularity. Incomplete monthly reports by the physician at the newly established Grand Ronde reservation (Kalapuyans, Takelmas, and others) in the Willamette Valley in 1856–58 show (among chronic diseases) 14 deaths from syphilis, 10 from scrofula, and 19 from consumption (Henry 1856–58). The most complete and accurate description of scrofula was made by James Swan, who had lived on the lower Columbia in the early 1850s and was Indian agent at the Makah reservation on the Olympic Peninsula in the early 1860s. Concerning the Makah he said:

The whole tribe are pervaded by a scrofulous or strumous diathesis which shows itself in all its various forms, enlargement and suppuration of the cervical glands, strumous ulcers in the armpits, and swelling and suppuration in the groin and thigh. The strumous bubo is of common occurrence in infants, children of all ages, and adults. These are invariably cut, I cannot say lanced, for the instrument in all cases is a knife, and the wounds are allowed to take care of themselves. . . . I think I can safely assert that there is scarcely an individual in the whole tribe but what has had strumous buboes or ulcerations of the cervical glands at some period of life. (Swan 1870: 79)

16. George Simpson used the word in 1825 among Chinook (1968: 99) and in 1841 among Kwakwaka'wakw (1847: 1.123), but it appears that in each case he confused the condition with complications of syphilis.

Dr. Comrie, surgeon on the H.M.S. *Sparrowhawk* in 1869, found both consumption and scrofula general among British Columbia coastal Indians:

They are very prone to pulmonary complaints. . . . a specific form of bronchitis ending in the softening and breaking up of the lung tissue the formation of cavities and all the symptoms of galloping consumption. . . . loss of flesh night sweats cough . . . purulent expectoration. . . . In other cases . . . glandular enlargements and suppurations most especially of the neck and in many cases a form of Labes muyituca [?] and ulceration of the glands of the small intestine.

In summary: Tuberculosis of some form might have been present on the Northwest Coast in precontact times (although as of 1994 there is no paleopathological evidence of it). The pulmonary form ("consumption") was introduced with the first explorers but did not take hold among Indians until they came into sustained contact with Whites by the 1830s; the cervical form ("scrofula") was first reported by midcentury. In the early reservation period of the late 1800s, tuberculosis of both forms became prevalent, and even epidemic, in many Northwest Coast reservations.

4 / The "Fever and Ague" of Western Oregon

Beginning in the summer of 1830, and recurring each summer for several years thereafter, the lower Columbia and Willamette River valleys were visited by yet another "new" disease, called "fever and ague" (by the Americans) or "intermittent fever" (by the British). Although there has been some controversy over the identity of this disease, current consensus favors malaria (see appendix 2 for a summary of the clinical and epidemiological characteristics of malaria). Cumulatively, the "fever and ague" epidemics had a devastating impact on the Chinookan and Kalapuyan peoples of the area. From a total population something under the 15,545 estimated by Lewis and Clark and the Hudson's Bay Company in the early decades of the 1800s, numbers for these two groups dropped to around 1,932 by 1841, a decline of 88% (see chapter 9). By 1850, the population of the region had rebounded to what it had been in 1829, but its composition was radically different: English-speaking Americans had almost totally supplanted the Native Americans who had occupied the area a mere 20 years earlier (Bowen 1975). The fever and ague epidemics probably constituted the single most important epidemiological event in the recorded history of what would eventually become the state of Oregon.

Fever and ague had been present for some time in regions that were developing ties with the Columbia River, and scattered cases were reported in the Pacific Northwest before 1830. The disease was endemic to virtually all the southeastern United States plus the mid-Atlantic, Ohio Valley, Lakes Michigan and Erie, and the lower Missouri Valley (Drake 1850; Boyd 1941a). An "epidemic of 'miasmatic' disease" killed 80% of the population of Pike County (Missouri) in the 1820s (Ackerknecht 1945: 23). There were also several febrile ports of call along the Latin American sea route to the Northwest. San Blas (in Nayarit State, Mexico) in particular was called the "most insalubrious place on the west coast of Mexico" (Langsdorff 1814: 123).

Chronic cases of fever and ague could have come from either the east or the south or both. Mountain men with roots in the Missouri Valley were present in western Oregon by the 1820s. Northwest Coast explorer James Colnett, imprisoned at San Blas in 1789, came down with a case of fever (1940: 75, 79). And there were cases of "Ague and low Fever" among the members of the Astor party, who arrived at the mouth of the Columbia in July 1811 after circumnavigating South America (Thompson 1962: 359). But none of the early cases "took" in the region until the summer of 1830. The Indians attributed the introduction of the disease to the "Boston" trading ship *Owyhee*, which lay at anchor at St. Helens on Multnomah Channel for almost a year between 4 August 1829 and 21 July 1830. According to the ship's log, one crew member (a "Mr. Jones") spent seven months at Fort Vancouver recuperating from an unspecified illness (Dominis 1827–30).

THE EPIDEMIC YEARS

Year 1 (1830–31): The Epidemic around Fort Vancouver

The first appearance of fever and ague at Fort Vancouver, the focus of the first year's outbreak, appears to have coincided with the departure of the *Owyhee*.[1] Hudson's Bay trader Peter Skene Ogden recalled (some years later) that he saw the first cases of "intermittent fever" among Company employees on 6 July 1830 upon his return to Fort Vancouver after an "absence" (Barker

1. Eyewitness accounts come particularly from people associated with the Hudson's Bay Company's Fort Vancouver, near the geographical center of the epidemic. Important names include Dr. John McLoughlin, Peter Skene Ogden, David Douglas, James Douglas, George Roberts, William McKay, John Work, John Tod, Francis Ermatinger, and James Harriott in 1830, joined by George Allan, Dr. William Tolmie, Dr. Meredith Gairdner, and the Americans John Ball, Dr. John Townsend, Hall Kelley, Nathaniel Wyeth, Jason Lee, and Cyrus Shepard in succeeding years. The single most important source of information is the correspondence of Dr. John McLoughlin, chief factor of the Company's Columbia District and virtual ruler of the Pacific Northwest during the period of his tenure. His letters consistently contain references to the fever from its inception in 1830 until its decline four years later.

1948: 137). Botanist David Douglas, writing on 11 October, stated that the fever "broke out in the lower parts of this river about eleven weeks ago" (i.e., ca. July 26) (1905: 292).

The circumstances of the disease's appearance are best stated in Ogden's own words:

I found a few of the servants suffering under an attack of intermittent fever. Two medical men [Drs. James Kennedy and John McLoughlin] being resident there at the time, its first appearance caused no serious apprehension to those in health. But some alarm began to arise when it was found that, instead of disappearing before the remedies applied, the malady fast increased both in virulence and extent. In twenty days after the first symptoms of its appearance, the whole garrison, with the exception of two [David Douglas and Francis Ermatinger], amounting in all to five gentlemen and eighty servants, had successively undergone the ordeal, and still remained subject to the influence of the pestilential fever. Those who remained in health were, of course, unable to attend properly to so many invalids, and this increased the inconvenience under which both men and officers suffered in common. The annual ship soon after arrived from London [the *Dryad,* on 16 August; Barker 1948: 38], bringing a seasonable supply of medicines, the recent demand for bark[2] and other tonics having speedily exhausted the limited supply we possessed. (1933: 68)

On 25 September, Chief Factor Dr. John McLoughlin said (in two letters): "Have so many sick I am quite harassed. We have now 50 laid up with the intermitting fever." "[T]he Intermittent Fever is making a dreadful havoc among the natives & at this place half our people are laid up with it" (Barker 1948: 132).

It appears that the "intermittent fever" attacked both Whites and Indians at approximately the same time. Ogden recalled what he saw at adjacent villages, which must have been Multnomah and Clannaquah (see map 13), on the Columbia bank of Sauvie Island opposite Vancouver.

In close contiguity with our clearances was a village containing sixty families of Indians; a few miles lower down was a second, of at least equal population. . . . A short month had passed away. . . . All, all was changed. Silence reigned where erst the din of population resounded loud and lively. . . . Why linger these foul birds around the spot, gorged? . . . Let these unburied carcasses resolve the question. . . . the fever-ghoul has

---

2. Cinchona bark; see appendix 2.

wreaked his most dire vengeance; to the utter destruction of every human inhabi-
tant. . . . Dreading lest the putrified remains of the dead should occasion some more
dreadful pestilence. . . . they were collected in heaps, and the whole point of wood
where they lay set on fire. (1933: 68–70)

The "point of wood" was undoubtedly Reeder Point, adjacent to Multnomah
village. In Lewis and Clark's time Multnomah's winter population was 200,
swelling to 800 for the spring fishery; that of Clannaquah was 130. The story
of the burned village, recalled here by an eyewitness, became part of the local
mythology and was retold (with elaboration) in several later accounts.[3]

Multnomah and Clannaquah were not the only abandoned or burned villages. Two other eyewitnesses, William McKay and George Roberts (both
youngsters at the time), recalled that a village on the Multnomah Channel
side of Sauvie Island (Lewis and Clark's Cathlanaquiah; population of 150)
met the same fate. According to McKay, nothing had been heard from the
village for several days, so a runner was sent and found all dead "except two
infants" (1878: 6); Roberts recalled that McLoughlin ordered trapper Michel
LaFramboise, who passed through the town on 19 or 20 October on his way
to the Umpqua, to burn it as well (Roberts 1880; Barker 1948: 152). Excavations
at Cathlanaquiah by the Oregon Archaeological Society uncovered a charcoal layer overlying all culture-bearing deposits (Strong 1959: 31).

The epidemic was not limited to the Indians of Sauvie Island. The
Chinookan village on the Columbia just downstream from Vancouver
(*gałákanasisi*), headquarters for "chief" Cassino, was also hit. In 1847,
Hudson's Bay people told American Paul Kane that Cassino's "own immediate family, consisting of ten wives, four children, and eighteen slaves, were
reduced in one year to one wife, one child, and two slaves" (1971: 91). In 1841
Charles Wilkes was told that Cassino had formerly been able to "muster four
or five hundred warriors" (from several villages) (1845: 4.395).[4] Despite the
elaboration of these after-the-fact accounts, *gałákanasisi* had definitely
suffered severely; in 1838 its population was censused at 37 (Hudson's Bay
Company 1838). Another village whose abandonment probably dated to summer 1830 was Cathlapootle, at the mouth of the Lewis River, across from the
downstream tip of Sauvie Island. In May 1833 Dr. William Tolmie visited it;

---

3. E.g., Townsend 1978: 222–23; Blanchet in Landerholm 1956: 18; De Smet 1906: 122–23.
4. A number that in 1847 had inflated to 1,000 (Kane 1971: 91).

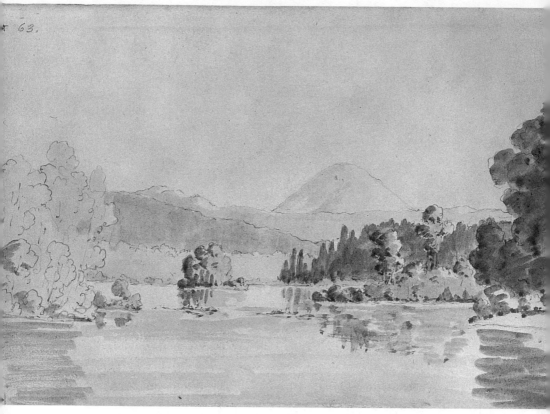

FIG. 2. *View of Mount St. Helens from the Mouth of the Cattlepoutal River,* by Paul Kane, 1847. Cathlapootle (Quathlahpohtle, *gałápuẋx*) village, at the mouth of the Lewis River, was depopulated by "fever and ague" (virgin-soil malaria) in the early 1830s. (Courtesy of the Royal Ontario Museum, Toronto, no. 80 ETH 85, 946.15.329.)

he stated that "a few years ago" it had 200–300 occupants (in fall 1805 it had 300), but now "only its superior verdure distinguished the spot from the surrounding country" (1963: 183) (figs. 2–3).

On 11 October Dr. McLoughlin stated: "The Intermitting Fever . . . has carried off three-fourths of the Indn. population in our vicinity" (Rich 1941: 88). The "vicinity" apparently was not limited to villages in the "Portland Basin," however, but included those west to the entrance of the Columbia and east to The Cascades rapids. Also on 11 October, David Douglas wrote (at the mouth of the river):

A dreadfully fatal intermittent fever broke out in the lower parts of this river about eleven weeks ago, which has depopulated the country. Villages, which had afforded

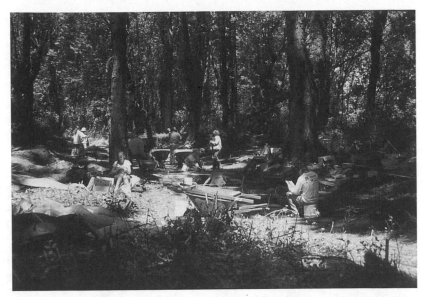

FIG. 3. Members of Portland State University's 1996 summer archeology field school at the site of Cathlapootle village, which was rediscovered in the early 1990s. (Courtesy of Kenneth Ames, Dept. of Anthropology, Portland State University, Oregon.)

from one to two hundred effective warriors, are totally gone; not a soul remains. The houses are empty and flocks of famished dogs are howling about, while the dead bodies lie strewn in every direction on the sands of the river. (1905: 292)

Among these villages were those of the Chinook people at the Columbia's mouth. Another eyewitness, Francis Ermatinger, said of them (in a letter dated 16 February 1831): "It carried off King Comcomly with most of his subjects and those of the tribes about him. It is no unusual thing to see two or three dead bodies, in a short excursion along the river. Some of the villages were entirely depopulated" (1980: 140). At Cowlitz, Simon Plamondon recalled "in 1830, the first ague summer, the living sufficed not to bury the dead, but fled in terror to the sea coast, abandoning the dead and dying to the birds and beasts of prey. Every village presented a scene harrowing to the feelings" (Douglas 1931: 8).

The following oral tradition, collected from Clackamas informant Victoria Howard (fig. 4) in 1930 (by Melville Jacobs), probably dates to 1830:

I do not know how long a time after then [tuberculosis deaths; see p. 79, above], and then again they were announcing, they said, "The ague (fever and shivering) is on its way here. Dear oh dear! Now another thing!" Soon but I do not know just how

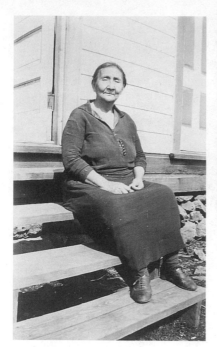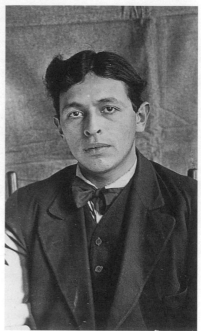

FIG. 4. Two important Indian informants on introduced diseases. Victoria Howard, interviewed at Oregon City in the 1930s by Melville Jacobs, was the major source of Jacobs's *Clackamas Chinook Texts*. William Beynon, Tsimshian translator and informant for Marius Barbeau and other anthropologists, was the primary author of the Beynon Manuscripts. (Left: Courtesy of Melville Jacobs Collection, University of Washington Archives, Seattle. Right: Courtesy of Canadian Museum of Civilization, Hull, Quebec, photo no. 21045.)

long after, then some one person got the ague. He lay with his back to the fire, he got only colder. They threw covers over him, but the ague got worse. His whole body shook. So long a time and then it stopped. Now he got feverish, he got thirsty for water. They gave it to him, he drank it. So many days, and then he died.

Then some other person too, and also I do not know how many others got the ague. Soon then a great many of them, I do not know how many. Their village was a large one, but they all got the ague. In each and every house so many of the people were ill now. They said that when they had fever, they would go to the river, they would go drink water, they would go back home, and directly as they were proceeding (back), they would drop right there, they would die. When some of them were feverish, they would run to the river, they would go and swim in it, they would go ashore, they would drop right there, they would die. . . .

The (Clackamas) people died (from the introduced sicknesses), I do not know how many. Only a few did not die. It (the epidemic of ague) quit even before they gathered them (the corpses that were lying around), they buried them. They were at last through with (burying) them all, and then they (the survivors) lived there. (Jacobs 1958–59: 2.546, 547)

Not everyone died. Some fled to the seacoast, as the Cowlitz account says; some to the mountains, according to a Klikitat account (see below); and others to the perceived safety of Fort Vancouver. Here, as McLoughlin admitted later in the fall, they did not find relief: "the Indians, who frightened at the Mortality amongst them came in numbers to camp alongside of us giving as a reason that if they died they knew we would bury them" (Barker 1948: 166). But "we were obliged to drive the Indians away instead of affording them the assistance they implored of us by our having as many of our people on the sick list as we could possibly attend to" (175).

On 12 November McLoughlin recorded the last new case at the fort (Barker 1948: 166), and on 28 January 1831 he was finally able to say "the fever has disappeared at this place" (181). Six months after it began, the first season of fever and ague on the lower Columbia ended.

One striking characteristic of the epidemic noticeable in the McLoughlin papers was that only Indians died in any great numbers, although fever struck both White and Native indiscriminately. Whites, after a long struggle and frequent relapses—"Some had three attacks and some even four" (Barker 1948: 216)—generally recovered. At one time in 1830 there were 75 Hudson's Bay people ill at the fort. Of this number 24 died, the majority of whom were Indian wives of the White trappers and traders (Harriott 1907: 260). In 1831, after two months of illness, McLoughlin reported no deaths at the fort (Barker 1948: 216). In 1832 (according to David Douglas) 137 out of 140 people at the fort contracted intermittent fever (1905: 306). He does not mention fatalities, but it is safe to assume that there were few.

One reason for this differential mortality was, of course, that the Whites had medicine for the disease (Ogden's "bark," see above). But probably more important in the long run was the explanation given by Peter Skene Ogden:

It may be inquired how such fatal effects arose from a cause not generally productive of them. This may easily be accounted for in the trust which the[y] . . . reposed in the juggling mountebanks with whom the science therapeutic solely rests among them, and the total neglect of the precautions that were recommended by us for their adoption. Maddened by fever, they would rush headlong into the cooling stream, where in search of relief, they found only the germs of dissolution. (1933: 97)

The accounts of corpses strewn on the beaches (Douglas and Howard; see above) back up this last observation.

Year 2 (1831–32): The Epidemic Spreads

In July 1831, "intermittent fever" appeared again at Fort Vancouver (Rich 1941: 232); McLoughlin first reported it to his superiors in London in a letter dated 13 August (Barker 1948: 208). On 18 August, the annual trapping expedition to the interior left the fort; when they reached Fort Nez Percés, the expedition leader, John Work, recalled:

An intermittent fever was raging at Vancouver when I left, this scourge was carrying off the few wretched natives who escaped last year, it had also attacked several of the people about the establishment. My people did not escape it several of them were taken ill, and some of them remained so badly that I am obliged to leave them here as they are not able to proceed. (1907: 264)

Work's party introduced fever carriers into the interior (map 5): four were sick on leaving; two more became ill the same evening; while ascending the Columbia Gorge they became weaker and Work worried that he should have sent them back and that his "medicines" would run out; just upstream from The Dalles a seventh came down with fever (1923: 71, 77).

On 20 October, McLoughlin stated: "Every man on this Establishment except seven has been ill at One time there were sixty three Patients on the sick list. . . . some had three Attacks and some even four" (Rich 1941: 233). On 1 March 1832, he wrote: "the fever and ague [note the use of the synonym] . . . raged with greater violence in 1831 and for a time put an entire stop to all our Business" (McLoughlin 1908: 40).

In its second season, the fever was worse, not better, than in the first. There were more overt attempts to prepare for and explain its prevalence. As far as medicines for fever were concerned, on 27 October McLoughlin placed an order with his supplier on Oahu to replenish the supply of quinine; for every

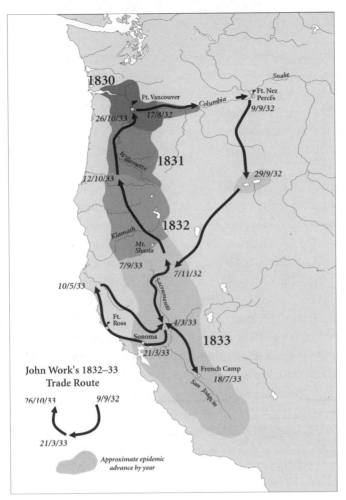

Map on map:
1830
Ft. Vancouver
Snake
Ft. Nez
Percés
Columbia
9/9/32
26/10/33
17/8/32
Willamette
1831
12/10/33
29/9/32
1832
Klamath
Mt.
Shasta
7/9/33
7/11/32
10/5/33
Sacramento
Ft.
Ross
4/3/33
Sonoma
1833
21/3/33
French Camp
18/7/33
San Joaquin

John Work's 1832–33
Trade Route

26/10/33   9/9/32

21/3/33

Approximate epidemic
advance by year

MAP 5. Spread of Fever and Ague, 1830–33, and John Work's 1832–33 Trade Route

pound not available, he requested that "30 pounds powdered Peruvian bark" be substituted (Barker 1948: 225).

Peter Skene Ogden speculated on the origins of the epidemic:

It is a question of some interest where this epidemic had its first origin; and upon the whole, I have little doubt that it came from the direction of the Spanish settlements. . . . To suppose it contagious from personal contact would be very erroneous. . . . the most plausible mode of accounting for the generation of this malady is to attribute it entirely to foul exhalations from low and humid situations . . . it doubtless proceeds from miasmata pervading the atmosphere whose virulent qualities are elicited only by certain coincidences of local origin. (1933: 71)

This is an important passage. Note that Ogden specifically *discounts* the possibility that the illness was contagious—passed from person to person—and instead invokes a purely environmental explanation. The "miasmatic" theory was the favored explanation of the cause of certain illnesses in Europe at the time. It was mentioned several times in later writings (e.g., Lee and Frost 1844: 94; Allen 1848: 75, who gives appropriate "preventive" measures; De Smet 1906: 147).[5]

In addition to attacking the Indians of the core area a second time and (as John Work said) "carrying off" those "who escaped it last year," the 1831 epidemic appears to have spread over a larger geographical area. The 18 October entry from the Fort Nez Percés journal for that year stated: "The fever at Vancouver is subsiding, but it is raging at the Dalles among Indians, and many are dead" (McGillivray 1831–32). Two days later, at Vancouver, McLoughlin wrote that "the Mortality has been very great among the Indians from Oak Point to the Dalles" (Rich 1941: 233). The Columbia Gorge, the stretch of river above The Cascades to The Dalles, had been specifically excluded from having suffered from the 1830 outbreak by Francis Ermatinger (1980: 140); now it experienced the disease too. Cases were eventually reported as far east as the John Day River (McGillivray 1831–32, entry for 23 October 1831).

Downstream from The Cascades, Indians (like Whites) were beginning to search for meaningful cultural explanations for what was happening. From the lower Columbia a disease-induced vision, "Cultee's Grandfather Visits the Ghosts," told to Franz Boas in 1894 by his Chinook-speaking informant,

---

5. Hudson's Bay governor George Simpson, in his annual summary report for 1831, waxed eloquent on the miasmatic theory as applied to the Columbia: "The disease is supposed to be occasioned by the putrid exhalations and penetrating damps which issue from stagnant water left in the neighboring swamps when the river overflows its banks at the height of the season. While the river was confined within its own channel the complaint was unknown but it has been unusually high both last and the preceding years, overflowing a great part of the lowlands in the neighborhood of the establishment and to this cause do we ascribe the late very unhealthy state of the country" (1832). Before this century's dams and resultant flood control, the water level on the lower Columbia varied greatly. With the late spring melting of mountain snows, it peaked in the annual June freshet; when the waters retreated during the next few months from low-lying areas such as Sauvie Island, the Columbia slough, and Lake River regions, they left behind swamps and intermittent ponds and organic debris. The fumes, or "miasma," arising from the swamps and rotting vegetation were assumed to "cause" fevers. In his 1831 report, faced with the possibility of a third year of fever and realizing that these environmental conditions would not change, Governor Simpson stated ominously that it might become necessary to move the Columbia Department's headquarters from Fort Vancouver to a healthier location, such as Baker's Bay at the mouth of the river.

Charles Cultee, probably dates to this time. Cultee's grandfather was a Willapa (north Columbia bank Athapascan) speaker.

> My grandfather wanted to take a woman from Oak Point [Clatskanie, or south bank Athapascan] for his wife. . . . Then an epidemic came. . . . he heard that the girl whom he wanted to have for his wife had died. The epidemic took the people away. Two days they were sick, then they died. Sometimes they died after three days' sickness. Now his people also were attacked by the epidemic. Several died each day, sometimes three died, sometimes four. Now my grandfather felt sick. After three days he died [the grandfather visited the land of the ghosts and revived]. . . . Then the seers learned what he had seen when he went to the country of the ghosts and saw everything there. (Boas 1901: 247, 251)[6]

Cultee's grandfather, suffering from the fever, shakes, and mental disorientation associated with this new disease, appears to have interpreted his experience, in aboriginal fashion, as an altered state of consciousness during which he entered the spirit world and received a vision.

Finally, in 1831 fever was reported for the first time among the Kalapuyan peoples of the Willamette Valley. McLoughlin's letter of 9 September stated: "Indians report that the mortality among the Indians of the Wallahamette has been very great" (Barker 1948: 213).

Year 3 (1832–33): An Endemic Focus

The third fever season began on 5 July, the day of departure of the interior fur brigade, when a single case was reported at the fort (McLoughlin 1832); by the 17th there were four cases (Barker 1948: 289). In mid-August, McLoughlin judged this year's outbreak not "as bad as last year" (Barker 1948: 295), but things apparently changed rapidly after that.

On 12 September, the doctor wrote: "The fever rages here with at least its usual violence; & it is only these two days that I have been sufficiently recov-

---

6. Contemporary upstream events are probably linked to the appearance of fever on the lower Columbia. These include an analogous vision by the Upper Chinookan chief Tilki at The Dalles and an increase in "Sunday dancing" by Indians at Fort Nez Percés. Tilki's vision predicted the spread of fever to the Columbia Gorge and prescribed dancing to stop it (McWhorter 1918). Details of Tilki's vision and Plateau Sunday dancing are given in Boyd 1996b: chaps. 4 and 7.

ered to be able to write" (McLoughlin 1832). Fort Vancouver in 1832 was without a full-time medical doctor.[7] While McLoughlin was ill, medical duties were assigned to his clerk, George Allan, who recalled:

In the fall of the year 1832, the fever and ague was very prevalent at Vancouver, and at one time we had over forty men laid up with it, and great numbers of Indian applicants for La Médicine, as they called it; and as there was then no physician at the fort, Dr. McLoughlin himself had to officiate in that capacity, although he disliked it, as it greatly interfered with his other important duties, until he himself was attacked with the fever, when he appointed me his deputy, and I well remember my tramps through the men's houses with my pockets lined with vials of quinine, and making my reports of the state of the patients to the doctor. (1882: 79)

The 1832 outbreak was tenacious: on 3 October McLoughlin optimistically announced, "I am happy to inform you fever is on the decrease," but a week later, "I am sorry to say the Fever is still raging among us. Five of our men were taken ill to day" (1832). Most of these were relapses: some people experienced up to four (Rich 1941: 104), and the hospital had "several" men in it throughout the winter (Rich 1941: 104). McLoughlin could not say that the disease was gone until 20 March (of 1833); three weeks later David Douglas reported, "Only 3 individuals out of one hundred and forty altogether escaped it" (1905: 306).

The 1832 outbreak was severe for the Indians too. For the third year in a row, Chinookan speakers "from the Cascades to Fort George" were attacked; "in the Willamette" Kalapuyan speakers suffered a second outbreak (McLoughlin 1832). In separate letters, McLoughlin said that "it has made dreadful ravages" (1832) and "the mortality has been very great" (Rich 1941: 104) among the Indians. In a letter dated 24 October, David Douglas gave a better idea of the cumulative mortality from three years of disease: "human heads are now plentiful in the Columbia, a dreadful intermittent fever having depopulated the neighborhood of the river, not 12 grown-up persons remain of those whom we saw when we were here in 1825" (1905: 303).[8]

---

7. James Kennedy transferred to Fort Simpson in 1831, and Drs. Meredith Gairdner and William Tolmie would not arrive from Britain until May 1833 (Larsell 1947: 68).

8. This passage was intended for Douglas's friend Dr. John Scouler, who, during his 1824–25 visit to Oregon, had attempted to collect an artificially flattened Indian skull for phrenological study.

The Santiam Kalapuya myth "Coyote, Turkey Buzzard, and the Disease," collected in 1928 from informant John Hudson, probably dates to this year.

A sickness came toward here. All those who were persons were frightened. . . . "What shall we do now? Now a sickness is coming toward here. . . . it is well if we go up above." [Birds carry them.] . . . Coyote and the disease met one another. And coyote said, "Where do you come from? Have they not all died where you have come from? . . . Here from where I come, they have all died. I am a disease too. I eat up people." . . . when it was becoming dark, coyote sent off mice to steal the disease. . . . coyote said, "It (the disease) is not (any longer so) strong now." (Jacobs 1945: 89, 90)

Jacobs added in a footnote: "Coyote stole only some of the disease substance, so that when its bearer continued on his journeying, his disease power was not as potent as before, and so people along the route did not get the disease as badly as they had before coyote weakened it." Several clues in this myth— awareness of the disease in an adjacent area before it spread, moving up (to a higher elevation) to escape the disease, and weaker expression of the disease when it was experienced a second time—are consistent with what is known about "fever and ague."

Year 4 (1833–34): Spread to California

By the fourth year of fever, few Indians were left in the focal areas to be infected. In his annual report, Governor Simpson said:

The Establishment of Fort Vancouver has been more healthy during the past year than at any time since 1829 very few cases of fever having occurred. This favorable change has restored confidence among the people, and as there is no immediate necessity for changing the situation of the principal Depot, no step has been taken towards that object. (1834)

Trade had not revived, however, "owing to the great mortality among the Indians . . . whole villages having . . . been swept away" (Simpson 1834). Conditions at the fort were certainly ameliorated by the arrival of Dr. Meredith Gairdner, a recent graduate of the University of Edinburgh.

In 1833–34 the focus of the epidemic shifted south, to California. During this year the fever and ague appeared for the first time among the Indians of the Sacramento Valley. And it was probably brought there by members of the Hudson's Bay Company's southern trapping expedition, which originated at Fort Vancouver.

The journal of the leader of that expedition, John Work, has been preserved (1945a; map 5) and is the source for the following summary.[9] In April 1833, on the lower Sacramento River, party members experienced relapses of fever and "several" were "laboring under . . . a very severe cold (1945a: 44). In early June they were plagued by "Muscatoes like to devour us" (56), and on 6 August, in Maidu Indian lands, Work noted ominously:

Some sickness prevails among the Indians on the feather river. The villages which were so populous and swarming with inhabitants when we passed that way in Jany or Febry last seem now almost deserted. . . . The few wretched Indians who remain . . . are lying apparently scarcely able to move. It is not starvation. . . . We are unable to learn the malady or its cause. I have given the people orders to avoid approaching their villages lest it be infectious. (1945a: 70)

Symptoms shortly appeared among expedition members: "pains in their bones & a violent headache—there are also two people ill with ague." On 14 August, more abandoned villages and corpses. On the 15th, 30 ill "with the fever"; on the 17th, 42; on the 18th, 51; on the 20th, 61; on the 24th, 72. The symptoms—"trembling fits," "fits of hot fever," "weak . . . helpless"—recurred regularly throughout the next six weeks.[10]

The party struggled back overland to Vancouver, arriving in late October. Four months later, after he had recovered, Work wrote to Edward Ermatinger:

9. Work's journal was used by both medical historian Olof Larsell (1947: 25–28) and ethnohistorian Sherburne Cook (1955: 311–12). The 100 members of the Work party were gone over a year, from August 1832 to October 1833. When they left Vancouver on 2 August 1832, some were already sick, but these initial cases disappeared in a few months, thanks to the supply of "medicine" carried from the fort. At The Dalles, Work noted a second disease among the Indians, a "cold which is very prevalent around the place and seems to be infectious" (1945a: 2). The party traveled south along the western periphery of the Great Basin and was in the Sacramento Valley by December.

10. Before reaching California Work reported a case of fever that had relapsed after bathing in cold water. In the fall of 1833, a similar case culminated in death: "C. Groslui had nearly recovered [from the fever], but exerted himself . . . and imprudently went in the water, has therefore relapsed again, and is worse than at first, during last night and today he bled profusely at the nose and throat" (1945a: 77). Two days later Groslui was "too weak to be moved" and after a few

24 February 1834

My last expedition . . . to California . . . the fever broke out among my people (near 100 in number) and spread so rapidly among them that in a short time more than three fourths of the party . . . were attacked with it. A number of us were soon reduced to a most helpless state, indeed wretched, without medicines (for my stock had all been expended) or any kind of necessaries for people in such a condition, having to pass through hostile tribes . . . and a month & a halfs march to get here . . . by persevering and with much difficulty we got this length. Two men an Indian & two children belonging to the party died on the way. I was so much exhausted by this debilitating disease that I was reduced to a perfect skeleton and could scarcely walk. . . . Ah! Ned, the dangers among the Blackfeet are bad enough God knows, but them and all the other troubles in . . . this savage country are not to be compared to the calamity of a whole party being thus attacked with sickness in a wilderness. . . . God keep me from experiencing the like again. (1908: 164)[11]

The expedition was preceded at Fort Vancouver by a letter to McLoughlin: "Mr. Work writes me that nine-tenths of the Indian population from here [Vancouver] to there (the Valley) is mostly destroyed" (McLoughlin 1833b). The area affected by fever and ague in 1833 had extended beyond the Willamette to include the upper Umpqua, upper Rogue, Sacramento, and San Joaquin Valleys as well. It *may* have occurred around Klamath, Harney, Malheur, and Pyramid Lakes in the Great Basin too.[12] Historical demographer Sherburne Cook estimated the population loss in the California valleys from fever alone at 50,000 (1978: 92).

1834–35: Doctors Deal with the Fever

Due to the efforts of the three trained medical doctors in Oregon between May 1833 and May 1836,[13] more specific diagnoses of the fever were made, and

---

more days, he was dead. "[F]or some days he refused all sustenance, and had to be carried on a kind of litter on horseback" (78).

11. Work would, unfortunately, have a very similar experience in 1848, when his ship, *Beaver*, introduced a measles epidemic to the peoples of the North Coast. See chapter 6.

12. Support for this possibility includes a contemporary reference to the spread of the disease to "the numerous Snake nation" (Gairdner 1834) and a traditional account from Malheur Lake Paiute dated to around 1830, "The Mean Old Witch Doctor and the Great Death" (Couture 1978: n. 23).

13. William Tolmie and Meredith Gairdner arrived at Fort Vancouver first; Tolmie soon left for Fort Nisqually; Gairdner relocated to Honolulu with a case of tuberculosis in September

better treatments became available. In November 1834, the American John Townsend provided the first coherent clinical description of fever and ague. "The symptoms are a general coldness, soreness and stiffness of the limbs and body, with violent tertian ague. Its fatal termination is attributable to its tendency to attack the liver, which is generally affected in a few days after the first symptoms are developed" (1978: 197). "Fever" and "ague" literally mean heat and shaking; "intermittent fever" refers to the periodicity of the hot attacks. John Work's "fits of hot fever" and "trembling [or "shaking"] fits" are the equivalents of "fever" and "ague"; his "pains in the bones" correspond to Townsend's "coldness, soreness and stiffness of the limbs." Along with a general weakness and a tendency to relapses, these symptoms form a common denominator which recurs often in later accounts.

Medicines used by the British and Americans have been noted incidentally in the preceding discussion. In 1830 Ogden stated that "bark" was in short supply until the arrival of the *Dryad* (1933: 68); in late October 1831 Dr. McLoughlin placed an order through Honolulu for quinine and "Peruvian bark"; and in August–September 1832 George Allan talked of both "La Médicine" and "vials of quinine" used at the fort. "Peruvian bark" was cinchona, from which quinine is distilled.[14]

Allan also noted that, given the scarcity of quinine in 1832, McLoughlin was "obliged to use the dogwood root as a substitute" (1882: 80). Dr. Tolmie (fig. 5), fresh out of the University of Glasgow medical school, was interested in alternative medicines. The day after his arrival at Vancouver, McLoughlin introduced him to this quinine substitute:

5 May 1833

In traversing pine wood the Govr. pointed out to me a tall slender tree having a profusion of large syngenesious flowers called here Devil's Wood. Having being informed that the root was employed in the U.S. for the care of the Intermittents, Mr. McL. used it here last season in doses of 3 1/2 drm of dried root in powder & succeeded in subduing diseases without cinchona etc. (Tolmie 1963: 171)

1835. American John Townsend was present until June 1836, following Tolmie's return to Vancouver.

14. The recipe for treating "Ague" or "Intermittent Fever" used by Dr. Forbes Barclay, physician at Fort Vancouver between 1840 and 1850, was "chiefly confined to the administration of Sulphate

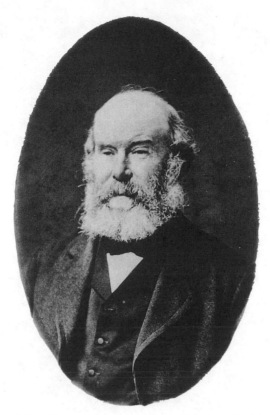

FIG. 5. Hudson's Bay Company doctor William Tolmie arrived in the Northwest in 1833. (Courtesy of Oregon Historical Society, Portland, negative no. CN 008712.)

Four days later Tolmie gathered and prepared some "Devil's Wood" himself, which he thought must be *"Cornus florida"* (dogwood) "used as a petrifuge in the U.S. . . . sometimes substituted for Cinchona in the dose of 1 oz. or 2 oz. powdered bark." A "petrifuge" is a medicine to subdue fevers.

Tolmie did not use dogwood medicine immediately. According to his journal, 15 May, when Dr. McLoughlin had a relapse, he bled him (during the cold stage), and on 19 May near Cathlapootle (Quathlahpohtle) village, he gave "doses of Quinine & emetic doses of Ipecacum" to "a boy in the hot stage of Intermittent" (1963: 180, 183). When he arrived at Nisqually, the only cases of fever were among people who had acquired it at Vancouver, but in

---

of Quinine, which seldom or ever fails in checking the disease. . . . In prescribing Quinine, Dr. Barclay recommends it to be administered early in the disease, and in small doses during every stage as there is more time lost than advantage gained by waiting till the cessation of the hot fit" (Dunn 1846).

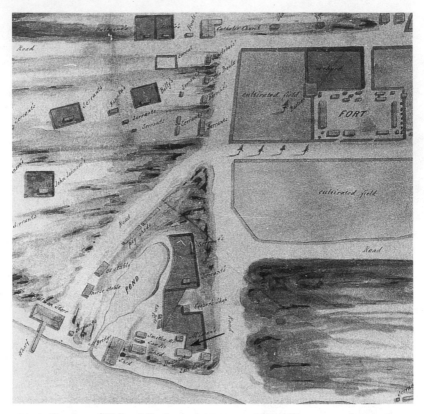

FIG. 6. Portion of Richard Covington's 1846 map of Fort Vancouver showing location of the hospital (arrow), where malaria and dysentery patients were treated. The area shown is just east of the I-5 bridge crossing in present-day Vancouver. (Courtesy of Washington State Historical Society.)

late August Tolmie went "to Mt. Rainier to gather herbs of which to make medicine, part of which is to be sent to Britain & part retained in case intermittent Fever should visit us—when I will prescribe for the Indians" (230).

Almost three years to the day later, and again near Cathlapootle, Townsend treated "a very pretty little girl, sick with intermittent" (1978: 233), with

an active cathartic, followed by sulphate of quinine, which checked the disease, and in two days the patient was perfectly restored. In consequence of my success in this case, I had an application to administer medicine to two other children similarly affected. My stock of quinine being exhausted, I determined to substitute an extract of the bark of the dogwood (*Cornus Nuttalli*), and taking one of the parents into the wood . . . I soon chipped off a plentiful supply, returned, boiled it in his own kettle, and completed the preparation in his lodge, with most of the Indians standing by, and staring at me, to comprehend the process.

While stationed at Vancouver, Gairdner prepared a report on the fever (Rich 1941: 129), which is apparently not extant.[15] During the summer of 1833 he "had an hospital erected" (see fig. 6), where by mid-November he had "treated 2 to 300 cases" (Tolmie 1963: 250). Gairdner was also probably responsible for yet another treatment (or more properly preventive measure) which was used at Fort Vancouver through most of the 1830s. Archeological work at Fort Vancouver in the 1970s uncovered several excavated pits, mostly around the hospital site, which contained charcoal, burned soil, unburned wood, and miscellaneous debris. Given the prevailing theory on the origins of intermittent fevers—that they were caused by "marsh miasms"—a frequent treatment of the time was the construction of smoke-producing fires, which "served to 'purify' the contaminated air of the miasmata" (Carley 1981: 32). The largest of these pits (F.127) was neatly stratified, in seven layers, some of which contained datable ceramics (Carley 1979: 70–76). The time frame for F.127 should have been 1834–41, give or take a year or so either way. It was probably constructed during Gairdner's 1833–35 tenure.

Nearing the end of his second (1834) fever season, Dr. Gairdner made the following statement on fever and ague (in one of his few surviving letters):

Since my arrival I have treated upwards of 650 cases chiefly Ague which is endemic here from July to November every year since 1830. This epidemic has swept away nearly all the natives on the lower part of the Columbia, & from its late extension among the numerous Snake nation & the tribes in California threatens to become the scourge of the whole southern division of the Columbia territory. (1834)

Supplementary Accounts
by American Settlers and Missionaries

Throughout the 1830s the Hudson's Bay Company was the dominant Euro-American presence along the lower Columbia. But there was a regular trickle

15. A search of Gairdner's letters in the Kew Gardens Herbarium Archives has not uncovered it.

of Americans as well, who, for various reasons, attempted to settle the area. Most commented on fever and ague. John Ball, who tried to start a farm near Salem in 1833, had to abandon it because of fever; Nathaniel Wyeth's Fort William on Sauvie Island, started in 1834, was shut down too. The Methodist founders of Willamette Mission were continually plagued by the disease from 1834 on.

First to arrive, in autumn 1832, was John Ball, who ran the school at Fort Vancouver that winter and, in June 1833, started a farm 50 miles up the Willamette. But the area he chose was sickly, and both he and his companion came down with fever and ague. Between trips to the fort for medicine and spells of fever when Ball "hardly knew whether it was day or night" (1925: 97), the strain was too much and the farm was abandoned. On 20 September, on the way back to Vancouver, the two men passed the Chinookan villages of Willamette and Clackamas:

[W]hen I got to the falls an Indian boy of perhaps eighteen assisted us in carrying our boat by. On inquiring of him how his people were he said they were sick and dying, and when we came back, as he expected we would, he should be dead. Asking the chief of the band below the falls for two of his men to row us to the fort, for I was feeble and had with me only my friend, Sinclair, he answered that his men were all sick or dead, so he could not supply us. So we had wearily to paddle our own canoe. (1925: 99)

In September 1834, explorer and entrepreneur Nathaniel Wyeth arrived overland from Boston and built Fort William at the site of Cathlanaquiah on the now depopulated Sauvie Island. Of the latter he said: "a mortality has carried off to a man its inhabitants and there is nothing to attest that they ever existed except their decaying houses, their graves and their unburied bones of which there are heaps. So you see as the righteous people of New England say providence has made room for me" (1899: 149). As it turned out "providence" was not quite ready to allow resettlement of the island: fever was still prevalent, and Fort William was destined to go the way of John Ball's Willamette farm. On 20 September Wyeth wrote: "Our people are sick and dying off like rotten sheep of billious disorders . . . one third of our people on the sick list continually, 17 dead to this date. . . . I am but just alive after having been so bad as to think of writing up my last letters" (153). Within a week Fort William was abandoned.

Also in 1834, the first contingent of Methodist missionaries, under Jason Lee, arrived in Oregon. They initially considered Scappoose, across Multnomah Channel from Sauvie Island, as a mission site, but as it was "subject to Fever & ague" (Lee 1916: 263), they looked elsewhere. Willamette Mission (north of Salem) was established in October, but (as John Ball had discovered less than a year earlier) this area was pestilential too. Two early letters from the mission reported:

23 December 1834

My brethren and myself were severally sick, and for several weeks, were afflicted by severe pain in the head, back, and limbs, attended with high fever. (Shepard in Mudge 1848: 138)

10 January 1835

The ague and fever have carried off numbers of the Indian population in this vicinity, and there are many poor destitute orphans, that have none to take care of them, whom we shall endeavor to gather in as soon as circumstances will permit. (Shepard 1933: 55)[16]

The missionary documents are the source for the two most detailed descriptions of individual fever and ague cases. The first case occurred near Willamette in 1840 and was described by the Methodist Henry Perkins; the second case occurred at Cowlitz in 1844 and was reported by the Catholic missionary Jean-Baptiste Bolduc.

Toward fall [1840] . . . I took a trip with my family to Willamette [from Wascopam Mission at The Dalles]. It was the sickly season of the year, and most deeply were we called to repent of the visit. . . . about the time we were ready to leave, one of my Indians began to show symptoms of the prevailing fever. . . . The heat was intense, and the poor sick native was obliged to lie down in the bottom of the canoe in great distress. When we reached our evening encampment he was burning with a high fever. . . .

16. These quotations introduce two themes that recur repeatedly in the history of Willamette Mission: the missionaries were routinely attacked, every summer, by fever and ague, which seriously compromised their ability to perform their duties; and the Willamette Mission school, attended by orphans of fever, chronically lost students to fever and other diseases. Endemic fever and ague contributed to the eventual abandonment of both the mission and the school in the 1840s. There are copious records on this history, but a full investigation is beyond the scope of this book.

The darkness and damp, chill miasma of the Willamette soon closed over us, and under their cover the poor fellow, being unable to endure the pains of fever longer crawled to the river's brink and tried to allay the burning inward heat by large draughts from the running stream. . . . In the morning our patient was a picture of disease and distress. We were obliged, however, to proceed, and by noon had nearly reached the Lower Settlement of the Willamette, when the violence of his pains obliged us to put ashore under the shade of some low willows. In a few minutes violent retchings of the stomach commenced, accompanied at intervals with short spasms and in less than an hour he lay stretched upon the grass before us a frightful corpse! . . . At length my second man died in the same manner. (Perkins 1843; Boyd 1996b: 263–64)

15 February 1844

It was during the few weeks passed at Walamette that I caught the ague (trembling fever). This illness, unknown in Canada, starts with a violent headache accompanied by pains in the limbs and a high fever. After a few days one begins to shiver. This is a chill that comes suddenly and no heat relieves it. If one were to put himself in a hot oven it would not do any good. Then one trembles from head to toe and to try resisting is futile. One feels just as hot now as one felt cold before and it lasts much longer than the chills. This sad illness sometimes lasts two months if one is not careful to stop it in the beginning. It is epidemic and remains in the blood. A person once visited by this illness is sure to experience it again during the ensuing years at the same period of time. Usually it is during the months of September and October. White people do not die from it, but it almost always affects their health. The Indians die very frequently because they cannot resist the temptation of drinking cold water, and when the fever overcomes them they at once run and dive into the river which causes instant death. (Bolduc 1979: 118)

RESEARCH ON FEVER AND AGUE

Despite the historical importance of the epidemics of the 1830s, within a century they had been virtually forgotten. People who remembered them were dead and so (apparently) was the disease that caused them. By the 1940s, even the identity of "fever and ague" had been called into question: it was called typhus (Larsell 1947: 28) or influenza (Taylor and Hoaglin 1962); even scarlet fever and cholera were mentioned. But a consistent body of research (Cook 1955; Hodgson 1957; Boyd 1975) maintained that it was malaria, a disease that (in the mid–twentieth century) was known in Oregon only from imported cases.

The key to identifying the disease was its epidemiology, or its distribution in time and space. Each year fever and ague followed a regular schedule, arising in midsummer, with no new cases after the advent of cold weather, and disappearing by midwinter. This timing did not fit the characteristics of any of the other candidate diseases, but it matched the breeding schedule of mosquitoes in temperate zones quite well (Craig in Boyd 1941b: 131). Similarly, the geographic extent of fever and ague, along the Columbia "from Oak Point to the Dalles" and in the "Wallahamette Valley," corresponded closely with that part of Oregon where *Anopheles freeborni,* the only local vector, is most common (Gjullin and Eddy 1972: 100). The species does not breed in brackish water and is uncommon in arid areas. Although nineteenth-century observers made the connection between malaria and swampy areas, they did not realize the disease was transmitted by mosquitoes.

A few other key pieces of information support the epidemiological evidence for malaria. Primary was the use of quinine or "bark" (of the cinchona tree) as the treatment of choice (then as now) for cases of malaria. Quinine does not act on any of the other candidate diseases. Quinine attacks the plasmodium; dogwood bark (the Hudson's Bay Company fallback treatment) alleviated the fever only.[17] Finally, malaria itself *was* endemic in western Oregon in the second half of the nineteenth century. The term "malaria" ("bad air" in Italian) was not coined until 1822 and did not supplant "fever and ague" in Oregon until the 1850s. In that decade army doctors stationed at both Fort Astoria and Fort Steilacoom recorded cases of "malarial fever," both "quotidian" and "tertian." At both forts the cases were relapses, mostly among "men who had suffered from the disease at Fort Vancouver" (Moses 1855: 45; Suckley 1857: 211). In 1928 at the University of Oregon Medical School Dr. C. J. Smith surveyed the "ten oldest physicians in the state about the prevalence of malaria in pioneer days." All reported cases, particularly in the Portland Basin and lower Willamette Valley. But malaria declined after the turn of the century, associated with swamp drainage and agricultural reclamation.

Of the other candidate diseases, both influenza and typhus may have (at different times) accompanied malaria. The global influenza pandemic of the early 1830s *may* have reached Oregon and contributed to the high mortality (Taylor and Hoaglin 1962), though local evidence for influenza itself is

---

17. Cornin is the active antifebrile ingredient in dogwood bark (Krupski and Fischer 1942: 128).

sparse. Typhus (carried by lice) mimics malaria symptoms and was certainly present in later years (Smith 1928).

The high mortality of the early "fever and ague" years was undoubtedly the result of a combination of factors. Several observers (independently and otherwise) commented on the counterproductive way Indians reacted to the fever. Early accounts include those of Peter Skene Ogden (from 1830; see above), John Ball (from 1833, see above), and the Reverend Samuel Parker, from 1835:

A more direct cause of the great mortality was their mode of treatment. In the burning stage of the fever they plunged themselves into the river, and continued in the water until the heat was allayed, and rarely survived the cold state that followed. (Parker 1838: 178)

Sweat bathing, the indigenous treatment for aches and pains and lice, had its own artificially induced febrile state. Wherever practiced in the Northwest, it was *always* followed by a plunge in cold water. For Chinookans: "An individual took a twenty to twenty-five minute sweat bath in a small beehive-shaped hut beside a stream; after steaming—using water poured over hot pebbles—he dashed into the stream" (M. Jacobs 1959: 14). The records also note that Indians reacted to the cold (ague) stage by taking sweat baths. Harmless in precontact times, the sweat bath treatment became deadly with the introduction of the new class of febrile diseases. It may have induced pneumonia (Hodgson 1957: 8; Harold Osterud, pers. comm., 1975) or shock (Taylor 1977: 58). Both the cold plunge and sweating were used with equally disastrous results in later measles and smallpox epidemics (chapter 6).

EPIDEMIOLOGICAL RECONSTRUCTION OF EVENTS

In summary, what seems to have happened on the lower Columbia in the year 1830 was the following. It was a hot and humid summer. After the retreat of the June freshet, many temporary lakes and pools were formed, some of which had deteriorated to swamps by late summer. Around Fort Vancouver, it is possible that runoff from newly plowed fields had made surrounding still waters murkier than ever and more attractive to breeding mosquitoes.

The Indians were engaged in their traditional pursuits. During late summer they came from places like the Tualatin Valley to gather wapato bulbs from the productive lakes of Sauvie Island. The Indian women waded in the water, stirring up the muck and separating the edible roots with their toes (Lewis and Clark 1991: 30). Most Natives abandoned their wooden dwellings to camp in the open by lakesides, where they were more subject to attack by hungry mosquitoes.

Epidemics of both malaria and influenza were raging in other parts of the world. The Indians believed that it was the "Boston" ship of Captain Dominis that brought the fever—in a vial that was opened on them because they refused to give him all their beaver pelts or from items associated with his ship, such as survey sticks or beads. Probably, some new migrant to the Oregon country from an endemic region brought with him a chronic case of malaria. He was bitten by local anopheline mosquitoes, which, when they attacked other humans, injected the malarial parasite into their blood. And so the fever spread among a dense population that had never experienced it before and that had no immunity, genetic or acquired. The Whites recognized that this illness could be arrested by quinine and used their meager supply on themselves. The Indians, without medicine, tried to allay the fever by plunging into cool water, which only encouraged the development of pneumonia or shock and hastened death. Frantic survivors gathered around the fort, where they were driven away by an overworked and distressed chief factor. In all probability, most of those who did not die fled to the forests and highlands—at least a mile away from the shallow breeding pools of the deadly mosquitoes. Eventually, these survivors probably joined neighboring villages that had not been affected.

The next year, when the mosquitoes bred again, the malarial parasite was present in the blood of those who had recovered from the initial attack and the stage was set for another epidemic. This time it spread beyond the vicinity of Fort Vancouver to all the villages and encampments of the lower Columbia and Willamette Valleys. Survivors from the focal area, who had relocated in settlements where they had relatives, became the vehicles by which the disease spread to all the Indians of Chinookan and Kalapuyan stocks. The plague reappeared yearly until there were few left to be infected, and only then, without victims, did cases of fever and ague become fewer.

THE MAKING OF A MYTH

At the end of chapter 2 we reviewed Northwest Coast mythological themes, region by region, concerning the origins of smallpox. On the lower Columbia

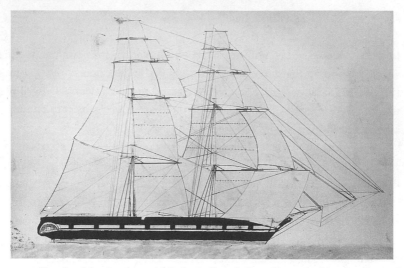

FIG. 7. Sketch of the *Owyhee*, which the Indians believed brought "fever and ague," from the frontispiece to the ship's manuscript log. (Courtesy of Templeton Crocker Collection, California Historical Society, San Francisco, FN-30750.)

there were similar attempts on the part of the Indians to explain the origins of "fever and ague." But with this disease, the oral accounts were written down at a much earlier stage in their development, and it is possible to link them with the specific, preceding historical events upon which they were based.

Historical Background

All of the lower Columbia traditions attribute the origins of fever and ague to Captain Dominis of the ship *Owyhee* (fig. 7). And each incorporates and interprets historical details drawn from the ship's time on the Columbia. Relevant information includes the following. The *Owyhee* was a "Boston" (American) ship, present on the Columbia between 4 August 1829 and 29 July 1830 and part of an effort by Boston entrepreneur Josiah Marshall to wrest a portion of the Columbia salmon and fur trade from the Hudson's Bay Company (Morison 1927). A second Marshall ship, the *Convoy* (Captain Thompson), arrived later, and a party of traders (under a former Hudson's Bay Company employee named Bache) was sent to The Dalles, where they set up a temporary trading station (Boyd 1996b: 14).

According to the *Owyhee* log (Dominis 1827–30; Howay 1934), the ship was usually anchored near the downstream tip of Sauvie Island, at the mouth of Multnomah Channel, or up Scappoose Bay. The anchorage was close to the large Chinookan villages at Cathlapootle and Clack Star, as well as at least three lesser settlements. A launch moved between this location and the river's mouth, trading. The entrance to the Cowlitz was a favorite location. The *Convoy* arrived in March 1830 and in June moved upstream to Willamette Falls, where it remained for two weeks.

There appears to have been much activity ashore at Scappoose Bay: wood-cutting is mentioned, involving the making of "spars & boards"; the entry for 6 November says, "Recd of Dr McLochlan 71 boards 12 ft by 1 ft." Journal entries note "burning coal . . . making a coal pit . . . making coal"; and on 18 May 1830 "moveing the armorers establishment on higher ground on account of the inundation of the low land on which it stood." The armorer's activities included "making traps" and "repairing musket locks for the natives." In early March trade items are mentioned, "bound up the river" or "for the falls": muskets, beads, blankets, crimson cloth, and cotton cloth. Beaver skins were preferred in return; in addition, the crew salted salmon: 53 barrels would be shipped to Boston.

The *Convoy*'s sojourn at Willamette Falls was marked by troubles. According to the reminiscences of a Hudson's Bay official, the retreating summer waters of the Willamette left the ship stranded, and Thompson "lost control" to the "Indians who . . . at that season in the vicinity of the Falls . . . were very numerous" (Rees 1880: 61). McLoughlin sent a dozen men, who retook the ship and compelled the Clackamas Indians to restore the stolen or extorted property (61).

The Marshall parties had both economic and political motives. The American traders attempted to win over the Indians by offering higher prices for their goods; when this failed (according to the Indian traditions), they resorted to threats. McLoughlin—as was his wont with outsiders—was, on an individual basis, cordial and even at times helpful; but economically, he fought back. A rival trading party was sent upstream to compete with the Americans at The Dalles, and the Company played its part in a bidding war to keep the Indian trade. The American venture ultimately failed on the economic level, and all parties were gone from the river by July. July, of course, was when fever and ague cases began to appear. After leaving the Columbia, the *Owyhee* and *Convoy* sailed north to the Strait of Juan de Fuca, where, between 6 August and 20 September, they traded with Indians.

In 1837 an American visitor claimed, in a report to Congress, that the Hudson's Bay Company had actively encouraged the Indians' belief that the

Americans had brought fever and ague to the river (Slacum 1972). Although there is no direct proof of this, and McLoughlin vigorously denied it, the fact remains that all surviving Indian sources attribute the disease to the "Boston" men, not to the "King Georges." One contemporary upriver source stated that "Canadians" (i.e., French-speaking rank-and-file Company employees) "encouraged" the rumor (McGillivray 1831–32, entry for 23 October 1831).

Origin Myths

As with smallpox, the Indians had no prior experience with malaria, and nothing in their traditional belief system to explain it. So they fell back on explanations that were standard for other diseases, or grasped at straws. Traditional theories of disease causation on the lower Columbia emphasized the supernatural: diseases were caused by intrusion of small foreign objects into the body; individuals with strong spirit powers could both "cure" and "cause" disease; powerful (and even disease-causing) spirits could reside in inanimate objects. In lieu of an understanding of the role of plasmodia-carrying mosquitoes in malaria causation, Indian theories on the origins of fever and ague were just as culture specific and plausible as the Euro-Americans' prevailing "marsh miasms" theory.

The earliest recorded tradition, interestingly, comes not from the lower Columbia but from Cape Flattery, home of the Makah people, who were visited by the *Owyhee* and *Convoy* after the ships left the Columbia in late summer 1830. In late September 1833, Dr. William Tolmie, then at Fort Nisqually, was visited by "a Sinnamish hunter & chief" who related "a long story of the arrival of two American ships at Cape Flattery & that the Chiefs threaten to send disease amongst them if they do not trade beaver. It appears that an American Captain who lay for some time in the Columbia the season intermittent fever first appeared is considered by the Indians to have left the malady in revenge for his not receiving skins" (Tolmie 1963: 238). Independent documentation from the Makah, 20 years later, appears to verify this account. In 1853, just offshore from Cape Flattery, a missionary from Victoria wrote: "A few years ago the Captain of a fur trading vessel, finding a tribe refractory assembled the chiefs and producing an empty bottle corked up, told them that it was full of 'skin sick' and unless his terms were agreed to he would uncork it and destroy them all; which so frightened them that he had his own way without further trouble" (Hills 1853). Out of historical context, this quotation might appear to refer to the "disease in a bottle" episode which occurred at Fort Astor in 1811. Considered along with Tolmie's 1833 note, however, it more likely recalls Dominis's modus operandi when dealing with recalcitrant Indians, Makah or Chinookan. Dominis certainly got his idea from the McDougall/Fort Astor "disease in a bottle" tale, passed on to him either by word of mouth or by reading records from the Boston-based Pacific Fur Company.

Three variations on the "Dominis brought fever" theme have been recorded from the lower Columbia. The earliest repeats the "disease in a bottle" story. It comes from the pen of the Methodist missionary Jason Lee, in 1840, apparently when he was near the mouth of the Cowlitz:

22 May

[C]amped near a small village of Indians. . . . We collected them together, and I spoke to them. . . . Some came to our tent and began to talk about their former numbers and the causes of the great decrease which they said had taken place since their remembrance. The small pox they said had carried off nearly all their people, many years ago; and that the "cold sick" (the fever and ague) had killed the rest, so that there were *"halo tilicum ulta"* no people now. The cold sick (they said) was brought by Capt. Dominis; that King Georges people told them to give them all the large beaver and salmon, and to give Capt. Dominis the small ones; and that he became very angry, and told them that they would see by and by, and that they would be all dead before long. Accordingly, when he was about to leave, he opened his phial and let out the "cold sick"! I told them that the small-pox could be carried in a phial, but not the ague. They seemed a little staggered in their belief; but of course, could see no good reason why the one could not be carried in a phial, as well as the other. (1841)[18]

A second variant was collected in 1854, apparently at Chinook village (but possibly at *gałákanasisi,* the refugee settlement near Vancouver), by William Tappan, Indian agent for the Columbia River district of Washington Territory:

An American vessell traded in the river all summer. . . . The Captain . . . had some triffling difficulty with a band of the Chinnooks, and when near one of their villages

---

18. Daniel Lee and Joseph Frost, also American Methodist missionaries, gave essentially the same story (1844: 108).

he set some stakes in the river. An Indian a few hours after chanced to pull up one of them and took it with him to the village, but he had scarcely reached the shore when a strange feeling came over him, and trembling, he complained of the cold, a fire was kindled and enlarged again and again. Still he was cold. Skins and blankets were heaped upon him, but yet his teeth chattered.

The medicine men and prophets were called. They examined the patient but could not understand the case. Suddenly to their great surprise the cold was followed by a heat as excessive and ungovernable as its opposite.

At length the stick was examined and found guilty. A shell had evidently been fixed upon it by the wicked captain. It was beaten with clubs, by means of long strings it was dragged over the rocks and through the water: finally it was placed over a fire and slowly reduced to ashes, which were carefully gathered and thrown upon the water, which precautions, as they supposed, utterly destroyed the evil spirit which inhabited the stick.

But alas for human hopes! The dreaded spirit had gained a firm foothold in their midst in spite of all their opposition. The man after a long sickness died and many others followed him. . . .

As may be supposed the ballance of the innocent stakes which the voyagers had placed to mark the channel, were left unmolested by the poor savages, who past them allways at a distance, and with fear and trembling. (1854)

The *Owyhee* logbook describes the making of "spars & boards" onshore at its Scappoose Bay moorage, and one of its crewmen, in 1889, repeated the attribution of the disease to survey sticks (Victor 1901: 39–40). Chinookan Indians did indeed believe that spirits might reside in "stakes"; "tamanous sticks," infused with supernatural power, were used by shamans in winter ceremony performances (Boyd 1996b: 123–24).

Yet a third variation of the Dominis tale was recorded from a Klikitat informant, William Charley, in 1910. It probably refers to events upstream on the Columbia from Fort Vancouver, in the area of Nechacokee and Washougalles villages (see map 13).

They saw two big black canoes, the largest they had ever seen [the *Owyhee* and *Convoy*]. . . . came opposite to the cabin at Vancouver and there stopped in the middle of the river. . . . Runners were sent to the other villages and all the Indians came to see . . . the Indians all gathered around them. . . . The boat people talked to the Indians, who could not understand them. They finally came out with many things. . . .

they gave hands-full of beads to the women. . . . Indians came from other villages. . . . They furnished them with deer meat.

It was not long after this that the Indians took sick. Those Indians who were given beads first, took sick first. They had never known to be sick before. The Indians were settled thick up and down the river and all the streams—about as thick as the whites are now [1910], not counting big cities. This sickness broke out and they did not know what it was, nor know what to do about it. They knew not how to take care of themselves. Everyone who took sick, never got over it. All died. They came to find out that this sickness was taken from the things given them by the people from the big boats. Some found that the sickness came from the beads and they threw them and the other objects from the strange people into the river. Those beads are still found at *Wachuga* [Washougal]. But this did not stop the sickness. The disease was already spreading among the villages. Every house or village would have sick people who died and nothing could save them. Some tried to get away by going to the mountains, but many had already taken the disease and died far away in the wilderness. But those not yet taken made escape to the mountains and saved themselves. This was the only way to escape the death. My grandmother and her people heard about the sickness and went out into the mountains and escaped. They went before they were taken and thus they were saved. (William Charley in McWhorter 1910)

5 / Becoming Part of a Broader
Disease Pool, 1835–1847

By 1835, all Northwest Native peoples had experienced major epidemics of introduced disease: on the North Coast, at least one smallpox epidemic; in the south, two or more smallpox visitations and the introduction of malaria in an endemic focus. Native populations had suffered major declines commensurate with their disease histories: less in the north, a great deal in the south.

The dozen years covered in this chapter were most notable, historically, for increased and improved transportation and communication links, both within the Northwest and with the outside world. During the 1830s the Hudson's Bay Company expanded northward from its original location on the lower Columbia and established forts in western Washington and coastal British Columbia, all linked by sea. By early 1835 missionaries had arrived and set up shop on the Willamette (Jason Lee's Methodists) and at Sitka (the Russian Orthodox Father Ivan Veniaminov). And in the early forties the great overland migrations from the American heartland to the Willamette Valley began.

The new and intensified links to the outside permitted the entry of several "new" diseases (and one "old" one) to the Northwest Coast. Between 1835 and 1847 the region saw localized epidemics of meningitis, smallpox, influenza, mumps, and dysentery. The epidemiological isolation of the Northwest from the rest of the world was rapidly breaking down.

THE SMALLPOX EPIDEMIC OF 1836–1837

The third of the five major Northwest smallpox epidemics began in Tlingit territory in late 1835 and ended in southern Oregon in summer 1837. It apparently skipped the entire central portion of the coast, between about 44° and 52° north latitude, which had experienced the disease in the first decade of the century. Records kept by Russian and Hudson's Bay Company eyewitnesses allow a fairly good reconstruction of the progress of the epidemic as it spread from place to place in the north. In the south, however, data are scarce, and it is necessary to resort to hypotheses.

Origins in the North

Tlingit. Smallpox first appeared in the Russian fortress at Sitka (fig. 8), in November or December of 1835, in a "Creole" (mixed-blood) boy (Kupreanov 1836, letter of 26 March 1836; Veniaminov 1836).[1] Although Russian eyewitnesses maintained, "It is impossible to determine where it came from" (Veniaminov 1836: 29), there are two possibilities. The first was an oceangoing vessel, several of which were docked at Sitka that fall. Likely candidates include the *Diana,* from China, the *America,* from Kamchatka and points east (Ivashintsov 1980: 115); and the Russian-American Company ship *Sitka,* which arrived in port on 29 October from Spanish America carrying the colonies' new governor, Ivan Kupreanov (Bancroft 1886: 554). There is also a good chance that the disease was accidentally introduced through contaminated vaccine, introduced and "tested" at Sitka in November 1835.[2]

Once established at Sitka, smallpox spread rapidly (see map 6). By the

1. The primary sources for smallpox among the Tlingit peoples of southeast Alaska are the writings of two Russian eyewitnesses: Governor Ivan Kupreanov and the Russian Orthodox priest Ivan Veniaminov. Kupreanov's letters are preserved in the Records of the Russian-American Company in the National Archives, Washington, D.C. Veniaminov's writings that discuss the 1836 epidemic among the Tlingit include a letter of 24 April 1836 and two 1840 works, "The Condition of the Orthodox Church in Russian America" (1972) and his "Notes on the Atka Aleuts and Koloshi [Tlingit]" (1981). Veniaminov, in particular, was the major source for two later reviews of the 1836 epidemic in Alaska—Tikhmenev 1978: 198–99 and Bancroft 1886: 560–62 (written by Ivan Petrov).

Two researchers, using original Russian documents, have studied the 1836–37 smallpox epidemic among the Tlingit. See Gibson 1982–83; Fortuine 1984a, 1989: 230–38. These works are highly recommended.

2. The fort's doctor, Eduard Blaschke, received three lots of the medication, from different sources, and apparently administered them in November 1835. Vaccine was later disseminated from Sitka to other parts of Russian America, and in at least two additional locations (Kodiak

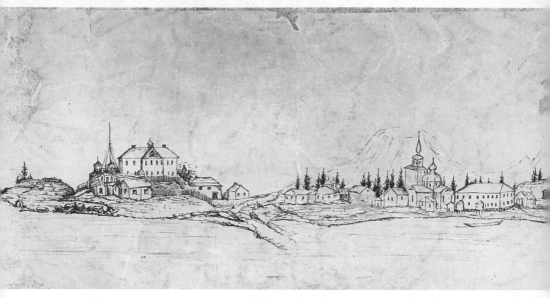

FIG. 8. The Russian-American Company headquarters at Fort Sitka, ca. 1829, pen and ink drawing, artist unknown. In late 1835, smallpox was introduced at Sitka and spread to much of the West Coast. (Courtesy of Hudson's Bay Company Archives, Provincial Archives of Manitoba, Winnipeg, HBCA Picture Collection, P-193 [N5380].)

beginning of January 1836 it was general among the Aleut and mixed-blood population of the fortress and had begun to appear among the "Kolosh" (Tlingit). As had happened before and would happen again in the Northwest, differences in treatment between Whites and Indians led to considerable differences in mortality. "Because of the care and attention given to those who fell ill," no Russians died of the disease, and of the more than 100 Aleuts and persons of mixed blood who were afflicted with it, only 14 succumbed (Veniaminov 1836). In the Tlingit village at Sitka, on the other hand, between 300 (Veniaminov) and 400 (Kupreanov), or half the population, perished. Only 50 Indians who caught the disease recovered. Father Veniaminov stated that during the peak of the epidemic 8–12 perished every day.

Most died because they did not take those precautions which we took, that is, avoiding chills. Quite the contrary, they threw themselves into the sea or ate ice and snow

and Aleksandrowsk Redoubt on the lower Nushagak River), smallpox outbreaks followed. The coincidence of vaccine introduction and smallpox appearance in these three areas has led researcher Don Dumond (1996) to hypothesize that "the subcutaneous introduction was of variola virus rather than vaccinia [cowpox]."

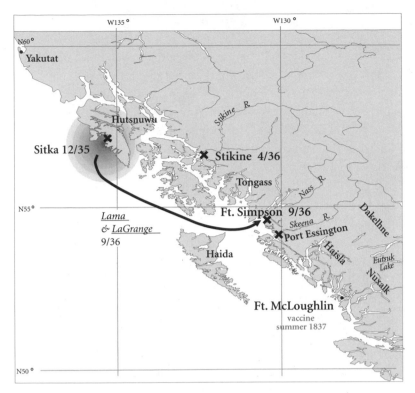

MAP 6. Smallpox Epidemic of 1836–37: Origins in the North

when they had a fever. (Veniaminov letter of 24 April 1836 in Veniaminov 1972: 47 n)

When the pox first appeared, they thought their shamans could drive it away. They raised the alarm and began to "shamanize" (that is, cast spells) every day.... They beseeched their spirits (eky) to deflect the scourge from the Koloshi to the Russians. (Veniaminov 1972: 47)

The Russians reported significant variations in Tlingit mortality: relatively few children and slaves but a disproportionate number of elderly, "who would not give up their ignorance [and] superstitions," died (Veniaminov 1972: 47).

The smallpox outbreak in Sitka lasted for four months (January to April), though cases were reported as late as September 1836. During this period and after, ships were coming and going from Russia, California, Kodiak, and the Tlingit villages. On 23 March a trading ship arrived from the Stikine River and on 26 March another was dispatched to "Stikine and the south Kolosh's fiords" (Kupreanov 1836, letter of 26 March). Despite preventive measures taken by the Russian traders,[3] letters dated April through June imply that the epidemic was spreading and becoming general among the Tlingit population. "Rumor has it that the pox is doing its work in the inlets but nothing is known for certain" (Veniaminov 1972: 47 n). "Among the Kolosh the epidemic wasn't equally strong everywhere, for example in Stikine it was quite small, but in Khutznov [Hutsnuwu] and other villages in the fiords it cleaned some families down to the last person" (Kupreanov 1836, letter of 4 May). "Smallpox is especially hard on our ships returning from the fiords" (Kupreanov 1836, letter of 6 June).

Shamans, using supernatural methods, "removed" disease objects and dealt with disease spirits. Although most could not cope with smallpox, a very few, by sheer chance, benefited from the epidemic. Veniaminov reported the case of a Yakutat shaman who was "so strong that . . . he prevented smallpox from harming his fellow tribesmen and relatives" (1981: 39). This may be the same individual, QAłax̣etł, whose encounter with disease spirits was recorded by ethnographer Frederica de Laguna in 1954:

[QAłax̣etł] became a shaman after visiting "Disease Boat." This happened in Dry Bay, when sickness or smallpox killed everyone. He "died" from that sickness for 4 days. His children were crying and his wife watched the body. The next day he made a noise, and the next day he made a noise. And in 4 days he came back. That's yek [disease spirit] business. . . . When he was dead, he was on shore, and he saw a big black boat with sails. . . . There were lots of people on it. A small canoe with four black men came to the shore to get him. . . . He went close to the big boat, but he was so lonesome for his wife and kids that he turned back against the shore. The men in the boat told him, "You try the song [spirit song]. . . . You are going to be yek yourself.". . . When he came back to the shore and came alive, that was the end of the sickness. No more died. He just waved his hand—no more sickness. (1972: 2.713–14)

Again, as in the case of lower Columbia Indians suffering from "fever and ague" (Cultee's grandfather; Tilki; see chapter 4), illness led to an altered state

3. On 3 March Governor Kupreanov, apparently acting on the advice of Dr. Blaschke, gave specific instructions to Captain Kashevarov of the ship *Kvikhpak*, bound for Kodiak, on how to avoid the spread of the disease. The ship was to wait in port at Kodiak for two days before unloading its cargo; no one onshore was to come onboard; the crew was not allowed shore leave. If any crew member came down with the disease, he and all his personal effects were to be quarantined from contact with all others (Kupreanov 1836, letter of 3 March).

of consciousness, a visit to the spirit world, and a return with a message or new powers. QAłax̣etł's vision incorporated the concept of a "spirit of pestilence" (chapter 2), which arrives in a disease boat. In the Yakutat Tlingit version, spirits claimed those who died in the epidemic and took them to the Land of the Dead. Only powerful shamans were able to see the boat coming, and only they had the power to stop it from landing (de Laguna 1972: 2.710, 769–70).

It was apparently during the spring or summer of 1836, as the disease was advancing, that the Russian authorities began to send medical personnel to the outlying Tlingit villages in an attempt to vaccinate the Indians. Here they encountered great resistance. Vaccination, in itself a suspicious operation, certainly did not fit the aboriginal concepts of disease causation, which attributed illness to the intrusion of foreign objects into the body or witchcraft by malevolent individuals (Veniaminov 1981: 50). Veniaminov believed that before the outbreak if "anyone had tried to vaccinate one of the Kolosh by force, I am certain that the Indian would have cut and ripped out the place where he had received the vaccine" (92). The activity of the vaccinators also played into a very real suspicion many Tlingit had of ultimate Russian designs on their own independence. In at least one case, a local shaman accused the vaccinators of attempting to produce through vaccination the very disease they had set out to prevent and forced them to flee for their lives (Sokoloff 1878).[4] Only after the Tlingit had had the opportunity to see for themselves the difference in susceptibility between vaccinated and unvaccinated individuals were they willing to submit in any significant numbers to the procedure.

A second wave of smallpox hit Tlingit lands in early 1837. This time, according to the Russian records, one out of four Sitka and Stikine Tlingit died, and mortality was also heavy among the Chilkat, Kake, Tongass Tlingit, and Kaigani Haida (Prince of Wales Island) (Gibson 1982–83: 68). The second wave is probably what Bancroft (or his writer, Ivan Petrov) was referring to when he stated that the epidemic originated in the southern British possessions and spread north to Sitka. Bancroft/Petrov also stated that 250 out of 900 Tongass (and Sanya?) died of smallpox, and that 3,000 unvaccinated Tlingit perished (1886: 560–651).

Tlingit stories from Sitka and Wrangell which note villages depopulated by "some disease" or "smallpox" may well recall the 1836 epidemic. Traditions

---

4. Vassili Sokoloff's reminiscences were dictated to Ivan Petrov in 1878. An excerpt appears in Bancroft 1886: 561 n.

from Chilkat and Yakutat relating the abandonment of partially depopulated settlements and the consolidation of the survivors into a few remaining villages certainly refer to 1836.[5] Well over a century after the fact, Yakutat informants told Frederica de Laguna:

Smallpox came after the Russians. There were people living all the way from Summit Lake, Second Summit Lake, to Lost River. And they all died. They died where they were sitting, mothers with babies in their arms. A few people were left alive at Lost River and some were left at Situk also. All the rest died. They didn't try to burn them that year [the Tlingit cremate their dead], but next year the survivors burned them. All the way from Summit Lake to Lost River, they were burning so many bodies, the air was thick with smoke. My father showed me the charcoal all along the ground. They moved from Nessúdat to Khantaak, and there the tribes all lived together in one village. From Khantaak, they moved to the Old Village at Yakutat. (1972: 1.278)

Father Veniaminov maintained that the epidemic was a turning point in the religious history of the Tlingit: the beginning of their "enlightenment." Differential mortality removed traditionalist elders, who "had a strong hold over the thoughts of the others"; vaccination, once proved to be effective, showed "that the Russians had a greater and more perfect knowledge"; and finally, the epidemic "shattered their faith in the shamans who, despite their guardian spirits, died together with those who sought their help" (1972: 47). After the epidemic, the Tlingit people were more willing to convert to Christianity.[6]

Fort Simpson. In 1836–38 there were two Hudson's Bay Company posts on the coast between the Russian possessions and Vancouver Island (see map 6). For the northernmost of the two, Fort Simpson, a manuscript journal (kept by Duncan Finlayson and John Work) survives in the Hudson's Bay Company

5. The Sitka and Wrangell stories are "The Origin of Iceberg House" and "The Duck Helper" in Swanton 1909: 51–52, 208–9; the Chilkat and Yakutat traditions are recorded in Sackett 1979: 59–60 and McClellan 1950: 40–41.

6. Despite the quarantine and vaccination programs of the Russian-American Company, smallpox appears to have spread in all directions from Sitka. In late 1836 it appeared on the Kenai Peninsula (Bancroft 1886: 561 n); from July to December 1836 it was reported on Kodiak Island; and from there, in 1838, it spread to the Aleutians (Sarafian 1977). Between 1836 and 1839, the carefully censused Native population of southwest Alaska dropped 38%, from 9,067 to 5,589 (Fedorova 1973: 276–77). The epidemic spread further north, up the Nushagak and Kuskokwim Rivers (VanStone 1967: 99–100; 1979: 58–61), along the Bering Sea coast as far as the Seward Peninsula (Ray 1975: 126–27, 178), and into the interior via the Yukon River (Zagoskin 1967). It seems to have died out before reaching the Kutchin of the upper Yukon (Krech 1978: 713). See map 7.

Archives in Winnipeg. It provides a day-by-day account of the appearance and spread of smallpox among the Tsimshian and their immediate neighbors.

Fort Simpson was a hub of trading activities for the entire Northwest Coast between the 53d and 56th parallels. The Simpson district embraced the territories of the Tsimshian peoples of Kitkatla, Port Essington, Fort Simpson itself, and the Nass River; the Skidegate, Masset, and Kaigani Haida of the Queen Charlotte and Prince of Wales Islands; and the Sanya and Tongass Tlingit. The Hudson's Bay Company ships *Lama* and *Beaver* stopped regularly at Fort Simpson, as did many American coasters. It was an ideal situation for transmission of infectious disease.[7]

September was an optimal month for trading, and Indians from throughout the district converged at Fort Simpson:

About the month of September, various tribes, who are friendly with the Nass Indians, visit the fort, and encamp around it: then the fort is surrounded with hundreds of Indians. [The visiting tribes are named, as above.] At this time there are all kinds of dancing, singing, and feasting amongst them. Trade is kept up at a brisk rate at the fort, which is made in a manner a lively show booth. (Dunn 1845: 189)

On 15 September 1836, two ships, the *Lama* and *La Grange,* arrived at Fort Simpson from Sitka. The first case of smallpox at the fort itself was reported on 28 September. Between 20 and 27 September seven canoes of Tongass (southern Tlingit) Indians arrived; all "went direct to the La Grange," where they "got drunk on the La Granges Liquor."[8] On 10 October, "2 Canoes of Tumgoss Indians returned home with 5 or six of them in the Small Pox." This

7. The first mentions of smallpox in the Fort Simpson journal (Finlayson and Work 1834–38) describe its occurrence among Indians to the north.

19 May 1836: "The Barque La Grange of Boston Capt. Snow arrived here from Sitka where she has disposed of a part of her cargo. . . . Capt. Snow informed us that the Small Pox was raging to the North (Sitka & Stikine) and carrying off great numbers of the Natives."

6 August 1836: "[T]wo Canoes of Stikine Indians arrived but have not brought many skins, according to their account . . . owing to the Small Pox being among the Indians from whom they procure the Furs."

The "Indians from whom they [the Stikine] procure the Furs" would have been the Athapascan Tahltan of the upper Stikine River. All mainland Tlingit, by the 1830s, were serving as middlemen in a flourishing trade between the fur-trapping peoples of the interior and the fur-trading Euro-Americans of the coast (McClellan 1950).

8. The Hudson's Bay Company had a no-liquor policy in the Indian trade; the independent American coasters were not bound by such limitations.

documentary evidence, plus the normal smallpox incubation period of two weeks, suggests strongly that the *La Grange* (and perhaps the *Lama* as well) introduced smallpox to Fort Simpson from Sitka.

During the next two months the Simpson journal dutifully recorded the progress of the epidemic both at the fort and in neighboring regions. At the fort, on 11 October, 13 cases and 2 deaths were recorded; a week later, with 3 new cases in one day, the journal stated the pace of the epidemic was "getting rather alarming." Men, probably due to their active role in trading, contracted the disease before women did. On 19 October "four of the Men's wives [who would have been Indians] and children started for Nass they have got allarmed of the Small pox . . . we could not prevail on them to remain in the Fort." The 4 December entry states that the women had returned with the news that "the Small Pox has reached the lower part of the Nass but has not yet got to the upper part of it, and that only one death has occurred."

Reports from the south, in the Skeena River valley, indicate that the epidemic there peaked in November:

2 November 1836
[A] canoe arrived from Skinna, the first . . . since 2nd Oct. They report that a great number of Indians are dying of the Small Pox.

15 November 1836
2 Large Canoes arrived from Skinna. . . . The Indians say that they have made a number of offerings to the Sun to stop the Small Pox, but the Sun will not accept of these nothing will satisfy him but the sick or human beings.

27 November 1836
[A] large [canoe?] arrived from Skinna, but have not brought anything for trade, have come to encamp alongside of the Fort in hopes of escaping the Small Pox.

29 November 1836
Port Essington [middle Skeena] They report that the Small Pox is not abating but is still raging with all its violence and carrying off vast numbers.

After three months' duration the epidemic at Fort Simpson gradually died out. Entries from April and May 1837 indicate that the disease was working its way up the Nass River to the interior. "The Smallpox has been very severe among . . . the Nass people . . . and carried off great numbers" (Work, 14 April 1837). "[T]hey state that in ten houses there is not a man left alive only some women and children have escaped" (30 April). True to form, smallpox spread along normal lines of communication "as far to the interior as they usually go to trade" (15 May).

A Nisga'a tradition, "TsEgu'ksk^u," collected by Franz Boas in 1894, includes a possible reference to the "offering to the Sun" mentioned in the Fort Simpson journal:

After a short time [following a Haida attack on Lax-anLôE village] an epidemic of smallpox visited the villages. TsEgu'ksk^u placed a pole, which he had painted red, in front of his house to ward off the disease. But, nevertheless, he became sick. . . . Then he made a bow and four arrows, which he painted red. He ordered one of his friends to shoot the arrows up to the sun. His friend did so, and the arrows did not return; but every time he shot, blood began to flow from TsEgu'ksk^u's forehead and from his cheeks. . . . Then he asked for a coffin box. He crawled into it and died. Then the people took the skin of a mountain-goat, cut ropes out of it, and tied the box tightly. Then they placed it on a large bowlder behind the village. On the fourth night after the burial a noise was heard proceeding from the box. When the people went out to see what it was, they saw that TsEgu'ksk^u had broken the thongs, and that he was sitting on the box. He had assumed the shape of a white owl. . . . [The owl said] "Nobody will be left.". . . [then] suddenly fell back into the box, and the thongs were replaced by magic. The staff which TsEgu'ksk^u had raised in front of his house fell to pieces and was seen to be rotten all through. . . . The epidemic continued for some time, and all the people died. (1902: 233)[9]

A year after its disappearance, a letter from Fort Simpson head John Work to acting Chief Factor James Douglas summarized the progress of the epidemic:

20 October 1838
The smallpox broke out to the Northward somewhere about the Russian Establishment

---

9. Other North Coast tales, associated with the later smallpox (1862) and dysentery (1888) epidemics, repeat the themes of a protective pole, arrows to the sun, and a white owl spirit (see chapter 7; Swanton 1905b; Beynon n.d.: MSS 53 and 84).

spring 1836 reached Fort Simpson end of September where it spread rapidly and committed dreadful ravages among the Natives during the fall and winter and did not
abate till the spring and finally shortly afterward disappeared. Its Southerly progress
ceased at Canal di Principe. The mortality was very great it was estimated to have carried off nearly one third of the Chimsyans, the tribe who inhabit about Fort Simpson
and from all accounts its ravages among the neighbouring Tribes were still more
destructive. The consequence was the Natives became so disenchanted that they exerted
themselves little early part of the season either to hunt or trafic and the Trade most
part of the winter was very slack but afterward it revived and attained an amount,
that from the unfavourable beginning, exceeded our expectation. The Smallpox did
not reach Fort McLaughlin on the Southward where the Steamer [the *Beaver*] chiefly
cruised and did not effect their Trade. Our American opponent Mr. Harris [super-
cargo of the *La Grange*] . . . made very little . . . principally owing to the prevalence
of the smallpox.

Fort McLoughlin. Fort McLoughlin was situated some 200 miles SSE of
Fort Simpson (and 125 miles SSE of Canal di Principe), on Milbanke Sound
on the central British Columbia coast. It is impossible to corroborate (historically) the Hudson's Bay Company's contention that the epidemic did not
reach Fort McLoughlin, as no journal and very few letters survive from this
post from the late 1830s. A second line of evidence on the southern extent of
the epidemic comes from two documents on the Native population of the
Fort McLoughlin district: an estimate of the various local groups made in 1835
(Tolmie 1963: 319–20) and a census of the same units that dates from 1838
(Kane 1859; Douglas 1878). A comparison of these two documents reveals only
slight population differences for the northernmost and southernmost *coastal*
peoples (Kitkatla and Kitkiata "Sabassas"),[10] the Heiltsuk peoples, and the
Oweekeno; see map 11), moderate differences (20–35%) for peoples just north
of the fort (Haihais, Istitoch, and Kitlope Haisla), and significantly varying
figures (50%) for the Kitasoo Sabassas[11] and the interior peoples Kitamaat
Haisla and Nuxalk. Even after taking into account the possibility that the 1835

10. "Sabassas" was the nineteenth-century term for the peoples of the three coastal villages
Kitkatla, Kitkiata, and Kitasoo, who spoke the language currently called "Southern Tsimshian."
"Sabassas" will be used in the remainder of this book.

11. A possible reference is the Haida myth "The Sleep Power," in which all the people of the
town of the "Gitadju" chief were struck dead in their houses because "they had killed the small
bird . . . Sleep-Power" (Swanton 1908: 428–29).

figures are overestimates and those for 1838 are underestimates, the remaining differences seem to be best explained as being due to disease mortality. Ethnographic support for the presence of smallpox along the spine of the central British Columbia Coast Range comes from Jenness: "the Bulkley [Dakelhne or Carrier] people incorporated the Eutsuk Lake area into their territory after the earlier inhabitants, who seem to have formed a distinct sub-tribe, were destroyed by an epidemic of smallpox about 1838" (1943: 475).[12]

There is no documentary evidence that smallpox spread to any Native peoples immediately south of the McLoughlin District at this time. It was specifically denied for the Kwakwaka'wakw by George Simpson, governor of the Hudson's Bay Company, in the account of his 1841 trip to the Northwest Coast:

Port McNeill
Curiously enough, they [Quakeolths] have been exempted from the small-pox, though their brethren, both to the south of the Columbia and in Russian America, have suffered severely from that terrible scourge. To secure them a continuance of this happy immunity we begged permission from the chiefs of the Quakeolths, to vaccinate the children of the tribe; but as they neither did, nor could, appreciate the unknown blessing, we preferred leaving things as they were, knowing well, from our experience of the native character, that our medicine would get the credit of any epidemic that might follow, or perhaps of any failure of the hunt or the fishery. (1847: 1.114)

Whether the Haida of the Queen Charlotte Islands were affected by this epidemic is, on present evidence, unclear. Researchers who have dealt with the issue at all are split right down the middle.[13] Despite the considerable data on Tlingit, Tsimshian, and other coastal peoples, there is not a single unambiguous citation documenting Haida participation in the 1836–37 epidemic. My previous position on this problem was that, considering this lack of data,

12. McIlwraith (1948: 1.16) notes that the adjacent upper Dean River territory, historically Dakelhne, may have been Nuxalk in the past.

13. Margaret Blackman's historical research on the Haida failed to discover any evidence for their participation in this epidemic (1981: 23). According to James Gibson (pers. comm., 1996), there is no documentation in Russian-American Company records for smallpox in the Queen Charlottes. George MacDonald, however, states that smallpox was present throughout the North Coast in 1836 (1983: 17). Robert Galois (pers. comm., 1996) notes that given the continuing trade and other interactions of the Haida with their Tlingit and Tsimshian neighbors, it seems unlikely that they could have avoided the 1836 epidemic. Epidemiologically, this makes eminent sense.

it was safest to assume that the Haida were spared (1990: 140, 143–44; 1992b: 252). But, epidemiologically, it is hard to understand how the epidemic could have missed them. As the Fort Simpson journal shows, there was constant canoe traffic and trade between the Queen Charlottes and the mainland, and hence ample opportunity for disease transmission. Hecate Strait was not a barrier to the spread of smallpox in other epidemics, and there is no reason to suppose that the situation in 1836 was any different. This, plus the following ambiguous historical citation, suggests to me that Haida participation in the 1836–37 epidemic was more likely than not.

In 1876, Haida chief Weah of Masset village told Anglican missionary William Collison:

The smallpox which came upon us many years ago killed many of our people. It came first from the north land, from the Iron People who come from where the sun sets [Russia]. Again it came not many years ago when I was a young man. It came then from the land of the Iron People where the sun rises [Canada]. . . . brave men have fallen before the Iron Man's sickness. You have come too late for them! (1981: 67–68)

The visitation from Weah's youth was certainly the epidemic of 1862 (chapter 7). The earlier outbreak could be either the epidemic of the 1770s *or* the epidemic of 1836, but the chronological closeness and presumed place of origin make it more likely that it was the later epidemic that Weah was referring to. Future research may provide more evidence on this problem.

Smallpox in 1837 in Northern California and Southern Oregon

The above quotation on the Kwakwaka'wakw from George Simpson notes the presence of smallpox in 1836–37 "south of the Columbia." Simpson was speaking in retrospect, four years after the fact, and from his wide knowledge, as governor of the Hudson's Bay Company, of events in the western portion of the North American continent. There was, indeed, a major smallpox epidemic in northern California and southern Oregon shortly after the outbreak on the North Coast. Moreover, despite the geographic gap, there was probably a direct connection between the outbreaks in the two regions (see map 7).

Northern California. Since 1812 the Russians had maintained an outpost on the coast of California, 60 miles north of San Francisco Bay. Fort Ross

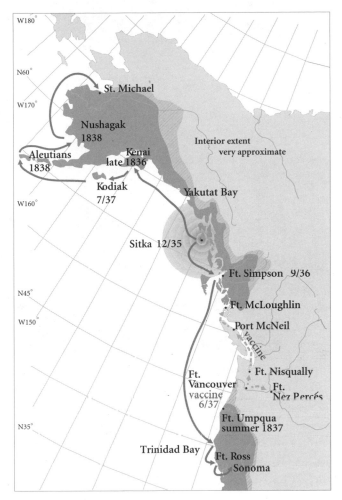

MAP 7. Smallpox Epidemic of 1836–37: Spread from the Focal Area

(fig. 9) was an agricultural station, which supplied the Alaska settlements with grain, vegetables, and meat (Gibson 1976). A company ship made an annual voyage between Ross and Sitka. In late 1837 there was a smallpox epidemic in Mexican California. Mexican records describe how it spread to the Central Valley:

Late in 1837 General Mariano Vallejo sent to Fort Ross a corporal of cavalry named Ignacio Miramontes to bring back a cargo of cloth and leather goods for the troops stationed at Sonoma. When Miramontes and his men returned they also brought with them the smallpox. How the disease got to Fort Ross or how much damage it did there is entirely unknown. (Cook 1939: 184)

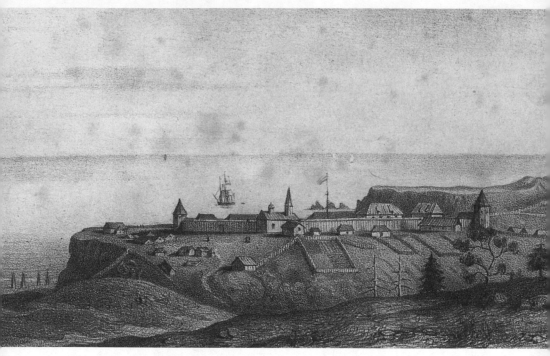

FIG. 9. Picture of Fort Ross, dated 1828, from Bernard du Haut-Cilly's *Voyage autour du monde* (Paris, 1834–35). Fort Ross was a possible point of entry into California for smallpox in 1837. (Courtesy of Bancroft Library, University of California, Berkeley.)

The ultimate origin of the disease most certainly was the Russian colonies to the north. As has happened many times in the historic epidemiology of the Northwest Coast, the carrier of the disease was probably an oceangoing vessel. The identity of this vessel remains unknown, however. Assuming a direct transmission of smallpox from Alaska to Ross itself, the most likely candidate would be the Russian-American Company supply ship *Sitka*. But there is a strong possibility (as later evidence will show) that the disease was initially introduced on the California coast north of Fort Ross sometime in late 1836 or early 1837 by one of the American vessels which traveled between the North and California coasts in search of sea otter (Ogden 1941).[14] From the north California coast smallpox would have moved to the interior and south

14. Possible landing sites are the mouth of the Klamath or Trinidad Bay. The *Diana, Joseph Peabody, Lama,* and (perhaps) *La Grange* are recorded as visiting both the North and California coasts in 1836–37 (Ogden 1941: 178–79). The log of the *Joseph Peabody,* which is extant, does not mention smallpox at all.

to Ross itself.[15] The disease spread through most of California between San Francisco Bay and Mount Shasta and was definitely recorded among the Patwin, Coast and Lake Miwok, Wappo, and Pomo (Cook 1939: 185). Estimates of deaths, given the lack of good contemporary population statistics for the area, probably provide only a rough approximation of reality.[16] In 1974 Sherburne Cook stated "the mortality may have reached 10,000" (1978: 92).

Southern Oregon. Another eyewitness to the California outbreak was Commander Edward Belcher of H.M.S. *Sulphur*. He had also been at Sitka in September 1837, where he noted the effects of the late epidemic (1843: 98). From Sitka he traveled via Nootka Sound to Point Reyes and the Farallon Islands, arriving at San Francisco on 19 October.[17] In November Belcher made an excursion up the Sacramento River and again observed the effects of small-pox on the Native population. His report states, "The later visitation of the small-pox was communicated by an American or Canadian" (1843: 129).

There were indeed both Americans and "Canadians" (Hudson's Bay Company trappers) in the Sacramento Valley in 1837.[18] The Americans may have been the aforementioned "coasters" involved in the sea otter trade or

15. From Fort Ross, Corporal Miramontes carried smallpox to General Vallejo's ranch at Sonoma, where perhaps 3,000 missionized Indians were concentrated (Alvarado n.d.: 162). Exactly one-half of Vallejo's Suisun and Napahoe (Patwin) infantry, who guarded the settlement from the hostile Satiyomes (Wappo), perished (Vallejo n.d.). In the vicinity of Sonoma the Indians "died daily like bugs" (Botello in Cook 1939: 184). Pits were dug to bury the dead (Richardson 1874: 8).

As in the north, California Indians used the sweat bath and cold-water plunge, with equally disastrous results: "The Indians immediately sought their sweat houses or 'temescales' where they exposed themselves to great heat and then plunged into cold water. Salvador Vallejo says that 'the death of so large a number of Indians is to be attributed to the fact that no sooner did they feel the attack of the smallpox than they went to the riverside and took a bath. I would not advise this method of curing smallpox, for as soon as an Indian took a bath death intervened.' Similarly Carrillo states that 'as they had recourse to sweating in their temescales, this mode of cure proved fatal to countless thousands'" (Cook 1939: 185).

16. Eyewitness estimates include 60,000 and 100,000; "over half" or three-fourths dead (Cook 1939: 185; Camp 1966: 148). These figures all imply a mortality much greater than the one-third loss documented for the 1836–37 outbreak on the North Coast and are likely excessive. They probably incorporate mortality from "fever and ague" in 1832 and later.

17. As he arrived late and bypassed the northern California coast, his ship could not have been responsible for the transmission of the disease to California.

18. By November 1837 smallpox was raging among the Indians of the Great Plains, introduced in June on the upper Missouri by a supply boat of the American Fur Company dispatched from St. Louis (Ray 1976: 155). But the Plains outbreak was probably not known to Belcher, and it most certainly was not related to the epidemic in California.

perhaps the Ewing Young party, who had come to California by ship in February 1837 from (smallpox-free) Fort Vancouver and driven a herd of cattle north through the Sacramento Valley in July and August (Edwards 1932). The Canadians were the annual Hudson's Bay Company fur brigade, headed by trapper Michel LaFramboise, also out of Fort Vancouver. Traveling overland, LaFramboise's party had been "south of the Umpqua" and in the "Valley of the Bonaventura [Sacramento]" from September 1836 through June 1837. They returned "to hunt the Feather River" in August 1837 and were probably in that vicinity at the same time Belcher was cruising the lower Sacramento.[19]

The importance of the American and Canadian parties in California is that they were involved in long-distance economic activities and thus could have transmitted diseases into regions that might otherwise have remained free of them. In 1833 one of the earlier "Bonaventura" parties had introduced fever and ague into the California valleys from its initial West Coast focus around Fort Vancouver (see chapter 4). Now, four years later, another trapping party apparently carried smallpox into Oregon from an earlier focus in California. The evidence for this connection comes from the Umpqua River region in southern Oregon, where a small Hudson's Bay post had been established in 1832. The Umpqua Indians believed that the Hudson's Bay people had brought first malaria and, later, smallpox to their country, and their consistent warlike behavior toward Euro-Americans reflected this belief.[20] In late 1838, Sir James Douglas, acting chief factor at Fort Vancouver, was forced to send a punitive brigade to the Umpqua to bring the Indians under control (Rich 1941: 261). From 1841, a member of the overland party of the U.S. Exploring Expedition reported a second threat to the fort:

19. McLoughlin letters of 15 November 1836 and 14 July 1837 in Rich 1941: 158, 187; letter of 30 August 1837, cited in Nunis 1968: 156–57.

20. Two quotations from Fort Vancouver describe what happened: "About two hundred miles southward, the Indians are said to be in a much more flourishing condition, and their hostility to the white people to be most deadly. They believe that we brought with us the fatal fever which has ravaged this portion of the country, and the consequence is, that they kill without mercy every white man who trusts himself among them" (August 1835; Townsend 1978: 224). "[T]he Umpqua Indians the fiercest, most untractable and vindictive of all the lower Columbia Tribes. . . . lately carried their daring so far as to menace their Post with distruction. . . . The sole cause I believe of this irritation was the prevalence among the tribe, during the latter summer months [1837] of an unknown and fatal disease attended by alarming mortality which they charitably ascribe to our ill offices" (18 March 1838; Douglas in Rich 1941: 282).

16 September 1841
Noticed on my way from the River to fort many Indians skulking about among the
bushes & upon enquiry was told by Mr Gangnia [Gagnier] that an unusual number
had encamped in his neighborhood and had lately threatened to attack him & burn
his fort—their hostility arising towards the Co. and Whites generally from their losses
by the small pox which was first introduced among them by the H.B.Co. Party under
Michael [LaFramboise] or [Thomas] McKay. . . . This being the state of affairs Mr.
G. had not ventured out of the Fort for many days & had kept up a vigilant watch
both night & day & of late had become so much alarmed by the increasing numbers
& menacing attitude of the Umpqua Indians that he was about dispatching a mes-
senger to Fort Vancouver to inform Dr McL. of his situation. . . . they were "terrible mauvaise savage" he frequently repeated while I was taking a bad cup of tea.
(Emmons 1841)

Sometime during 1837 (probably in June, as the party was returning to Fort
Vancouver from California, and prior to the "latter summer months" outbreak of disease among the Umpqua), LaFramboise and his men had apparently introduced smallpox into southern Oregon (or at least into the Umpqua
River valley). It should be noted that, according to the sources, smallpox at
Umpqua seems to have predated (slightly) its appearance at Fort Ross, suggesting that the origin for both was at some intermediate point, perhaps along
the northern California coast.

There is no indubitable documentation of smallpox at this time for the
"intermediate" peoples between the Sacramento and Umpqua Valleys. The
major reason for this may simply be a lack of contemporary records. Smallpox,
however, was the reason given by Indian informants for the abandonment
of some villages by the Yurok people of the lower Klamath (Cook 1956: 85);
and a record from one of the earliest agents to the Tututni of the lower Rogue
River indicates they also experienced the epidemic:

Port Orford, 10 July 1854
They show evident marks of small-pox having been among them about thirty years
ago; also the measles, about eighteen years since [the dates of 1824 for smallpox and
1836 for measles should be reversed on the basis of ethnohistorical information]; both
of which were very destructive to them from their mode of treatment. . . . They, like
all the other tribes along the coast, and in the interior, practice sweating in houses
built expressly for that purpose, and invariably, when they sweat themselves by this

process, they immediately plunge into cold water; and in consequence of treating small-pox and measles in this manner, it proved fatal to most of them. (Parrish 1855: 498)

It is possible that smallpox was present elsewhere south of 44° north latitude at this time: known distribution and epidemiology suggest as much. Comparison of 1805 (Lewis and Clark) and midcentury population statistics from the central Oregon coast (Coosan and Siuslawan) indicate considerable decline, some of which may be explained by mortality from this epidemic.

Central Coast

The central portion of the Northwest Coast, from approximately 44° to 52° north latitude, was bypassed by smallpox in 1836–37. One reason for this discontinuity was epidemiological: Indian populations had already diminished to the point where there were many breaks in their geographic distribution; in addition, a large proportion of that segment of the Indian population of the Central Coast over 35 years old was probably immune to smallpox. The 1836–37 epidemic did not spread to populations that are known to have suffered from the 1801–2 epidemic. Second, beginning in the summer of 1837, the Hudson's Bay Company seems to have made a concerted effort to block the spread of smallpox with smallpox vaccine, disseminated from Fort Vancouver to major Hudson's Bay posts in districts threatened by the spread of the epidemic. Although present in California by 1806 (Langsdorff 1814: 2.125) and at Sitka by 1808 (Tikhmenev 1978: 161), vaccine had not been used in earlier Northwest smallpox outbreaks, and there is no evidence that it was present in quantity or that any Indians were vaccinated prior to 1836. Hudson's Bay Company records do not even mention it until 1837.

Shortly after the return of the LaFramboise party from "the Bonaventura" in June 1837, however, this situation changed quickly. Indians were being vaccinated by Dr. William Tolmie at Fort Vancouver in June 1837, and by 10 July the post head at Fort Nisqually stated, "To day we have inoculated all the women and Children of the place" (Huggins: entries of 9 and 10 July 1837). On 3 July McLoughlin wrote to Fort Nez Percés (Walla Walla) offering to send vaccine if needed.[21] A 29 August letter from McLoughlin noted: "The

---

21. Hudson's Bay Company Archives, MS B. 223/b/17, fol. 31. Chance (1973: 120) cites this as evidence for the presence of smallpox on the Columbia Plateau at this time. Other than Splawn's

smallpox was still raging at Fort Simpson. . . . but it had not reached Port McLoughlin and as we have sent them Cowpox I hope the Indians will allow themselves to be vaccinated." On 2 October, the Reverend Herbert Beaver stated that he had vaccinated "about an hundred and twenty . . . Klickatack" Indians near Fort Vancouver, some 80 others having been previously inoculated by Dr. Tolmie (1959: 58).

Although one Company employee recalled that "all the indians that could be got at were vaccinated" (Roberts 1878), it is not likely that this amounted to any great number. In addition to logistical problems, the British (and the Russians too) had to surmount a large barrier of suspicion (note the comments of both Veniaminov, p. 121, and Simpson, p. 127). The Hudson's Bay program seems to have been limited to the most tractable Indians with closest ties to the Company itself. Many of the Klikitat vaccinated at Fort Vancouver were employed by the Company in various capacities; the Fort Nisqually journal suggests that the vaccination effort was limited to local Indians, trading partners, and prominent men. Purposeful or not, there was a selective process involved in this differential treatment. The most acculturated segment of the Indian population was given an edge in survival and future increase that was not shared with the unacculturated majority.

After the 1836–37 epidemic had run its course, the Hudson's Bay vaccination program apparently ceased. The Russians, however, to their credit, continued vaccinating Tlingit and other Alaskan Natives well into the next decade (Romanowsky and Frankenhauser 1962). Although we cannot be sure of the dimensions of the Russian program, it certainly contributed to the failure of the 1862 epidemic to spread very far into Alaska, whereas the former Hudson's Bay lands in British Columbia were devastated.

Mortality from the 1836–37 Smallpox Epidemic

Details on mortality from the epidemic of 1836–37 are presented in chapter 8. The common wisdom among Hudson's Bay officials was that the epidemic claimed one-third of the population of the North Coast (from the Aleutians to central British Columbia) (Douglas letter of 18 March 1838, in Rich 1941: 271; Simpson 1847: 1.123). The 1868 report to the U.S. Congress *Message on*

---

certainly misdated Sahaptin account (see chapter 2), I find no contemporary record indicating that the epidemic had spread to this area.

Russian America stated: "In 1838 ten thousand persons are reported to have fallen victim to this disease" (U.S. Congress 1868: 159). Adding the 10,000 deaths estimated by Sherburne Cook for northern California, the 3,500 from southwestern Alaska estimated by Fedorova (1973: 276–77), plus those from the unenumerated areas of southern Oregon, between 25,000 and 30,000 Indians must have died from the 1836–37 epidemic on the West Coast.

CENTRAL COAST INFLUENZA, 1836–38

Although there is no solid evidence for smallpox on the coast between Fort McLoughlin and the central Oregon coast in 1836–37, extant documents *do* mention a second disease, influenza. Influenza was recorded at Fort Nisqually on Puget Sound, Willamette Mission near Salem, and Waiilatpu Mission near Walla Walla. The disease was prevalent in much of the Old World in 1836 and epidemic in northern and western Europe from December 1836 through February 1837. There were three outbreaks at Nisqually, in March and April 1836, May 1837, and May 1838. The Willamette outbreak occurred in February 1837, and the Waiilatpu outbreak in April of that year. The 1837 outbreaks were probably part of a more extensive epidemic in the Central Coast. The contemporaneity and apparent exclusivity of smallpox and influenza in 1837 are remarkable. In none of the documents on smallpox are any symptoms of flu mentioned, and in the documents on influenza, smallpox is mentioned only in the context of vaccination. If, of course, the two had existed together in any one place, the mortality rate would have been much higher than it otherwise was.

The 1836 outbreak at Nisqually appears to have been limited; only five Indian deaths were recorded, and the journal entries are most interesting for what they say about treatments, aboriginal and White.[22]

The 1837 outbreak is first recorded at Willamette, in the (Methodist) Mission Record Book entry for 21 February:

Have been greatly afflicted with sickness in our [mission] family for a week past an unusually severe cold or influenza having suddenly seized most of the [Indian school] children—seventeen of them have been nearly confined to their beds for several days

22. The first mention of sickness in the Fort Nisqually journal for 1836 was on 2 March; on the next day it was identified as "the sore throat." On the third day five people in one family

requiring care both night & day so that we are nearly worn out with labour and watch-ing. Some of them are now getting better. This evening died Mosley Dwight infant son of Welaptulekt [Cayuse] and Marie age five months and fifteen days—his disease appeared to be croup several of the other children have also to appearance had a touch of that disease. (Carey 1922: 253)

"Croup" was a contemporary synonym for influenza, usually applied to chil-dren. The disease apparently spread to Forts Vancouver and Nez Percés, and in early April attacked the Cayuse Indians who had gathered around Waiilatpu Mission to plant crops. Here as elsewhere there were no deaths among those "to whom medicine was administered," and the missionaries were thankful that no blame for the disease was ascribed to them (Hulbert 1938: 272–73, 280).

At Nisqually the 1837 outbreak first appeared the second week of May; within a week Dr. Tolmie arrived from Vancouver to aid the sick. Although the disease was only mentioned briefly in that year's journal, it must have claimed several lives. The 1837 trade at Nisqually was poor and James Douglas attributed it to "the prevalence of disease among the natives, and the wars existing between several of the Tribes" (Rich 1941: 280). An outbreak of "sore throats" among Indians recurred at Nisqually in May 1838.

Influenza, unlike smallpox, mutates rapidly, and recovery from one attack does not provide immunity to a second. The regular yearly patterning of the

---

were ill; an 18-year-old girl died that night; her sister died five days later, on the ninth. Post head Edward Huggins attempted to treat the ill family but had to compete with shamans.

6 March 1836: "The Indians are still gathering about the sick, but without success in their singing and blowing, the poor people are getting worse daily."

10 March: "I paid a visit to the sick, the eldest son very low the next getting bad, the latter came [and] put himself under my care. The complaint is an inflammation of the throat. I have-given him a dose of Dovers powders, put his feet into warm water and blistered his neck, then into bed well covered over."

Shamans might blow on the affected body part to remove the causative agent. "Dovers pow-ders" consisted of 10% each ipecac and opium and was used to produce a sweat and as a seda-tive; blistering, usually performed with a mustard plaster, served as a counterirritant. Needless to say, both treatments were quite culture specific.

11 March: "The Indian Doctors succeeded in killing the eldest son by improper application of cold water to the body."

15 March: "The Indians Doctor have given out that it was my Tobacco that made the Indians sick."

According to Huggins, the young man under his care recovered and brought his father in for treatment. By mid-April, the Indian family had lost five of its children to influenza. On 4 April, all of the fort employees were "unwell of colds and inflammations of the throat."

flu at Nisqually between 1836 and 1838 suggests introduction of new strains, at this relatively isolated post, from some contact with the outside world, either direct, through Whites, or indirect, through neighboring Indians. Similar annual outbreaks of respiratory diseases occurred at Columbia Plateau trading posts in the 1820s and 1830s. On both the coast and Plateau the respiratory outbreaks occurred during the lean season of early spring when the Indians were, nutritionally, at their weakest (see appendix 1). On the Plateau these diseases appear to have been brought when the isolation of the post was broken with the return of the last fur trappers in early winter (Boyd 1985: 344).

LOWER COLUMBIA DYSENTERY, 1844

Dysentery was the major epidemic on the lower Columbia in the mid-1840s. According to Dr. Forbes Barclay (see fig. 10), physician at Fort Vancouver throughout the decade, the disease was brought to the Northwest by sea from Hawaii. From a focus at Fort Vancouver, it spread up the Columbia, Willamette, and Cowlitz Rivers. Dr. Barclay's description, as recorded by a visiting British sailor, gives both clinical and epidemiological characteristics:

Previous to the year 1844 diarrhoea and dysentery of a mild character prevailed occasionally at Fort Vancouver. In August of that year, dysentery prevailed to a fearful extent. Dr. Barclay states that it raged throughout the winter, attacking all classes and sparing neither age nor sex. Four hundred Indians died of the disease in the vicinity of the Fort. The evacuations were incessant, and the torment most distressing—sometimes pure blood was voided by the patient, but more frequently the dyections [sic] consisted of mucus and blood, accompanied by severe tenseness, and in many cases, with violent spasms of the back, and drawing up of the lower extremity. In a great many cases, there was great relaxation of the rectum/prolapsis ani. & the disease was always attended with pyrexia and thirst. Dr. B. who appears to be a Contagionist, is inclined to believe that this aggravated form of dysentery was introduced into Oregon by a Merchant Vessel from the Sandwich Islands!! Calomel in large doses, and Castor oil, was found to be the most useful remedies during the acute stage of the epidemic disease. (Dunn 1846)

Barclay's 1850 "Memorandum of Medical Facts" adds the following details: "violent equal to . . . Tropical Dysentery . . . a great many cases approaching the cholera, vomiting, purging, cramp, spasm, coldness and tossing of the

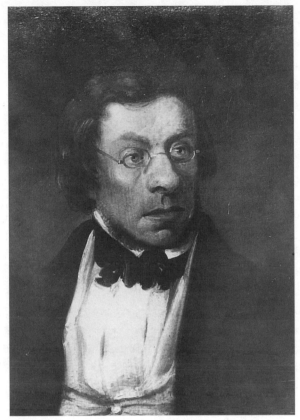

FIG. 10. Hudson's Bay Company doctor Forbes Barclay arrived in the Northwest in 1840. (Courtesy of Oregon Historical Society, Portland, negative no. OrHi 60534.)

body forcibly in every direction attended with Lock Jaw—loss of pulse. Clammy sweats terminates in death" (Larsell 1947: 90).[23]

Whether this particular outbreak originated in Hawaii, as suggested by Barclay, is not clear, though it appears that it most certainly was transmitted by boat from somewhere in the Pacific. Major outbreaks occurred in Tahiti

23. The doctor's "contagionist" theories, unfashionable in early-nineteenth-century America, were not far from the mark. The disease is transmitted via the fecal-oral route, commonly through contaminated water, and is associated with conditions of poor sanitation and crowding. The form of dysentery closest to Barclay's descriptions is shigellosis, caused by the bacterium *Shigella dysenteriae*. Symptoms include "fever, nausea and sometimes toxemia, vomiting, cramps and tenesmus. In typical cases the stools contain blood and mucus" (Benenson 1995: 421). Dehydration and shock are common outcomes, especially among children, and case fatalities have approached 20% in recent outbreaks. A second, less severe form of dysentery, caused by the protozoan *Entamoeba histolytica*, may be the form noted by Barclay before 1844 and in other sources in later years.

and the Cook Islands in 1843, and Samoa and the Marquesas in 1844 (MacArthur 1967), although no references in available contemporary sources from Hawaii itself have been located. Of three vessels docked at Vancouver in early summer, the *Modeste* seems epidemiologically the most likely culprit. It arrived on the Columbia in mid-July, traveled upstream to Vancouver, and its captain made a short trip inland to Willamette Mission. Within a month of these events, deaths were reported from Cowlitz, Vancouver, and the Willamette.

The course of the epidemic is well recorded in several contemporary documents, particularly those of the resident Catholic clergy.[24] Father De Smet, who arrived from Holland in early August on the *Indefatigable* with six Jesuit priests and the sisters of Notre Dame de Namur, stated:

We arrived in the Oregon Territory during the prevalence of a disease (bloody flux) which was considered contagious, though the physicians attributed it to the unwholesome properties of the river-water. Numbers of savages fell victim to it, especially among the Tchinouks, and the Indians of the Cascades, large parties of whom encamped along the banks of the river, on their way to Vancouver to obtain the aid of a physician. Those who could not proceed were abandoned by their friends; and it was truly painful to see these poor creatures stretched out, and expiring on the sand. The greater part of our sailors, and three of the sisters, were attacked by the pestilence; the Rev. Father Accolti also experienced its terrible effects; for myself, I was obliged to keep to my bed during 15 long days, and to observe a rigorous diet. (De Smet 1906: 167)[25]

The register of vital statistics kept by the priests at Vancouver and Cowlitz indicated a slight increase in deaths in late July and a sudden jump after 10 August: 43, regularly spaced, were recorded in the next seven weeks, and after 17 October, fatalities declined rapidly. Judging by the 44 whose ages were given, children under five and young adults were most susceptible (Munnick 1972, 1979). The vast majority of those registered were Indians. As far as *total* Indian

24. Fathers Norbert Blanchet, Modeste Demers, Jean-Pierre De Smet, Gregory Mengarini, the sisters of Notre Dame de Namur, and, especially, the records of baptisms, marriages, and deaths kept by Blanchet and Demers at Vancouver and Cowlitz.

25. The captain of the *Indefatigable* and three of the sisters of Notre Dame died (Evans 1981: 53); at Fort Vancouver three men expired (Lowe 1843–48); and at the Methodists' Willamette Mission Mrs. Lewis Judson passed away (Judson 1845).

mortality is concerned, we have only anecdotal and incomplete numbers. Dr. Barclay's total of 400 from the vicinity of Fort Vancouver is noted above; Father Point said a "tenth" died in the same area (Buckley 1989: 475). At Cowlitz, Father Bolduc (see below) said 30 died; Father Demers's wretched handwriting records an indecipherable number between Cassino's village and The Cascades (Demers 1844). And the Methodists at The Dalles recorded 30 deaths at a village which was probably *ninułdixdix̣* at the mouth of Hood River (Brewer 1845).

But this is certainly only a sample of the true total. We can only guess at what happened in the hinterland. A passage from Father Bolduc of Cowlitz Mission and a tradition recorded from Mary's River Kalapuya informant William Hartless give us a hint:

The natives inhabiting the country from the mouth of the Columbia up to Fort Vancouver were visited this year by a dysentery that has more than decimated them. . . . Of thirty . . . at Cowlitz . . . who became its victims, only four refused to become Christians. The epidemic lasted from the end of the month of August until the beginning of the present month [November]. During this time I did not have more rest than did the priests of Quebec during the cholera. In spite of my weariness, which was great— if one considers that I had to travel over an extent of territory of at least five leagues, without roads, through forests, with rivers to ford, being obliged myself to make coffins for the dead, as many as three a day; in spite of, I say, these fatigues I experienced great comforts, and I hope that the good God has pleased to bless my feeble efforts for the salvation of the dying [an example of a deathbed conversion follows]. (Bolduc in Landerholm 1956: 237–38)

Now a sickness came (it was some type of diarrhoea in which blood was passed), and the people then became ill. They never got well. All who had become ill died. When they doctored them they never got well, a great many of them died. . . . Half the people had died now. . . . So then the shamans indeed stood to their dance. They (then) said, "The disease came from nowhere (else). The disease started right here". . . . the shamans said . . . the child [a misbehaving orphan] has been killing us . . . they seized the child. . . . They buried him while he was still alive. Now indeed it checked (but it did not stop) the disease. (Jacobs 1945: 274)

Dysentery was an important epidemic. According to the records, the virulent form reappeared in subsequent summers at Vancouver and Cowlitz

(Lowe 1843–48), Wascopam, and Nisqually. At the latter location, the Indians claimed that "the Americans used magic to cause the distemper, in revenge for (the Indians) not trading their beaver skins with them" (Heath 1979: 39). Shades of Dominis and the fever!

CHILDHOOD DISEASES: TWO FOCI

Demographically, the fur-trading posts of the Hudson's Bay Company were unique—populated by Euro-American and half-blood adult males, sometimes with common-law Indian wives. There were no foreign-born women or, more important, children to import diseases prevalent among their age category in settled areas to the east. On the south coast this situation began to change with the first missions in 1834, picking up speed after the arrival of the first settlers over the Oregon Trail, starting in 1841. On the Columbia Plateau, mission stations were foci for several new diseases characteristic of children: chicken pox, scarlet fever, and whooping cough among them (Boyd 1992a). None of these, interestingly, spread to the coast. Two early foci for introduced childhood diseases on the coast itself were Willamette Mission, with a concentration of children at its Indian school (1835–44), and Sitka, with some Russian families and close ties to the Eurasian landmass. Two particularly well-recorded minor outbreaks, of meningitis and mumps, are described below.

Willamette Mission: Meningitis, 1835

The meningitis outbreak is known from only two contemporary sources. The Oregon Mission Record Book noted two Indian deaths, on 27 November and 13 December, from "a distressing pain in the head," which caused a "loss of reason" and death within a week (Carey 1922: 239–41). The Reverend Samuel Parker, visiting Oregon under the auspices of the American Board of Commissioners for Foreign Missions, was at Willamette in the midst of this minor epidemic, and his journal contains an explicit description of the disease:

26 November 1835
At the time of my continuance in this place, an epidemic prevailed among the Indians, of which several persons died. In some respects it was singular. The subjects of the complaint were attacked with a severe pain in the ear almost instantaneously, which soon spread through the whole head with great heat in the part affected; at the same

time the pulse became very feeble and not very frequent—soon the extremities became cold and a general torpor spread through the whole system except the head—soon they were senseless, and in a short period died. In some cases the attack was less severe, and the patient lingered, and after some days convalesced, or continued to sink until death closed his earthly existence. (1838: 165–66)[26]

The mission school, which was created to serve the many Indian children of the Willamette Valley who had been orphaned by fever and ague, was plagued by disease throughout the brief decade of its existence. Endemic malaria, tuberculosis (both consumption and scrofula), venereal disease, influenza, meningitis, and (perhaps) whooping cough were recorded (Boyd 1995). Dutifully, the mission's Record Book recorded the deaths of one after another of its students from disease. Between deaths and desertions, the school had trouble maintaining its membership; in 1843, the Reverend Joseph Frost, one of the more cynical members of the Oregon Mission, noted that there were "more Indian children in the mission grave-yard . . . than there were . . . alive in the manual labor school" (Lee and Frost 1844: 311). After a "strange fatality" (Hines 1868: 160; whooping cough?) descended upon it in 1844, the mission school was closed for good.

Sitka: Mumps, 1843–44; Influenza, 1845–46

Sitka, where some Russian families lived, picked up many European diseases earlier than the rest of the coast. But none of these is well recorded, and most appear not to have spread to the Tlingit Indians. According to Robert Fortuine, the authority on Alaskan disease history:

Dr. Blaschke . . . described several types of epidemic disease he saw at New Archangel [Sitka] in the 1830s. "Gastric fever," probably typhoid, was particularly common during the winter months. What he called "acute hydrocephalus" (probably meningitis)

---

26. Meningitis, an inflammation of the outer membrane of the brain, may be caused by any number of viral or bacterial agents. The most common forms result from infection by the bacterium *Haemophilus influenzae* or the meningococcus *Neisseria meningitidis* (Benenson 1995: 303); the symptomatology and epidemiology of the latter variety seem closest to Parker's description. Meningococcal disease is characterized by "fever, intense headache," sometimes followed by "delirium and coma"; it is most common in winter, among children and males, and "under crowded living conditions." It is spread by droplet infection and formerly had a case fatality exceeding 50% (303–4).

assumed epidemic proportions one winter. Diphtheria and whooping cough also were reported not infrequently among the children. (1989: 205)[27]

The mumps outbreak was limited to Native Americans (both Tlingit and Aleut). Russians, certainly because of immunity acquired from childhood attacks in the mother country, did not catch it. The epidemic began in October 1843 in the "southern Bays" and spread north, attacking Sitka in December 1843 and January 1844. Dr. Romanowsky, who treated the mumps outbreak, gave the following clinical description: "Parotitis is an inflammation of the salivary glands of the ear, occasionally accompanied by simultaneous affection of the submaxillary gland, which becomes obvious by a hard swelling of the above mentioned glands, difficulties in chewing and opening of the mouth, hindered deglutition [swallowing], and accompanied by severe inflammations" (Romanowsky and Frankenhauser 1962: 34). Individual cases lasted four to five days, rarely more.[28] Romanowsky used purgatives and ointments to treat mumps and reported no deaths at Sitka.

There was an epidemic of influenza ("croup") among children at Sitka in winter 1845–46. Symptoms included an inflamed respiratory tract, dry cough followed by expectoration of yellowish mucus, fever, rapid heartbeat, cold sweats, and weakness. Death came from "paralysis of the lung." Twelve died at Sitka; Dr. Frankenhauser said that in the "Colony of the Koloshes [Tlingit], there were also large casualties among the children" (1962: 63).

27. Of the above diseases, the localized 1835 outbreak of meningitis among the Indian students at the Willamette Mission school is described above. Typhoid first occurred among lower Columbia Whites in 1844, and whooping cough had been reported in February 1827 at Fort Kamloops and in January–February 1844 at Wascopam Mission—both in the Plateau culture area (Boyd 1992a, 1996b: 143–44).

28. Romanowsky's description is consistent with that in the American Public Health Association's *Control of Communicable Diseases Manual* (Benenson 1995: 347).

6 / Two Midcentury Epidemics

Measles and Smallpox, 1847–1848 and 1853

The mid-nineteenth-century measles and smallpox epidemics shared several characteristics, historical and medical. Historically, both were introduced from California and spread ultimately to Hawaii; both came via improved, rapid means of transportation (horses and steamships) involved in the exchange of new, valued economic goods (cattle and oysters); both spread throughout the Northwest Coast *and* Plateau culture areas; both were associated with a moderate mortality; and (in the States) both were followed by Indian-White hostilities. The one-two punch of these two deadly epidemics, a mere five years apart, was the coup de grace for most South Coast (U.S.A.) Indian peoples. Treaty making began in 1853, and by 1857 most surviving Indians in Oregon and Washington west of the Cascade Mountains had been herded onto hastily drawn reservations.

MEASLES, 1847–1848

Background and Origins

Measles, like smallpox, is a classic crowd disease. In many of its clinical and epidemiological characteristics measles is very similar to smallpox; it differs in the less severe nature of the rash, a predilection for children, and a lower average mortality (10%).[1] The epidemiological similarity of the two diseases has created some uncertainty about the identity of some early epidemics: as noted in chapter 2, the "mortality" of 1824–25 may have been either small-pox or measles.[2] Judging from the severity of the effects and relative paucity of evidence for acquired immunity, however, the 1847–48 epidemic appears to have been a virgin-soil visitation.

In 1846–47 measles was epidemic throughout much of Europe and North America; the direction of diffusion appears to have been generally from east to west (Hirsch 1883: 160). In Hudson's Bay Company lands, measles was first reported at the Red River headquarters (Winnipeg) in June 1846; from there it spread north, west, and south, reaching the Shoshone of present-day Wyoming by 1847.[3] As one of the overland emigrants of 1847 noted, "Measles was general that year on the Plains" (Jory in Lyman 1902: 283). Though most of the Oregon Trail migrants passed through areas where measles was epidemic, there are no reports in diaries of measles cases or fatalities among the overland migrants as they crossed the Rockies or before their arrival at Waiilatpu Mission near Walla Walla. Given the short incubation and duration of the disease and the length of time required to make the overland journey, it appears unlikely that the emigrants carried measles overland. Instead, measles was already present in Oregon by August 1847.

The source for this early appearance of the disease on the Columbia Plateau

1. For bibliographic sources on smallpox, see appendix 2. The data on measles are from Benenson 1995: 293–94 and Babbott and Gordon 1954. A limited but excellent literature on virgin-soil measles epidemics exists. Peter Panum (1940) discusses an 1846 Faroe Islands outbreak in a population that had not experienced measles for a life span; James Neel et al. (1970) review a 1968 outbreak among the Yanomamo Indians of the Brazil-Venezuela border; and Robert Wolfe (1982) describes a 1900 epidemic among Bering Sea Inuit.

2. In 1850 Dr. Forbes Barclay wrote: "The measles have been known to prevail in the Columbia in 1812—supposed to have been carried thither by the H. Bay Company Express from York factory where it prevailed at the same time" (Larsell 1947: 90). Barclay's "1812" may be a transposition of 1821, the year that the Hudson's Bay Company formally entered the Pacific Northwest, and the terminal date for a measles outbreak that spread through central Canada. Arthur Ray (1974: 106–8) discusses the 1820–21 epidemic in the Canadian prairie provinces. John Taylor (1977: 80) notes measles among Indians of North Dakota and Montana, and Shepard Krech (1981: 85) cites references to the epidemic among Subarctic Athapascan Indians. A measles epidemic spread among the missionized California Indians in 1827–28 (Valle 1973a).

3. Geographer Arthur Ray has reconstructed the spread of the disease throughout Hudson's Bay Company lands in central Canada (1976: 151–54). From the Red River, measles spread to Norway House (north of Lake Winnipeg) by midmonth; and from there to all other Company forts throughout the Canadian Shield in August. Boat brigades, which converged on Norway House in midsummer from all points north and west, were the agents of diffusion. To the south

was central California. How measles arrived in California is not yet known: conveyance via one of the southern overland routes from the Plains or by ship from Mexico are possible explanations.[4] However it arrived, the disease was epidemic around Sutter's Fort (or New Helvetia, near modern Sacramento) in mid-June 1847. August Sutter's diary for 17–19 June stated: "Great Sickness and diseases amongst the Indian tribes, and a great Number of them were dying notwithstanding of having employed a doctor to my hospital" (Sutter 1939: 40). References to illness (never specific as to type) continue from mid-June through late July; the diary also notes the presence of "Walla Walla" Indians in the vicinity, between 26 May and 26 June. The Oregon Indians, on an unsuccessful trip to obtain Spanish cattle, left California just after the epidemic had started there (Heizer 1942).

The return of the California party to Fort Nez Percés on 23 July 1847 was recorded in a poignant passage in the journal of artist and explorer Paul Kane:

A boy, one of the sons of Peo-Peo-mox-mox, the chief of the Walla Wallas, arrived at the camp close to the fort [in advance of the party of 200]. . . . bringing the most disastrous tidings, not only of the total failure of the expedition, but also of their suffering and detention by sickness. . . . After describing the progress of the journey up to the time of the disease (the measles) making its appearance, during which he was listened to in breathless silence, he began to name its victims one after another. On the first name being mentioned, a terrific howl ensued, the women loosening their hair and gesticulating in a most violent manner. When this had subsided, he, after much persuasion, named a second and third, until he had named upwards of thirty. The same signs of intense grief followed the mention of each name. . . . the Indian's statement occupied nearly three hours. . . . The Indians . . . immediately sent messengers in every direction on horseback to spread the news of the disaster among all the neighbouring tribes. (1971: 116–17)[5]

---

the disease was present among all the Indian peoples of North Dakota and eastern Montana in 1846, and Wyoming in 1847 (Taylor 1977: 80–81).

4. Although the great Mormon migration did not occur until the summer of 1847, some emigrants preceded it. The "sick detachment" of Mormons spent the winter of 1846–47 at Pueblo, Colorado.

5. Anthropologist Robert Heizer was the first to note the epidemiological significance of this crucial passage (1942). Thirty years later Clifford Drury quoted much of it in his discussion of the causes of the Whitman Massacre (1973: chap. 22).

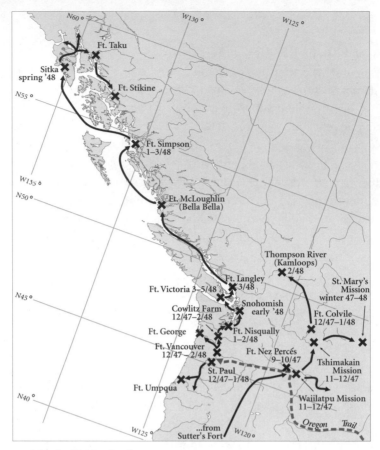

MAP 8. Measles Epidemic of 1847–48

Some of the "messengers in every direction" must have carried the measles virus with them. Given the disease's incubation period, we can speculate that within 10 days the messengers would have transmitted the virus to residents of their home communities, and that after another two weeks large numbers of Indians would have come down with the disease. By the last week of August, according to this time frame, people on the middle Columbia would have begun to die. In fact, the next recorded mention of measles comes from a 3 September diary notation, made at the "Umatilla crossing" of the Oregon Trail: "found in Camp Hodges & Taylor Co. with a man very sick with the measels" (Brown 1847). The man died on 4 September. The first Indian cases were recorded in early November; on 27 November frightened Cayuse killed 13 people at Whitman Mission (Waiilatpu), whom they blamed for the epidemic;

during the next two months measles spread the length and breadth of the Plateau culture area (see map 8).[6]

Measles in the Lower Columbia Region

Although emigrants from the United States were not responsible for introducing measles across the Rockies to the upper Columbia, there is no doubt that they carried the epidemic downstream from the middle Columbia to Fort Vancouver. In October and November, journals of overland migrants recorded measles cases on the trail between Waiilatpu Mission and Fort Vancouver (e.g., Lee 1847; Hastings 1847), well after the first cases were reported in the interior and preceding the earliest reports of illness at Fort Vancouver. Fort records, such as the following (by Peter Skene Ogden), are unanimous in attributing the introduction to the Americans.

10 March 1848
The Immigrants numbering upwards of 4000 Men women and Children made their appearance about the usual time and with [them] came Measles Dysentery and Typhus Fever, Cholera alone being wanting to complete the catalogue but still with the first three the deaths have been great at the French Settlement [Willamette] 65—Cowlitz 1—here 12 of the Servants and an equal number of Americans, but it would be impossible to form any idea of the Indian's population they were swept off by hundreds.

In a letter written just one week later, Dr. Barclay claimed that "the Indian population have suffered about a *ninth*" (Barclay 1848). His reference was to "the Columbia"—perhaps the entire Columbia District but more likely the environs of Fort Vancouver were meant.

Two remarkable documents kept by Catholic missionaries, the registers of baptisms, burials, and marriages made at Fort Vancouver and at St. Paul, on the French Prairie of the Willamette Valley (Munnick 1972, 1979), allow a reconstruction of the duration of the epidemic and its effects on different segments of the local population. Neither register gives causes of death, but

---

6. Details on the epidemic among Plateau peoples from Waiilatpu to as far north as Fort Alexandria in central interior British Columbia appear in Boyd 1994a. Robert Galois (1996) discusses the epidemic's spread into northern interior British Columbia.

the pronounced clustering of fatalities in a limited time frame suggests that the vast majority resulted from the newly introduced disease, measles. At Vancouver deaths clustered between the last week of November (the first casualty was a half-Cayuse child) and the third week of February, a three-month span. Thirty-nine deaths were recorded during this period, with a peak during the first week of 1848, when 11 died. Judging by the names, almost all of the recorded fatalities were local Indians, though one Iroquois and two Hawaiians expired as well. There was no significant difference between the sexes among those who died, but there was a marked pattern to the fatalities by age group. Of those whose ages were recorded, 17 were five years old or younger and 18 were between thirteen and thirty-five. No one between the ages of six and twelve died; 2 whose ages were estimated at thirty-seven, 1 forty-year-old, and 1 sixty-year-old died. The last two were Hawaiian and Iroquois, respectively.[7] At St. Paul in the Willamette Valley 17 deaths occurred between 15 December 1847 and 23 January 1848, within a French Canadian/mixed-blood population. Ten of the total were babies; only one of the dead was over thirty. In both these populations measles typically showed no favoritism by sex but hit infants and young adults disproportionately hard. A concentration of fatalities among the very young (as noted earlier) is usual for measles.[8]

Among Willamette Valley Indians, at least five accounts of the measles epidemic have survived. The most descriptive was collected by anthropologist Melville Jacobs from his Clackamas Indian informant, Victoria Howard, circa 1929–30:

I do not know how long after [the fever and ague] . . . they now got measles. Now they were again just like that, they died. They drank quantities of water in the same manner again, they died quickly. They were like that (one of the people after another

7. Thomas Lowe's journal (1843–48) first mentions measles on 26 November 1847; by 8 December, "Almost all our working hands are laid up with the measles"; and on 16 December, "Most of the sick are gradually recovering." Lowe recorded seven deaths at the fort between 11 December 1847 and 5 January 1848; *all* were Hawaiians.

8. The lack of recorded deaths among adults may be significant. Among elderly people with no acquired immunity to the disease, measles is deadly. The paucity of deaths in the over-35 age group at Vancouver and French Prairie could be related to several factors, but the most likely explanation is that most individuals over 37 had acquired immunity from a previous bout with the disease. Among those of White ancestry, the resistance was probably acquired in their homelands to the east. But it is also interesting to note that subtracting 37 from the year of the epidemic (1848) yields 1811, one year from Dr. Barclay's previously noted (n. 2) date of 1812 for the initial appearance of measles in the Pacific Northwest.

catching measles) for a considerable time. It (the rash) would come out on a child, he would get cold, it (the disease) would (because he had not been kept sufficiently warm) go in (into his heart or stomach), and presently he would die. Some of them went to sweat (in their sweathouse). It would come out all over on them, the measles would come out on their eyes. Some of them would come out (from the sweathouse), they would pour cold water on (themselves), they would die soon after that. Some came out, they lay down, they put covers over them, they would recover. After a long time then they did not die much more from that. But it was quite a while before the disease left. (Jacobs 1958–59: 2.547–48)

Mrs. Howard's account provides the most explicit record of the dynamics of death among South Coast Indians from the 1847–48 epidemic. It also points out the importance of treatments inappropriate for febrile diseases in increasing the fatality rate. Mrs. Howard notes the similarity of treatment for measles and the preceding "fever and ague" (malaria); significantly, the same methods were used again during the 1853 smallpox epidemic.[9]

How far south and west the epidemic spread from the Willamette is unknown. A few cryptic references point to its presence in the vast area beyond

9. A second Willamette Valley account that includes a description of a sweat lodge comes from an 1847 immigrant. The Indians in question were probably the Santiam band of Kalapuya; the location was their winter home "along the [Willamette] shore below the present town of Salem" (Clarke 1905: 1.131): "In the year 1847 the measels [*sic*] followed the immigration over the plains. The Indians contracted it. It was just as fatal to them as the smallpox. . . . In the lower part of Salem there was an Indian encampment containing 300 or 400 persons. The measels broke out among them & swept away at least one half of the Indian population of Willamette Valley. Their system of doctoring was: the Indians would make a wickeup. . . . They would take poles to 8 or 10 feet long & put them in the ground making a circle. Then they would gradually bring them together at the top & lash them with grass or straw & cover them all over with earth & make it entirely air tight like a potato heap except at one place they would make a door sufficiently large to crawl in. The Indians would gather in that place as thick as they could set in a circle & in the midst of them they would have their tin pans & drums. . . . and sing. . . . At the door they would have a fire with hot rocks in it & on these they would throw water to make steam. They would sit in there until they reeked with perspiration especially the sick ones affected with measels. Then they would all come out & plunge into a cold creek. The water would be ice cold in winter. The effect would be that most of them would die. One of them did not, getting out of the water alive. He only lived a short time after he got in. I do not think there was ever seen an Indian that ever recovered from that kind of practice. They doctor everything in that way, so they applied it to measels also. The Americans & missionaries attempted to prevent it" (Brown 1878).

Although Brown's mortality figures are certainly exaggerated, other information in his account is ethnographically accurate. Three other accounts which verify the presence of measles in the Willamette Valley are Lockley 1916: 369–70; Alderman 1957; and Elliot 1927.

the valley. A 16 March 1848 letter written by Hudson's Bay Company factor James Douglas stated: "The fur returns of the Indian shops of Fort Vancouver, Fort George and Umpqua River are inferior in value to those of last year, a result accounted for by the distressed state of the Natives, who have been suffering with measles since the month of December last, and have not recovered from the stunning effects of that severe visitation" (Douglas 1848a). A single statement in the *Oregon Spectator* in July 1848 noted: "It is said that all the lower Umpqua Indians except seven died with the measles and dysentery during the last winter."

North of Fort Vancouver measles spread quickly to the Hudson's Bay Company farm on the Cowlitz River, where progress of the epidemic was fully recorded in the journal of George B. Roberts (1962). Initial exposure must have occurred at the beginning of December; on 16 December, 11 individuals at the farm, Hawaiian and Indian, experienced symptoms. On 17 December, 20 people were ill; by the 21st, measles was "spreading thro the settlement." On the 27th, the first fatality, as well as several convalescents, was reported (again, the timing points to an early December infection). On 30 December, Roberts wrote, "The poor indians taking the measles fast & are suffering extremely." It appears that the Indian community was infected later than those at the farm itself and thus constituted a second wave of the disease at Cowlitz:

31 December 1847

The greatest alarm prevails on account of the still spreading disease. It assumes two forms here. Those in whom the fever subsides immediately after the eruption suffer but little comparatively & are quickly restored to health. On the other hand the most part have their sufferings increase after the breaking out of the measles & remain a long time in a sinking state. There is a languor, a want of appetite & dreadful thirst. The Owyhyees are nearly well but have been troubled with a bad diarreah, which I fortunately have the means of stopping by administering small doses of opium & Tonic mixture. (1962: 141)

The epidemic apparently peaked in mid-January, with three deaths in one day.[10] Belatedly, measles attacked a third group: On 30 January Roberts wrote,

---

10. 14 January 1848: "Poor William ended his suffering to day. His wife [who died two days later] with a babe in the month and two other very young children lie also in a most pitiable & helpless state. We have to feed & assist all the indians about us, draw fire wood for them & etc. 3 died to day. All hands either ill themselves or attending their sick families" (Roberts 1962: 141).

"Measels [*sic*] now very prevalent among the settlers." These were largely French Canadians, who had traveled overland in 1841 from the settlement at Red River.

Roberts last mentioned the disease on 21 February: "The dregs of the measles seem to hang about many." At Cowlitz the epidemic lasted roughly two months. As at Vancouver, there appear to have been minor waves within the total duration of the epidemic, as relatively discrete communities or subgroups were infected in sequence. Unlike Vancouver, though (and like most other places), other diseases accompanied or followed measles among the infected. In the same passage where Roberts noted the "dregs" of measles, he mentioned that some of the convalescents had "severe colds." These, however, were probably symptoms of yet another disease, typhus, which the journal identified by name on the next day. Several non-Indians subsequently acquired "camp fever," certainly brought with the overland migrants of 1847. And as if this was not enough, in mid-May influenza was introduced to Cowlitz Farm from Fort Vancouver.

Measles North of the Columbia

Extant records describe the measles epidemic at four more locations to the north of the Columbia: Forts Nisqually, Victoria, and Simpson—all Hudson's Bay Company establishments—and Sitka, a Russian outpost (map 8). The key to how the epidemic spread to these locations is contained in a letter from Company trader John Work, dated 10 February 1848. Work had been sent from Vancouver via the Cowlitz Trail and the Company vessel, the *Beaver* (fig. 11), to Fort Simpson, where he was to assume the position of post head:

I left Fort Vancouver 26th Nov (with the East side Otters for the Russians), and Nisqually with the Steamer 14th Dec. and Fort Victoria on the 20th and reached this place [Fort Simpson] 5th January. . . . As I passed the different establishments to the Southward all were well. The emigrants had brought Measles and dysentery to the Columbia and the Indians . . . were dying fast of these complaints. When I left Vancouver there were a few cases of Measles in the hospital. A Sandwich Islander who with other men for Fort Langley accompanied me across the Cowlitz portage brought the measles with him, he was ailing when we left him at Point Roberts and some days before, but it was thought it was the ague he had till about a week after when four men and two boys on board the Steamer were taken ill with the measles. On arrival here [Fort Simpson] the disease soon spread both in and outside the fort, four men

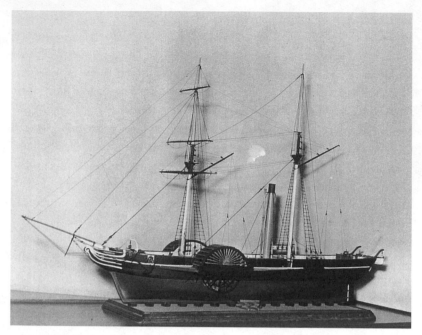

FIG. 11. The Hudson's Bay Company's steam-powered vessel *Beaver* carried personnel and equipment between the Company's coastal forts; it may have transmitted measles to coastal Indians in late 1847. This model shows the *Beaver* as it looked before remodeling in the 1880s. (Courtesy of Maritime Museum of British Columbia, Victoria, B.C.)

and most of the Women and Children in the fort have had the disease, two of the men's children have died of it; there have also been several deaths among the Natives, and from the almost utter impossibility of getting them to take proper care of themselves while under the disease it is to be feared it will prove fatal to numbers more of them. . . . Captain Dodd now starts with the Steamer for Sitka. . . . and then. . . . North to attend to the trade. (Work 1848a)

Work's route may be reconstructed with some detail from this letter and other sources. On 26 November he left Vancouver; on 1 December George Roberts recorded Work's arrival at Cowlitz Farm (1962: 136); he left on the 3d and reached Fort Nisqually on the 7th (Tolmie 1847–48). Embarking on the steamer on the 14th, landfalls were made on the 16th at Victoria; on the 21st at "Youcalters" (Lekwiltok Kwagiulth; probably the Cape Mudge or the Campbell River village); on the 22d at "Cogholes" (Kwakwaka'wakw); two days after Christmas at "Bellacolla"; on the 30th at "the forte" (probably McLoughlin); and on 5 January at Fort Simpson. Leaving Work at Fort

Simpson on 10 February, the *Beaver* proceeded to Sitka (on the 23d), to Chilkat (27th), to Cross Sound (28th), back to Chilkat (8 March), to Taku (15th), and then to the Stikine River (19th) (Thorne 1847–48). Measles subsequently appeared at all these locations for which records are extant.

At Fort Nisqually (on Puget Sound) post head Dr. William Tolmie recorded the first case at the fort on 27 December: "I am sorry to inform you that two of our Sandwich Islanders are laid up with Measles. No cases have yet been heard of amongst the Indians." The journal of Joseph Heath, a Steilacoom farmer, noted an Indian case on 7 January; on 8 January Tolmie wrote: "Measles, as yet I am thankful to say, of a mild type are prevalent here and at the present three fourths of our establishment are either on the sick-list, or employed in tending the sick" (Tolmie 1847–48).

By 31 January the epidemic had spent itself among the personnel at Fort Nisqually, but a second wave was in progress among the Indians. The first recorded cases were among the family of Lehalet, chief of the Sequalatchew Nisqually, on 17 January (Helen Norton, pers. comm., 1992). At Steilacoom Farm Heath visited and tended the Indians in their lodges, providing "provisions" (including venison and cow's milk for "the Indian babies, their mothers, ill with measles, having none"), administering medicine, and "preventing them getting into the cold water as well as drinking it." The number of sick increased until 14 February, when Heath reported, "All my people now laid up" (Heath 1979). After the measles had run its course, dysentery and pneumonia followed and claimed still more lives. On 11 March, Tolmie said: "Sickness still lingers in this quarter I am sorry to say, and Indians are occasionally dying of Dysentery, and Inflammation of the Lungs succeeding Measles" (1847–48). Since Nisqually was a hub of trade for most Indian peoples of Puget Sound, "the potential for spread of the infection was great. . . . From 12/8/1847 to 4/3/1848 Steilacoom, Nisqually, Puyallup, Snoqualmic, Snohomish, Suquamish, Sinuamish, Skagit, Cowlitz, Taweisomis (Prairie de Buttes), Yakama, Klikitat and perhaps Lummi were doing business at the fort" (Helen Norton, pers. comm., 1992).

No records survive from the northern part of Puget Sound or from the Hudson's Bay Company fort at Langley (near present-day Vancouver, British Columbia), but the epidemic certainly spread to this area as well, as it was present to the south, west, and north. Word of the Whitman Massacre, received on 20 December at Nisqually, "caused a great sensation" among the Indians. Thirty years later Dr. Tolmie recalled:

There were no stockades or bastions at Nisqually then. A fugitive Indian conjurer or curer of the sick, flying for his life from the Sinahomish country (on S. River Possession Sound and south end of Whidbey Island), arrived at Nisqually and stated that the Whites had brought the measles to exterminate the Indians, were coming to massacre the whites at Nisqually. . . . On this being reported at Ft Vancouver the Doctor was instructed to erect forts and bastions. (1878)

The Fort Victoria journal entry for 3 April 1848 noted the arrival of "a Canoe of Sinahomish" who gave "a woful account of the deaths amongst their tribe from measles & Dysentery." On 13 April the journal noted measles at Fort Langley; on 14 April, "to the North" (Finlayson 1846–50).[11] On 15 April the Fort Nisqually letterbook reported "the Klallum and Sinahomish ready to attack because of the measles" (Tolmie 1847–48).

Chronologically, the next place the epidemic reached was Fort Simpson (near present-day Prince Rupert, British Columbia), John Work's destination, where he arrived from Fort Nisqually on 5 January 1848. The epidemic among the local Tsimshian Indians began later in the month and continued through February and March. Work's family all came down with measles at the same time, and he nearly lost two of his four daughters to the "fever" (influenza) that followed (Work 1848b). Chief Factor James Douglas's summary report to Company headquarters in London, dated 5 December 1848, stated:

The natives of Fort Simpson were unfortunately attacked with measles in the month of January 1848, and that highly contagious disease spread with frightful rapidity among the neighbouring Tribes, producing an amount of destitution, wretchedness and mortality perfectly heart-rending. . . . Food, medicine and advice were liberally dispensed to the Indians living about the establishment, but these formed a small part of the suffering thousands who were crowded into distant villages beyond the reach of our aid. Some idea may be formed of the fatal effects of that disease among Indians, from the number of deaths which occurred at Fort Simpson alone, being estimated at 250

11. The presence of measles among the Kwakwaka'wakw is suggested by a tradition of "smallpox" just prior to the 1849 establishment of Fort Rupert by the Hudson's Bay Company: "lots of people died in the houses and then what Indians were left moved across the Bay, and when they came back the old village site was claimed by the Hudson's Bay Company's men" (Charlie Nowell in Galois 1996: 37 n). In 1849 a report from the new fort noted that the Kwakwaka'wakw had "greatly decreased" since 1841 (38).

in a population of about 2500 persons. The ignorant Indians in despair at the loss of so many of their dearest relatives, conceived a suspicion that the disease had been propagated through the Agency of the whites, and were at one time thinking seriously of attacking the establishment, but their better feelings prevailed over the passion of the moment. . . . The violence of the disease abated or more properly it had run its course, before the beginning of April, but the evil did not cease with the disease: it was impossible to efface so soon from the minds of the Indians the scenes of misery they had witnessed and the remembrance of whole families of their dearest friends swept off by the destroying pestilence. (1848b)[12]

Douglas's letter continued by noting the spread of the epidemic during spring 1848 to the Tlingit peoples of Fort Stikine and "the District wherein the Steam vessel carries on trade" (Douglas in Bowsfield 1979: 21–23). At Stikine "Old Seix [Shakes], the head chief" and "upwards of a hundred others" died about this time, though the sources are ambiguous about the cause ("sickness" or "the very severe cold"). Upstream on the Stikine, measles spread to the Tahltan peoples (Galois 1996: 40). Russian sources describe the epidemic's progress from Stikine to Sitka, where it was present until "mid-summer," and then to the Aleutians. About 300 deaths were recorded in the Russian territories, mostly among Aleuts (both in their homeland and at Sitka). Very few Tlingit or Russian fatalities were noted (Fortuine 1989: 206).

The last of the Hudson's Bay Company North Coast forts to be afflicted with measles was Fort Victoria. In this case, though, the Company vessel, the *Beaver*, was not responsible for its introduction. The ship had stopped at Victoria Harbour on 15 December, but cases of the disease were not recorded until 13 March. The disease probably came with Indians who crossed the straits in canoes. There are several possibilities: on 14 February four canoes of Makahs arrived at the Songhees village at Esquimalt; and on 20 February Indians from the Fort Langley area appeared at the fort. It is also possible that Indians from the island itself brought measles back from a trip to the mainland. Indian transmission of the disease to Fort Victoria is also likely in that the first "wave" of the epidemic occurred among Indians, not Whites.

The initial cases were reported at the Songhees village. Exactly one month

12. Belatedly, in 1848, measles was reported among interior Athapascan peoples in Hudson's Bay post journals from New Caledonia. The disease apparently spread from the coast along well-established aboriginal trade routes, or "grease trails" (Galois 1996).

later (on 12 April) the Fort Victoria journal noted that "Liealthae the Songes Chief who had been troubled with Dysentery after having recov. from the Measles, is now I am happy to say getting better" (Finlayson 1846–50), implying an end to the first (Indian) wave of the epidemic. At the fort itself the first non-Indian cases (four Hawaiians) were reported on 7 April. By 18 April two had died, and on the 19th all the Hawaiians were sick. On 2 May the fort head wrote, "The Measles . . . are now raging in this place and the neighbourhood" (Tolmie 1847–48). Throughout the remainder of the month, cases of dysentery, recoveries, and a few deaths were recorded at the fort, the epidemic spending itself by the beginning of June.

But measles lingered in other quarters. Workers at the Hudson's Bay Company mill were exposed later and were still ill in June. In addition, there was a resurgence of measles among the Songhees. Two deaths were recorded on 25 April; on the 26th, "Indians . . . are being daily laid up." Within a month (26 May) dysentery, one of the sequelae to measles, was present, with deaths recorded through 2 June (Finlayson 1846–50). Adding insult to injury, on 5 June a ship arrived from Nisqually carrying the missionary Father Auguste Veyret and influenza. The weakened Indians succumbed to this too, and more died. On 14 July the journal stated:

The Revd Monr Vegnet [sic] appears to be rather unsuccessful in making the Sanges attend his lectures; they appear to be impressed with the idea that he brought sickness amongst them, the influenza, with which some have died, having unfortunately broke out amongst them on his arrival here. (Finlayson 1846–50)[13]

Summary

Measles disappeared from the Pacific Northwest after June 1848, approximately 10 months following its introduction from California. But between late July 1847 and early June 1848 the measles epidemic proceeded from one location in the Pacific Northwest to another, lasting from 2 to 3 months at each place until the local pool of susceptibles was exhausted. Measles appears to have

---

13. Measles continued its march westward after it disappeared from the Northwest: "In September 1848, an American warship brought the disease known as measles to Hilo, Hawaii" (Kamakau 1961: 237–38). Mortality from the ensuing epidemic was high. Demographer Robert Schmitt (1970: 363) estimated 10,000 fatalities. In 1835–36 Hawaii's population was estimated at nearly 108,000; the 1850 census returned 84,165 (Schmitt 1968).

affected nearly every ethnolinguistic group in the Northwest Coast and Plateau culture areas, with the probable exception of those in southern Oregon.

Generally, the disease was transmitted from one location to another by means of transportation introduced by Euro-Americans and by individuals who were infected with the virus but did not yet show symptoms of the disease. For example, Indians mounted on European-introduced horses brought measles from California, overland migrants carried the disease from the middle Columbia to Fort Vancouver, a Hudson's Bay Company brigade transmitted it from Vancouver to Fort Nisqually, and the Company steamer *Beaver* carried infected individuals to several locations along the coast between Nisqually and Sitka. Purely Indian transmission occurred only incidentally and occasionally: for instance, by trading canoes venturing across the Strait of Georgia or the Strait of Juan de Fuca. Rumors of the role of Whites in the epidemic and their supposed intentions spread rapidly among the Indians of the Plateau and large segments of the coast, usually well in advance of the disease itself.

Recorded mortality from the epidemic varies widely from one location to another, dependent upon several variables. In most places dysentery or respiratory diseases accompanied or followed the measles. Mortality appears to have been lower at those locations where no such complications were noted. Among a few groups, such as those around Fort Vancouver, there may have been a small segment of the population (those over 37 years of age) with acquired immunity from an earlier outbreak. At all locations, as is typical of measles, fatalities appear to have been concentrated in the under-five-year-old segment of the population, surely resulting in a numerically diminished generation that persisted through the remainder of the century.

We will never know for certain the total number of deaths among the Indian peoples of the Pacific Northwest attributable to the 1847–48 measles epidemic. The best estimates, based on sources cited earlier in this chapter, are as follows: over 500 Indians, from various Northwest Coast groups, are *recorded* as having died from the disease. For some groups—the Willamette Valley tribes, for example—perhaps as much as 50% of the population was lost. For other groups—the Tsimshian of Fort Simpson and Aleuts resident at Sitka, for example—probably no more than 10% died. Chief Factor James Douglas, in his letter of 16 March 1848, estimated that, in the area "from Fort Hall to Nisqually," measles "destroyed about one tenth of the Indian population." Though this is only an estimate, it comes from the individual in the best position to know and is identical with (later) losses recorded from Fort Simpson and Sitka. In the absence of other documentation, it is the best estimate of total mortality we are likely to obtain.

A major, if not the most significant, factor in accounting for different mortality rates appears to have been variations in treatment of the disease. In areas where Indians persisted in exposing themselves to cold water (through either drinking or bathing) or where (as in the Columbia River drainage) Indians treated the disease by placing infected individuals in sweat lodges, mortality appears to have been higher. Differences in treatment were correlated with differences in survival among various groups and subgroups. The less acculturated and more traditional groups, who would not submit to proper treatment, seem to have experienced greater mortality than more tractable groups.

In several cases the mortality produced by measles created such fear among Indians that they were provoked to take more general aggressive actions. Marcus and Narcissa Whitman and the Snohomish curer who fled for his life to Fort Nisqually were assumed to have "caused" the new disease and were treated accordingly. At Forts Nisqually and Simpson, frightened Indians threatened to attack the White establishments, leading to construction of defensive walls at Nisqually.

THE 1853 CENTRAL COAST SMALLPOX EPIDEMIC

Introduction

At the very beginning of 1853, for the fourth time in less than 80 years, smallpox appeared among the Indians of the Pacific Northwest. The epidemiological patterns are by now familiar: the disease was introduced from outside the region by seagoing vessels; none of the peoples who are documented as having suffered from the 1836–37 epidemic were affected in 1853; the disease occurred among both Coast and Plateau peoples; and in a few places vaccination apparently prevented spread to susceptible Indian populations.

Washington Territorial Indian Agent E. A. Starling and Oregon Superintendent of Indian Affairs Joel Palmer summarized the geographic extent of the epidemic in their respective territories:

4 December 1853

The small pox appeared among the Indians this year and has proved very fatal with them. Its first appearance was among the Chinooks, at the mouth of the Columbia River; and from there spread among the Chehalis Indians, and to the Sound in the south. It was, also, a short time after communicated to the Macaw Tribe of Indians, at Cape Flattery, by a vessel; and to the Sock-a-muckes [Sauk], living in the headwaters of the Skagit River; and has since spread to almost every Tribe in the Sound. It has been most fatal among the Macaws, more than half of the Tribe being carried off by it. Large numbers of the Indians were vaccinated, when it was first known to be among them. . . . A large majority, however, remain unvaccinated. (Starling 1853)

27 May 1853
The smallpox has made fearful ravages among the Indians south of Clatsop Plains, and north of the Columbia as far as Puget Sound, entire families have been cut off and whole villages depopulated. Late accounts are received that it has made its appearance at the Dalles, and is making fearful progress in its fatal work among the Indians of that vicinity. The only hope of arresting the ravages of this terrible disease among the unfortunate natives appears to be vaccination. (Palmer 1853)

The two accounts are very accurate: smallpox appeared first at the mouth of the Columbia, from whence it spread north and south along the Pacific coast, and up the river to the Columbia Plateau. It entered northwest Washington via two routes: across the Cascade Mountains to the Skagit and Nooksack Valleys and from a second focus of origin among the Makah at Cape Flattery. Unvaccinated Indians suffered most; areas populated by Whites (Portland Basin, Willamette Valley, Puget Sound) had few cases. All locations appear on map 9. Documentation for this epidemic is presented in geographic order.

Smallpox at the Mouth of the Columbia

In January 1853 James Swan (author of the regional history *The Northwest Coast*) was homesteading at the mouth of the Bone River on the east bank of Shoalwater (Willapa) Bay, where he observed the beginning of the epidemic:

[T]he smallpox had broken out at Clatsop. . . . Several vessels had been wrecked on the coast north of Cape Disappointment. . . . old Carcumcum and her son Ellewa, the present chief of the Chenooks, with his wife and two or three slaves. . . . had been to the wrecks. . . . At supper time, I gave [Ellewa's wife] some tea and toast, and remarked that her face and neck were covered with little spots like fleabites. I said . . .

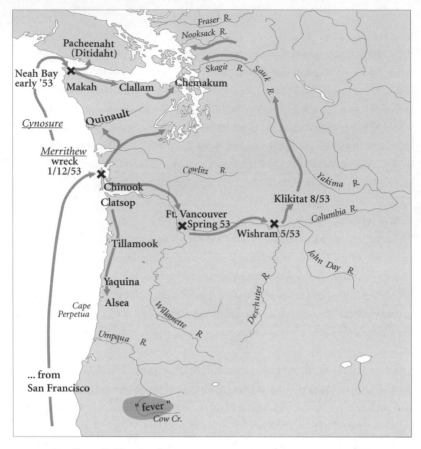

MAP 9. Smallpox Epidemic of 1853

"This woman has either got the smallpox or measles." . . . About nine o'clock . . . she was entirely dead.[14]

Besides Ellewa's wife, other fatalities included Cartumhays's wife and Que-a-quim (whom Swan buried in the sand, because no one else would touch him) (1972: 35, 54–59).

Smallpox had been communicated to the Indians from a shipwreck near the mouth of the Columbia. There were several shipwrecks in this area during the stormy December and January of 1852–53.[15] All ships disembarked from

14. Chinookans conceptualized trance states, comas, and other passages out of the normal state of consciousness as lesser varieties of the final state, true death. See chapter 6 in Boyd 1996a.

15. In 1853 Astoria was an important port, gateway to the interior of Oregon, and Shoalwater Bay, with its extensive beds of native oysters (*Ostrea lurida*), was the site of a burgeoning trade in shellfish.

San Francisco. On 13 December the *Bordeaux* was wrecked on Clatsop Beach; on 9 January the *Vandalia* sank, followed on the 12th by the *Mindora* and *Merrithew*. Corpses and wreckage from the latter three were strewn from Cape Disappointment to Gray's Harbor: what was probably the hull of the *Mindora*, bottom up, came ashore "on the beach near McKenzies' head" (on Cape Disappointment); the *Merrithew* washed in just north of modern Ocean Park; and the remains of the *Vandalia*, north of the bay, near Grayland. Six bodies were found; one close to Long Beach, two at the *Merrithew*, one near the mouth of Shoalwater Bay, and two more on the beach near Gray's Harbor. Whites stopped Indians from looting the *Mindora;* Indians salvaged an outboat with several trunks and money from the *Vandalia;* and when Whites arrived at the *Merrithew*, the ship's skeleton "had not yet been carried away," but the bodies were stripped.[16] It was certainly the *Merrithew* that Ellewa, Carcumcum, and the other Chinooks had salvaged prior to their coming down with smallpox. Most likely they caught the disease from clothing, but we cannot rule out the possibility that they picked it up from southern (Clatsop) Indians, who, as Swan said, apparently had it earlier.

Swan's is the only eyewitness record of this epidemic among the Chinook; other accounts date from after the fact. In mid-1854 at Chinook village the agent for southern Washington said:

But six or eight houses containing one hundred and twenty six souls now mark the place where a few years ago lived a great and happy tribe. The ruins of their houses are still visible for miles along the shore. As nearly as can be ascertained this tribe has been reduced within the last two years from three times its present population. Small pox swept off the mass of them. (Tappan 1854)

On the Long Beach peninsula: "Some lodges . . . were left without a survivor and the dead were found by the whites lying wrapped in their blankets as if asleep. Quite extensive cemeteries are scattered along the bay, the canoes in which the bodies of former generations were deposited having outlasted the race itself" (Gibbs 1855: 454).

It is difficult to say how many Chinook (and Clatsop) died of smallpox in 1853. Hudson's Bay records estimate 429 Lower Chinook in 1841 (Wilkes

16. The sources for this information (Wright 1895: 43, 48–49; Holman 1853) disagree on the exact locations and identity of the wreckage. My reconstruction relies most heavily on the primary source, Holman.

1925–26: 276). Two informants in the 1902 Chinook Claims case, Julia Russell and Silas Smith, estimated between 400 and 500 Chinook before 1853 and great losses from smallpox. The 1854 total (126 plus Clatsop and Shoalwater) is 238 (Tappan 1854). Even allowing a 10% loss from measles in 1847–48, a mortality of nearly 50% is probable. Of 19 original signers of the 1851 Anson Dart treaty, Julia Russell was able to recall that at least 5 died of smallpox.

Smallpox on the North Oregon Coast

To the south smallpox "killed off many . . . north of Cape Perpetua but south of that promontory its ravages were very limited" (Gibbs 1857: 12). Peoples north of Cape Perpetua included Tillamook, Yaquina, and Alsea. A few early settlers in this area recorded the effects of the epidemic. At the Necanicum River (Tillamook area) in 1854 Warren Vaughan met an Indian "badly scarred up" with smallpox who told him that "most of my folks caught the disease from me and are dead" (Vaughan n.d.: 24). On Yaquina Bay, 1852 homesteader George Boone had a supply of vaccine: "the Indians heard and swarmed to 'Big Medicine' to vaccinate them. The more it hurt the better they felt. Old Allopi's band of Klikitats came; for days and days we worked, attending to all" (1941: 226).[17] Lewis and Clark estimated 4,100 north Oregon coast Indians in 1805. A half-century later their destruction was almost complete. In 1854, the first complete census of the Tillamook returned 193 (Raymond 1854); the corresponding number for Alseans in 1866 was 155 (Collins 1866: 85).

Nineteen years after the smallpox epidemic, a West Coast version of the Ghost Dance spread from California to the remnant Tillamook and other western Oregon peoples.[18] The Tillamook belief was that one of their people, a man with a crooked leg, visited South Wind and brought back songs and their version of the Ghost Dance, which they called the South Wind Dance. In

---

17. Sahaptin Klikitat Indians had been permanent residents of the Willamette Valley since the late thirties. Some Klikitat were vaccinated at Fort Vancouver in 1837 (chapter 4), so they were aware of its benefits. The band that Boone treated was probably centered in Kings Valley, modern Polk County, from whence they had a trail down the Alsea River to the coast.

18. The 1870s Ghost Dance originated with the Paiute prophet Wodziwob and spread via disciples through Nevada, California, and western Oregon (Du Bois 1939).

Tillamook and Alsea mythology, South Wind was responsible for sending diseases to punish wrong behavior.[19] The Ghost Dance was a nativistic religion which held that if the proper religious activity (i.e., dancing) was performed, Whites would disappear and dead Indians would come back to life (Du Bois 1939: 25–26). Native American demographer Russell Thornton has pointed out that the Ghost Dance was most readily adopted by peoples who had recently suffered from introduced-disease outbreaks and rapid population decline. He interprets the dance as a ritual response to this devastation and an attempt by depopulated groups to regain control of their destiny (1986: 17–19, xi).[20]

Smallpox Travels up the Columbia and across the North Cascades

Smallpox appears to have passed through most of the Indian communities on the Columbia River from its mouth to Kettle Falls.[21] Fort Vancouver letters state smallpox "is making great havoc amongst the Indians"; "has already

19. In the "South Wind" myth, told by a Tillamook informant born about the time the dance was popular, South Wind (in her southern cave) called to her daughter (atop Saddle Mountain near the mouth of the Columbia): "When . . . too many of the people are being mean here, you will stand up on your mountain and raise your hand like this [palm outward], and you will say just one word. I will see you from the south and I will answer you with one word. Our words will fly to meet each other and everywhere they go there will be disease and people will die off" (E. Jacobs 1959: 142 43). See also the myths "Wind Woman" (Alsea) and "Wild Woman" (Tillamook) (Frachtenberg 1920: 33; E. Jacobs 1959: 158).

20. There are no contemporary accounts of smallpox among the coastal Indians south of Cape Perpetua, an area which had probably experienced the disease in 1837. But it is possible that there were *some* scattered cases, as well as transmission to peoples who had escaped the earlier outbreak. From the upper Umpqua River, settler George Riddle wrote of "an epidemic of some kind of fever during the winter of 1852–53" that "swept away two-thirds of the band" of Chief Miwaleta's Cow Creek Umpqua (Riddle 1920: 53–54). "I well remember my chum Sam and several other Indians who came to our house and said the Indians would soon all be gone, that Chief Miwaleta was dead. They had lost all hope, in fact they were dying so fast that they were unable to bury their dead, but placed them upon drift wood and burned them. . . . We boys were not allowed to go near the Indian camp at the falls of Cow Creek for fear of contagion. . . . the Indians who were not affected with the fever scattered into the mountains leaving some of the sick who were not able to follow to shift for themselves" (Riddle 1920: 36, 55). Nowhere is smallpox named or a rash mentioned, notable omissions. The Riddle family treated Sam in their home, and "after lingering about three months, he died."

21. Contemporary letters confirm its presence in Portland (e.g., letter of 13 June 1853 in Winthrop 1913: 250) and at Fort Vancouver, where between 15 May and 2 August, 16 "Servants," mostly Hawaiians, died.

carried off a number of the natives"; and "the Indian population is nearly extinct" (Peter Skene Ogden, letters of 15 June and 12 July 1853).

At the city of The Dalles smallpox was said to have "been virulent . . . the Indians dying in crowds—almost every one who was attacked" (Winthrop 1913: 250). The Indian fishery was hit during the last half of May: 257 are said to have died at Wishram (*nixlúidix*) village (Bolon 1854), and the Indians hanged a shaman who was believed to have caused the outbreak (Alvord 1884). On the Klikitat Trail between Vancouver and Yakima, a surveying party "met 3 or 4 parties of Indians who were suffering terribly from the smallpox . . . traveling like spirits of evil, urged by a feeling of [illegible] & despair, to spread the scourge still further among their brethren" (McClellan 1853: entry of 11 August). From The Dalles and Yakima smallpox spread through most of what is now eastern Washington. Vaccination by Jesuit missionaries at Kettle Falls and elsewhere apparently stalled its spread to points north and east.

As it had entered the Plateau in the south over mountain trails, so smallpox exited it in the north and reentered the Northwest Coast culture area and western Washington (see map 9). According to Skagit informant John Fornsby:

The Indians got smallpox from Nooksack. . . . One old man went to Nooksack, helped a woman sick with smallpox. He got the sickness. They left him on a little island below Mount Vernon. . . . They got killed from smallpox at Skagit City. Lots of Indians got killed. At Kikialos, at Fir they got killed there. Mr. Ball . . . a logger . . . brought smallpox. He married an Indian woman, Mrs. Joe Lish; he stayed with the Indians. That is the way the Indians died. (Collins 1949: 307)

Like the people on the Oregon coast, but independent of them, Puget Sound Indians responded to the new disease and the death it brought with ritual. The career of Ləx̌i'lbid, a Swinomish prophet, appears to have begun during the 1853 epidemic.[22] While singing alone in a canoe at daybreak Ləx̌i'lbid received a curing "power from the north, like measles," which

---

22. The assignation of Ləx̌i'lbid's disease experience to 1853 is provisional. Ləx̌i'lbid was a cousin of the grandfather of Wayne Suttles's informant Peter Charles, who was born in 1869. Although the date of Ləx̌i'lbid's spirit quest may well have been earlier than 1853 (in 1848 [measles] or even 1836 [smallpox]), the direction of spread of the epidemic ("from the north": Skagit and Nooksack lands) strongly suggests 1853.

allowed him to cure people of disease by "passing his hands over" their bodies (Peter Charles, from Wayne Suttles's 1948 field notes). When "everybody got sick," the village at Swinomish Slough was wiped out except for Ləx̌iʼlbid and his extended family, who stopped the disease by dancing and were saved:

> He gathered his people and told them that unless they prayed to their gods they would be overcome by some very powerful sickness, the like of which they had never seen before. It had been revealed to him in a dream that the Medicine Man would be powerless against the new sickness and that only group praying would save them. . . . his family group. . . . lined up in rows across the council house, facing south, with their hands in front of them making the motions of pushing something away. They sang and danced to a slow rhythm for many days and nights, stopping only to eat and sleep. . . . After many more days and nights the lines of dancers found themselves facing west. It was then that Lahailby ordered his people to stop, telling them that the sickness had passed and that their prayers had been answered. (Sampson 1972: 28)

Smallpox along the Strait of Juan de Fuca and in the Olympic Peninsula

Smallpox was introduced independently to the Makah people on the Strait of Juan de Fuca in early 1853, according to eyewitness Samuel Hancock, resident trader at Neah Bay. The source was the ship *Cynosure* from San Francisco: one White onboard was ill, and two Makah who were returning home on the vessel communicated the disease to those onshore.

In the densely occupied winter villages of the Makah people, smallpox spread rapidly and effectively. The Makah would "not allow vaccination, imagining it to be a charm of the whitemen to make the Indian women barren, and so by extermination to possess their lands" (Hills 1853). The results were "truly shocking": Hancock stated that within "a few weeks" after introduction, "hundreds of the natives became victims to it, the beach for a distance of eight miles was literally strewn with the dead bodies of these people" (1927: 182). Patterns typical of high-morbidity, high-mortality epidemics set in. When it became obvious that the disease was spread by contact, those with symptoms were abandoned: "so much alarmed that when any of their friends were attacked, all of the other occupants who lived in the house would at once leave it and the sick person with a piece of dried salmon and some water, laying all their personal effects by the sick person's, not intending to ever approach them again." People without symptoms panicked and fled:

[T]hose who had escaped became almost frantic with grief and fear, and conceived the idea of crossing the Strait and going to the Nitanat tribe living on Vancouver's Island. They crossed over to this place, carrying the infection with them, and soon nearly all those who fled from Neaah Bay, besides a great many of the native tribe, became victims to the epidemic. (Hancock 1927: 181)

And finally, they found a scapegoat to blame for the epidemic:

The remaining Indians, after reflecting and mourning over this visitation . . . apprehended the Indian who contracted the disease on the schooner, but recovered. As punishment he was taken out in the middle of the Strait of Fuca and placed in a small canoe, barely large enough to hold him, and set adrift, without a paddle or anything else. . . . he succeeded in reaching by morning Neaah Island, where he was discovered by the natives who went after him and shot him with their muskets. (Hancock 1927: 183)

Hancock notified Washington Territorial Indian Agent E. A. Starling of the epidemic, and the agent attempted to quarantine the affected. "[W]hen I learned it was among them, I immediately took measures to prevent the neighboring Indians from trading for blankets, shirts, etc., or from having any intercourse with them" (Starling, letter of 15 June 1853). The quarantine included the Makah's neighbors immediately to the east, the Clallam (Hills 1853: 137).[23]

The Makah apparently did, as Hancock claimed, carry the disease to their neighbors across the Strait of Juan de Fuca, the Pacheenaht of San Juan Harbour. Five years later Indian Agent William Bamfield said: "the smallpox . . . ravaged them some 8 [sic] years since. They were at that time nearly annihilated" (Arima et al. 1991: 295). Despite ethnographer Philip Drucker's

23. The Clallam tale "A Girl Gets Supernatural Power from a Steamboat" may date from this time. As told to Erna Gunther in the early 1920s: "she saw a big steamboat painted white. She looked at it and fell down dead. Her body was lying on the ground and her soul was in the boat. The man on the boat told her that the boat was full of sickness, smallpox and measles" (Gunther 1925: 154). The girl already had dancing power and a magic staff; this vision increased her power.

contention that this epidemic was general among Nuu-chah-nulth peoples (1951: 12), there is no evidence of smallpox farther north along the Vancouver Island coast until 1875 (see appendix 4).

Smallpox occurred among the other Indian peoples of the Olympic Peninsula in 1853. George Gibbs said that it spread along all of the Pacific coast between Shoalwater Bay and Cape Flattery (1855: 454). In 1926, 90-year-old Quinault informant Bob Pope provided independent confirmation of an epidemic about this time. He recalled that in his youth "came an epidemic (smallpox?) and most of the people of the village [t'o'nans] died, and only a few of their descendants are alive today" (Olson 1936: 182).

The year 1853 probably marked the demise of the Chemakum, the aboriginal inhabitants of the Port Townsend area. Two accounts suggest as much. The first is an oral tradition which speaks of an epidemic among the Chemakum and their relatives on the Pacific coast, the Quileute:

The People Kill a Medicine Woman
There was a bad medicine woman who lived among the Quileute. Every place she went a pestilence broke out. People would die by hundreds. She went away from Quileute. She went to Hoh. Soon there were many sick people there. Everybody was dying. She went away from Hoh. She went to Chemakum where Port Townsend is now. It was the same there as at Hoh and at Quileute. Soon many people were sick and dying. The people at Chemakum buried the dead. There were many funeral ceremonies. . . . the shamans all rose and said, "this woman is a witch. . . . " (Reagan and Walters 1933: 345–46)

This tradition, unfortunately, cannot be dated, genealogically or otherwise, so its association with the 1853 epidemic cannot be confirmed. But it does provide a comfortable fit with what Reverend Myron Eells was told in the 1880s about the decline of the Chemakum:

George Gibbs, in 1852, states that their number is ninety, but they are now virtually extinct, there being only ten left who are not legally married to white men or into other tribes. Of these ten there is only one complete family, four in number. With the exception of two or three very old persons, they now mainly speak the Klallam language. They say that their diminution was caused by small pox, but probably war had something to do with it, as Gibbs says they have been engaged in wars with the Makah,

Klallam, Twana, Skokomish and Duwamish Indians, by whom their power has been broken. (Eells 1889: 607)

With exposure to at least two and perhaps more smallpox epidemics between the 1770s and 1853, plus wars with almost all of their Salishan neighbors, it is no wonder that this small, strategically located non-Salishan group was driven to the brink of extinction.

Smallpox advanced on Puget Sound on three fronts: from the Pacific coast to the head of the Sound, from the Columbia Plateau down the Nooksack and Skagit Rivers, and from Cape Flattery along the northern perimeter of the Olympic Peninsula. In the more heavily settled areas of Washington Territory, at least some attempts were made to disseminate vaccine among the Indians:

Large numbers of the Indians were vaccinated, when it was first known to be among them by Dr. Haden U.S.A. at Fort Steilacom & by Dr. Tolmie, at Nesqually. Both of these Gentlemen deserve the thanks of the Community for their disinterested troubles. Numbers were also vaccinated by persons who fortunately could obtain vaccine matter. A large majority, however, remain unvaccinated and I would recommend that someone be employed to attend to this. (Starling, letter of 4 December 1853)[24]

Computing smallpox mortality in northwestern Washington is difficult, given the imprecision of contemporary population estimates. For the Puget Salish, near-complete Hudson's Bay estimates from the late thirties give 5,479 people; the total for the same population taken at temporary Puget Sound reservations in 1855–56 was 4,872 (607 fewer) (Boyd 1985: 470, 474, recomputed). The Clallam had 1,485 in the 1840s and 926 in 1855 (Douglas 1878; Gibbs 1877: 177). The Company estimated 1,200 Makah and 800 Ditidaht in the early 1840s (Douglas 1878); James Swan's careful winter 1861 enumeration of the Makah returned 654 (1870: 2); in 1881 there were 362 Ditidaht (Guillod 1882: 63), indicating a loss of about 50%, the same as that estimated for the other 1853 focal people, the Chinook.

The 1853 epidemic was shortly followed by treaty making. The new

---

24. When Dr. Tolmie sailed by "the Indian village of Kowitchin" in 1853, "a squadron of trollers . . . crowded about, praying to be vaccinated, and paying a salmon for the privilege" (Winthrop 1913: 28).

Washington territorial governor I. I. Stevens met in council with most western Washington tribes in the winter of 1854–55; dissatisfaction with the treaties and the general state of Indian relations contributed to the winter 1855–56 uprising under Nisqually chief Leschi (Marino 1990: 169–72). As Indian affairs began to be settled, Whites poured into the territory. By 1860 there were over 11,000 newcomers in western Washington, 11 times the number of a decade earlier, and 4,000 more than the Indian population. As had happened in western Oregon following the immigration of 1845, a population shift occurred. The only segment of the Northwest Coast culture area where Indians still constituted a majority was north of Washington Territory, in the British possessions.[25]

25. As with measles before it, smallpox was epidemic in Hawaii at the same time it was epidemic in the Northwest. It probably arrived on the ship *Zoe* from San Francisco, in port at Honolulu from 23 March to 7 April. The first case was documented on 13 May; deaths were recorded well into the autumn; and the total mortality has been gauged at around 5,000 (Greer 1965–66).

7 / A Final Disaster

The 1862 Smallpox Epidemic in Coastal British Columbia

As the "fever and ague" epidemics of the 1830s led to a demographic shift on the lower Columbia, and the 1848–53 epidemics had a similar effect in Puget Sound, so the 1862–63 smallpox epidemic served as a final blow to the Native peoples of British Columbia and paved the way for the colonization of their lands by peoples of European descent.[1] The epidemic was a major demographic disaster, by any measure. Wilson Duff estimated that 20,000 Indians, two-thirds of the pre-epidemic total in British Columbia, perished (1964b: 43); my own figures (see chapter 8) suggest that nearly 14,000 died on the coast alone.[2] What is worse is that this epidemic might have been avoided, and the Whites knew it. Vaccine was available, though in short supply, and the efficacy of quarantine was understood by well-placed Whites. But, for several reasons (lack of governmental authority, fear, and a regrettable degree of bias), neither was employed on the Indians in Victoria, where the epidemic started. Native peoples were treated only by a few heavily bur-

---

1. The smallpox epidemic began in 1862 on the British Columbia coast. In winter 1862–63 it spread over the Coast Mountains to the peoples of the western interior. Since the affected groups (Nlaka'pamux, Stl'atl'imx, Dakelhne, Tsilhqot'in, and some Secwepemc) belong to either the Plateau or the Subarctic culture area, their experience with smallpox will not be covered here.

2. It took almost 20 years for the Euro-American population to overtake the Indian population. In 1871 there were just over 10,000 non-Natives in what is now British Columbia; in 1881 there were 23,797, as opposed to 25,661 Native Americans (Barman 1991: 363).

dened missionaries, and instead of quarantining the infected in their camp on the outskirts of town, the colonial police expelled them from it, and canoes of infected Native peoples carried smallpox to their coastal homelands along the entire coast from Comox to the Stikine River. A vigorous program of vaccination by Oblate priests on the lower Fraser and by Anglicans due north of Victoria prevented the epidemic from taking hold among the Halkomelem peoples, and isolation spared (temporarily) the Nuu-chah-nulth (see appendix 4). But among the Kwakwaka'wakw, Oweekeno and Heiltsuk, Nuxalk and Tsimshian, Sabassas, Nisga'a and Gitxsan, southern Tlingit, and (most of all) Haida, the losses were large and the human suffering was great. Many families were wiped out; virtually everyone lost relatives. Bereavement and confusion as to why hung like a pall over nearly all of the First Nations[3] of the British Northwest. As in Oregon and Washington before, the 1862–63 epidemic was followed quickly by village abandonment and consolidation, hostilities with Whites, culture loss and replacement, and treaty making.

STAGE 1: ORIGINS IN THE SOUTH

On 11 March 1862, the *San Francisco Bulletin* printed a short notice on smallpox, buried in the fourth column of page 3 of the paper: "We understand that there are now 26 cases of small pox in the small pox hospital, most of them mild cases. There is a good deal of this loathsome disease in the city. Let no one neglect to employ all the precautions vouchsafed by vaccination." In the first six months of 1862, this small article was the only item the San Francisco papers devoted to smallpox.[4] The disease was apparently not unusual or considered newsworthy in this port city, already the hub of communications on the West Coast, in constant contact with Latin American, East Asian, and Atlantic ports. Once again, as had happened in 1853, a passenger on a ship from the Bay City introduced smallpox to the North Coast. The ship was the *Brother Jonathan;* the port of entry, Victoria (map 10). Unlike San Francisco, smallpox *was* news in Victoria: during three months of spring 1862, the *Daily*

---

3. Since the mid-1980s, the term "First Nations" has gradually become accepted as the preferred designation for most of Canada's Indian peoples (see Tennant 1990: 210–12 for a history of the term).

4. During the 1853 smallpox epidemic, when San Francisco was the origin point for two ships supposed to have carried the disease to the Northwest, the city's newspapers did not mention smallpox at all.

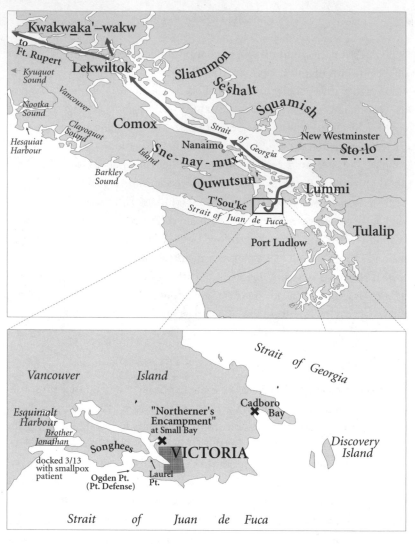

MAP 10. Smallpox Epidemic of 1862 in Victoria and Southwest British Columbia (with West Coast Vancouver Island Locations of 1875 Outbreak Shown)

British Colonist (*DBC*) and *Daily Press* (*DP*) printed over 60 articles on smallpox, providing the major sources for this chapter.[5]

After spending barely a week in San Francisco, the *Brother Jonathan* sailed

---

5. Previous discussions of the epidemic in Victoria include Yarmie 1968; Pethick 1978; Keddie 1993.

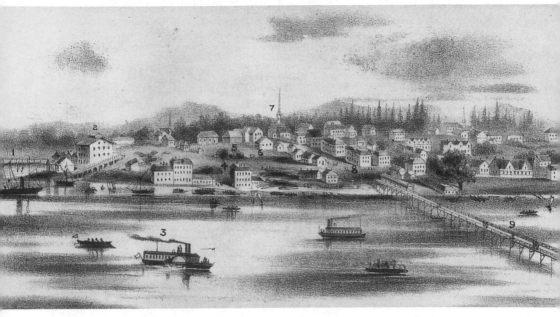

FIG. 12. An 1862 lithograph of Victoria (note the *Beaver* in the foreground), the year of the major West Coast smallpox epidemic of the nineteenth century. (Courtesy of British Columbia Archives, British Columbia Information Management Services, Victoria, catalog no. PDP00264.)

on 9 March and docked at Victoria's Esquimalt Harbour on 13 March. There were 350 passengers; 150 came ashore. On 18 March the *DBC* reported "*one case of varioloid.* . . . The patient . . . was attacked by the loathsome disease either just before reaching this port or soon after landing. The case is not considered a dangerous one by the authorities." Initially, no precautionary measures were taken: the sick person was housed "in a thickly populated neighbourhood, and in a house where several other persons reside" (*DBC*, 18 March 1862). He was soon removed "to a house in the suburbs," but it was already too late: on the 19th a second case was reported. The second infected person shortly departed on the *Otter* across the Strait of Georgia (*DBC*, 20 March) and was reported at New Westminster on the 22d (*DBC*). The stage was set. On 26 March the *DP* stated, "there is no doubt that some cases of this disgusting malady have occurred in the town, confined at present to new arrivals."

Victoria in 1862 (fig. 12) was not in a position to deal with public health crises. The city had not yet been incorporated and lacked a centralized government, and the regional government of the Vancouver Island colony had no coordinated public health agency to provide vaccine to residents. But James Douglas, employed by the Hudson's Bay Company since 1826 on the coast and now the colony's governor, knew from experience how devastating small-pox could be.[6] With the powers available to him, he enlisted the services of the Company's physician, Dr. John Helmcken, and took immediate action concerning prominent local Native people:

[A]ll the principal Indians of the various tribes now living here were summoned to the Police office to have a *"wawa"* [Chinook Jargon: "talk"] with his Excellency with regard to the small-pox. . . . It was pretty hard at first to convince them of the benefit arising from this simple operation, but after a while they were made to believe that the threatened sickness, the small pox, was far worse than their great enemy, the measles. This morning, accordingly, about thirty Indians, amongst whom were King Freezy, his queen, and the young princess [of the Songhees tribe], and all the Indian doctors, were brought to Dr. Helmcken's office and there underwent the ceremony of being vaccinated for the small pox. (*DP*, 27 March)

The next day the *DBC* reported rumors of "several" cases among children "at the main Songish village." On 1 April an Indian woman living near the bakery on Humboldt Street was "stricken down with small-pox" (*DP*, 1 April). And on the 16th Dr. Helmcken vaccinated 30 more Indians (*DP*, 16 April). But these efforts were too little and too late, because the disease had already spread to the main Indian concentration.

The "Northerners' Encampment"

Ever since the gold rush of 1858 there had been a sizable contingent of north-ern coastal Indians (Tsimshian, Haida, Stikine Tlingit, Heiltsuk [Bella Bella], and Kwakwaka'wakw ["Fort Ruperts"]) assembled for the purpose of trad-ing in a camp (called the Northerners' Encampment) on Small Bay just out-side Victoria. The "Northerners" were in regular communication with their home villages, and like trading centers elsewhere, the camp was a prime source for the spread of European diseases (Dobyns 1992). When a count was taken on 15 April 1859, there were 2,235 First Nations peoples in the Northerners'

---

6. Douglas was second in command at Fort Vancouver during the 1836–37 smallpox epi-demic (and in full charge during the 1847–48 measles epidemic) (see chapter 5).

Encampment. Of the 1,545 (in 111 "huts") whose tribal affiliation was given, 44% were Tsimshian, 26% Haida, 15% Tlingit, 8% Heiltsuk, and 7% Kwakwaka'wakw (*Victoria Weekly Gazette,* 29 April 1859).

Anglican missionary Reverend Alexander Garrett's "Reminiscences" record the first time he saw smallpox in the Northerners' Encampment, probably in mid-April:

[O]ne Sunday afternoon, no Indians appeared . . . the Missionary went to the village to see what was wrong. He found a large number gathered on the margin of the Bay staring at some object on the beach. Investigation revealed a white man's body dead of smallpox lying on the sand. The sight was most revolting. The first thing to be done was to dig a grave where it lay, cover up the dreadful sight, then the matter was reported to the authorities. Inquiry among the Indians revealed the fact of several cases. (F. A. Garrett n.d.)

Garrett and Bishop George Hills began attending to the stricken population. The entry for 25 April from Bishop Hills's journal reads:

I visited the Chymsean camp to-day, and found the poor people in a great panic. The small-pox was raging with virulence; twenty had already died; I saw eleven more cases in various stages of the disease. The patients were mostly removed to little tents or huts by themselves, and shut in as if left to die. There seemed readiness to do what was directed, and great patience in the sufferers; one dead body was lying, left because there were no friends; another in a coffin was also unburied. (1863)

The next day the *DBC* reported that Dr. Helmcken had "vaccinated over 500 natives," and that others were demanding it. An "old chief" at the encampment was selling "vaccine scabs . . . and expects to make a good thing by practicing as soon as the Northerners get down."

The lack of clear governmental authority continued to facilitate the disease's spread. On 27 April Garrett met with Augustus Pemberton, the colonial police commissioner, and asked for his help in disposing of the "two or three bodies left unburied on the beach adjoining the camp." Garrett was told that the commissioner "had no authority to interfere, and could not order the Police to bury the dead" (*DP,* 27 April). In a fit of fear and bigotry the *DBC* editorialized against the camp ("the moral ulcer that has festered at our doors throughout the last four years") and its Indians, who "have free access to our town day and night." The newspaper recommended that, given the inaction of the police chief and the absence of the governor in New Westminster, Victoria's "citizens improvise a Board of Health. . . , remove . . . the entire Indian population . . . to a place remote from communication" and burn "the infected houses with all their trumpery" (*DBC,* 28 April).

In response to this journalistic threat and without the permission of Governor Douglas, Pemberton reacted quickly: "The Tsimpsean tribe have one day given them to leave this portion of the island, and one of the gunboats will take up a position opposite the camp to expedite their departure. . . . men will be stationed at the bridge, and other main entrances to the town, to prevent any Indian entering" (*DP,* 28 April). The bodies on the beach were removed (*DBC,* 28 April), and those Indians in Victoria who did not live with Whites were warned to leave (*DBC,* 30 April).

The entire Songhees tribe was *"hiyou quash"* (Chinook Jargon: "very afraid") and abandoned their village east of the city on 29 April and removed to Discovery Island, just offshore from Victoria. In addition to the many Songhees already vaccinated, this voluntary act of self-quarantine saved the rest from further infection. As for the Tsimshians in the encampment, King Freezy "firmly believed" that they were "visited by the smallpox as punishment for their many sins" (*DBC,* 29 April).

On 1 May most of the Tsimshians left, following the orders of the police:

The Tshimpseans burnt their houses and blankets and other *"iktas"* [Chinook Jargon: "things"], without any compulsion from the police, and left this morning in their canoes. Only three huts remain standing, which are occupied by those of the tribe who have remained as nurses. Numbers of the Stickeen and Hydah Indians have also left in canoes, and those that remain have moved their huts to a greater distance from the camp of the Tshimpseans. (*DP,* 1 May)

By 29 April, apparently by order of the Colonial Assembly, a smallpox "hospital" ("two rough buildings") had been built at the Northerners' Encampment; six patients moved in immediately (*DBC,* 30 April; *DP,* 1 May). The hospital was operated by the Anglican missionaries; fear of infection appears to have kept everyone else away.

[W]ho should care for these poor savages amongst whom the plague spread like wild fire? They refused with very few exceptions to be vaccinated, nor was there vaccine enough within seven hundred miles to go around. . . . Neither doctors nor nurses were willing to take the risk involved in caring for Indians with small pox. An old Canadian sailor, badly marked with the disease, was engaged. He with a handy man as carpenter and cook, helped Mr. Garrett to care for the patients, but as the fever grew hot upon the patients, they left their beds and plunged into the sea to cool themselves, and returning shortly to die. The Missionary and his helper were little else than grave diggers, placing beneath the sod an average of four a day. (Garret n.d.)

The eviction of the Tsimshians did not end the epidemic in the Northerners' Encampment. On 5 May a remaining Tsimshian died, "[t]wo cases of a violent type" appeared in the "Fort Rupert" (Kwakwa̲ka̲'wakw) camp, "and a white man, badly marked, was admitted to the hospital on the same day" (*DBC*, 5 May).

Between 3 and 9 May, Bishop Hills visited the Indian smallpox hospital four times:

7 May 1862

There were ten cases; one had just died; it was a wretched sight. Two women had been forced out through some superstitious feeling, and were likely to die; indeed, one could not escape. I assisted in putting in some other bedsteads.

Poor Mr. Garrett is sadly worked. I saw there in succession, in the different lodges, fourteen more cases; some were concealed: in one place, about eight feet by four, were four poor creatures lying very ill, concealed for fear of being sent away. The filth and stench were intolerable. Mr. Garrett on Sunday was obliged to make a coffin; no one else would do it.

9 May

I visited the Indian Smallpox Hospital, found nine inside, one dying, and another dead outside. The Indians have a dread of a dead body and cast out the dying.

I went through the Hydah and Bella Bella camps, and found thirteen cases and one dead body. I have never witnessed such horrible scenes of death, misery, filth, and suffering before. (Hills 1863)

The 14 cases discovered by Hills were apparently all "Fort Ruperts"; of these, 3 died on 8 May. In addition to the 14 Kwakwa̲ka̲'wakw, the 10 Tsimshian in the hospital, and 13 sick Haidas and Heilksuks, there were 12 ill Stikines "at Ross' farm. . . . beyond Laurel Point." The *DBC* reported with alarm that one Indian woman "has arrived each morning for the last three mornings at the Indian small-pox hospital from the town, where they [*sic*] have been living with white men," and again advocated "banishing" "every Indian" to "some place remote from the whites, and that without a moment's delay" (8 May).

Initial Dispersal of the Northerners

By 11 May the smallpox epidemic in Victoria was a month old. Several groups of Indian evacuees had set up temporary camps to the east and north of Victoria. The Songhees had removed to tiny Discovery Island. Tsimshians and some Stikines were "encamped on small islands in the Canal de Haro"; other Stikines were north of Laurel Point. Haidas had set up a large camp at Cadboro Bay, four miles east of the city. On the morning of 11 May, the local authorities, backed by the newly arrived British gunboats H.M.S. *Grappler* and H.M.S. *Forward,* took further action:

Mr. Police Magistrate Pemberton, with Superintendent Smith and an effective force of policemen, repaired to Cadboro Bay and supervised the embarcation to their homes of about three hundred Northern Indians. Twenty-six canoes in all, containing about three hundred native men, women, and children, departed about 10 o'clock. One of the gunboats remained within hailing distance of the camp, in order to render assistance to the police should any obstreperous conduct on the part of the Indians occur. The poor creatures protested feelingly against the injustice of the procedure, but manifested no desire to resist the stern mandate of the law. Edensah, chief of the Hydahs, reported only one sick man in the tribe. Twenty of the canoes were nearly filled with Hydahs, five with Queen Charlotte Islanders, and one with Stickeens. The gunboat, at the urgent request of the chief, will accompany and protect the Indians until they have passed Nanaimo—the Indians of which place have many old scores to wipe out in consequence of outrages received at the hands of the Northern braves in years gone by when the latter were the terror of this coast. (*DBC,* 12 May)

With Cadboro Bay vacated, the police dealt with the remnants of the Northerners' Encampment. On 13 May they "destroyed all the lodges . . . by fire," leaving 200 Haidas "sitting upon their '*iktas,*' having no canoes wherewith to transport them from Victoria" (*DP,* 13 May). The stragglers were to be evicted, said the *DBC,* "to one of the islands in the Straits—there to rot and die with the loathsome disease which is now destroying the poor wretches at the rate of six each day" (13 May). On 14 May the police "dislodged" the Stikines at Laurel Point (*DP*, 15 May).

Remnant Camps near Victoria

The police activities did not by any means result in the removal of all the Northerners from Victoria. On 24 May three Indian corpses were reported "festering in the sun on the beach at the rear of the Government buildings." On 27 May the *DP* was informed that some Haidas had escaped eviction at Cadboro Bay. "The smallpox is raging amongst them, and several deaths occur daily from this cause. They have a tent erected apart from the rest of their dwellings, which they use for the purposes of an hospital" (*DP*, 27 May).

On the same day, the Reverend Mr. Garrett visited a detached camp of 70 Haida at Ogden Point and "found that . . . *thirty* were down with the small pox in its most virulent form!" (*DBC*, 27 May). Three days later Garrett and Hills found the survivors "hidden in the bushes." There were "seventeen cases, most of whom were very bad, and three corpses" (Hills 1863). The missionaries were approached by a woman who, with "shovel and axe," was attempting to dig a grave for her husband but could not lift him. No one, Indian or White, would help her. On 1 June the "10 or 12" surviving Haida at Ogden Point "stampeded" (*DP*, 5 June). Arriving three days later to evict them, the police found the camp abandoned:

[T]hey were soon informed by an Indian belonging to another tribe, who chanced along, that . . . the survivors . . . procured a canoe, put into it such of their *iktas* as could be accomodated, and started for the North, leaving several ["20," according to *DP*, 5 June] bodies unburied, but humanely taking all their sick with them. . . . The houses were left open, as if the late occupants had stepped out intending to return in a few moments. Guns, pistols, knives, tools, dresses and trinkets lay scattered confusedly on the floors of the lodges or on the ground hard by. . . . The lodges were examined by the policemen, and, sickening to relate, under the floor of each hut were found the bodies of at least one and sometimes four or five Indians—men, women, and children,—who had fallen victims to the small-pox! . . . Poor creatures!

The police set the houses aflame and covered the corpses with quicklime (*DBC*, 6 June).

Although on 6 June there were still 33 Indians in the smallpox hospital (*DP*, 6 June), and deaths continued to be reported in the newspapers for three more weeks, the epidemic in Victoria was now winding down. Starting on 13 June, the *DP* ran a series of excoriating articles on the way the epidemic had been handled and the need for more governmental structure.[7] Although we will never know how many First Nations peoples died in Victoria in 1862, in early 1863 the *British Columbian* (New Westminster; citing the *Victoria Chronicle*) said: "It is estimated that the bodies of from 1000 to 1200 Northern Indians, who have fallen victims to the small-pox, lie unburied in the space of about an acre of ground a little bit to the west of the reserve and a stone's throw from the school-house" (11 June).

7. Between 13 and 24 June, the *DP* ran four editorials ("The Spread of Disease," 13 June; "The Indian Mortality," 17 June; "The Small Pox," 19 June; and "The Board of Health," 24 June). The *DP* pushed the need for the incorporation of the city and the creation of an effective Indian Department and Board of Health, stressing what the absence of the latter had meant for the spread of the epidemic in the city. The articles also displayed a pronounced bias and hostility toward the Indian population (particularly the Northerners) for their perceived amorality and role in spreading the epidemic, though this was leavened by some recognition of the Whites' moral responsibility for the cruelty of the Indian expulsion and the direful effects it would have on all the Native peoples of the British Pacific. "The Indian Mortality" (17 June) was the strongest of these statements, attacking first the Northerners' Encampment and then the "policy" of "the authorities," which caused the smallpox epidemic to spread:

"For four years Victoria has suffered to an extent unknown in any civilized town in the universe from the residence of an Indian population. Time and again were the evils pointed out by the press, but no notice was taken of injunction or admonition. Thefts were committed. . . . murder was added to the list. . . . The place became a moral as well as physical pest-house . . . we had squaw dance-houses—no better than brothels—licensed last winter. . . . The justice of Nature could not allow such things to pass with impunity, and accordingly we are visited with a malady that clearly proves how rotten is the 'paternal guardianship' under which the 'poor Indian' reposed!

"'What will they say in England?' when it is known that an Indian population was fostered and encouraged round Victoria, until the small-pox was imported from San Francisco. Then, when the disease raged amongst them, when the unfortunate wretches were dying by scores, deserted by their own people, and left to perish in the midst of a Christian community that had fattened off them for four years—then the humanizing influence of our civilized Government comes in—not to remedy the evil that it had brought about—not to become the Good Samaritan, and endeavor to ameliorate the effects of the disease by medical exertion, but to drive these people away to death, and to disseminate the fell disease along the coast. To send with them the destruction perhaps of the whole Indian race in the British Possessions on the Pacific. . . . There is a dehumanizing fatuity about this treatment of the natives that is truly horrible—a callousness to suffering humanity that one can scarcely credit. How easy it would have been to have sent away the tribes when the disease was first noticed in the town, and if any of the Indians had taken the infection, to have had a place where they could have been attended to, some little distance from Victoria, until they recovered as they in all probability would have done with medical aid. By this means the progress of the disease would at once have been arrested, and the

The Spread of Smallpox beyond Victoria

Smallpox spread incompletely among Native villages outside Victoria. Acquired immunity—either from the 1853 epidemic or from vaccination (usually by missionaries)—was a decisive factor. The "first people" of the Victoria area, the Songhees, vaccinated and quarantined, "remained comparatively free from the disease" (Helmcken 1975: 187). Smallpox appeared at Sooke Harbour in early August, when "Charlicum, the big chief" was reported to have died, and "others of the tribe" were sick (*DBC*, 7 August). Three months later the disease was "still continuing its ravages [at Sooke] . . . several deaths having occurred of late" (*DBC*, 14 November). Smallpox was not reported from any of the Nuu-chah-nulth peoples; the closest band, the Pacheenahts, "thinned" by the 1853 epidemic and recent attacks by the Songhees, had recently "amalgamated" with the Ditidaht and moved over 20 miles west (Brown 1864).

None of the numerous Halkomelem-speaking peoples (Quwutsun' [Cowichan], Sne-Nay-Mux[w] [Nanaimo], Musqueam, Sto:lo) were much affected by the 1862 epidemic, due to vigorous programs of vaccination. Catholic missionaries had vaccinated the Quwutsun';[8] the Anglican missionary John Good had vaccinated the Sne-Nay-Mux[w] early in May,[9] and Oblate missionaries vaccinated the vulnerable Halkomelem-speaking peoples of the lower Fraser, as described by the New Westminster *British Columbian:*

---

population saved from the horrible sights, and perhaps dangerous effects, of heaps of dead bodies ying putrifying in the summer's sun, in the vicinity of the town. . . . The authorities have commenced the work of extermination—let them keep it up. . . . Never was there a more execrable Indian policy than ours."

8. One Quwutsun' died in mid-July: "He was vaccinated, but the matter wouldn't take" (*DBC*, 22 July). Reportedly, some fled in fear to the Straits islands (*DP*, 20 July). At least four, however, died in early December from a second outbreak (*DBC*, 3 December).

9. "Soon after we were actively at work in the District the dreaded pestilence small pox began to make havoc . . . some of the northern tribes . . . fleeing Victoria . . . left both the dying and the dead along the islands. . . .Two men of the Nanaimo tribe carried off the blankets left at the encampments and . . . fell victims to the deadly scourge. I assisted in burning their remains, and saw that all their belongings were burnt to stay the spread of the infection. I was kept vaccinating young and old for days, and with the aid of the new Coal Company we succeeded in removing the Nanaimo Indians proper to a new site within their own Reserve, white washing their dwellings, and instructing them in sanitary precautions to prevent any further spread of the disease. In this way they were saved from destruction; whilst in places beyond us, further north, where no such superintendence and aid could be rendered, whole villages were decimated and in some cases not one escaped. I had fortunately an abundant supply of medicine always on hand, and in my medical training at S. Augustine's served me in good stead" (Good

The Revd. Mr. [Leon] Fouquet, Catholic Missionary here, has visited Yale recently, calling at all the immediate rancherias and vaccinating the Indians. During the last twelve days he has vaccinated no fewer than *three thousand four hundred*, between this city and Yale inclusive. And in this place alone, during Monday last, he disposed of *one thousand cases!* The entire community is under obligation to the rev. gentleman for his philanthropic and praiseworthy exertions in this matter, as in the event of the smallpox breaking out amongst our native population, the result would be terrible indeed both to them and to the whites. (14 May)

Letters to the editor (24 May, 7 June) questioned Fouquet's (fig. 13) statistics, but the newspaper stood by its report: "A medical gentleman in high standing informs us that as many as 1,500 may be vaccinated by one person in a day . . . the rev. gentlemen. . . . visited 23 Indian villages or rancherias, most of them two and three times; and in this city he vaccinated Indians representing 17 villages, principally on the coast." The *Columbian* subsequently named the 23 Fraser Valley villages: 21 were Halkomelem-speaking and 2 were Nlaka'pamux. Of those vaccinated in New Westminster, 14 came from Squamish villages, 2 were from Se'shalt villages, and 1 was from a Stl'atl'imx village. Father Fouquet himself claimed to have put "at least 8,000 under the knife"; his partner Father Pandosy "vaccinated several thousand" (Fouquet 1862: 198).

Fouquet sent plenty of vaccine to Casimir Chirouse at Tulalip (in Washington Territory) for his parishioners: the missionary vaccinated many "two or three times." Among the vaccinated were Nooksack ("Mousak") who had suffered from smallpox 10 years earlier; Chirouse said that "they seem much more humble and more fearful of God than formerly." When smallpox finally appeared in early August, only three died at Tulalip, while those a few miles away who had not been baptized were "ravaged" (Chirouse 1862).

In December 1863, after the epidemic was over, Vicar Louis d'Herbomez made the exaggerated claim of having vaccinated "15,000 to 16,000" Native peoples around the Strait of Georgia.[10] According to him, "This outcome touched the Indians, who became more and more favorably disposed to our

---

n.d.). On 17 August 1864, Robert Brown noted in his journal that the northernmost village at Nanoose Harbor had been abandoned and the dozen survivors had joined the Sne-Nay-Mux[w] proper.

10. The numbers are too large for contemporary Native populations and probably include revaccinations.

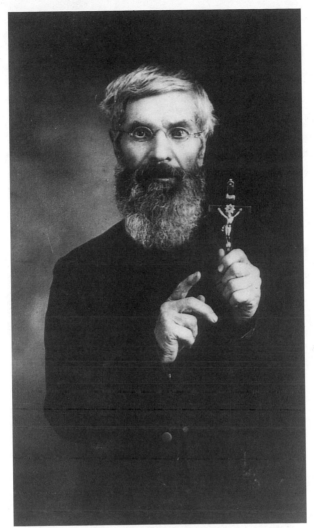

FIG. 13. Father Leon Fouquet, an Oblate missionary who vaccinated lower Fraser River Indians during the 1862 smallpox epidemic. (Courtesy of British Columbia Archives, British Columbia Information Management Services, Victoria, catalog no. I-51542.)

religion" (1863: 308). Despite the unrealistic numbers, the Oblates' activities stand in sharp contrast to those of the secular authorities at Victoria. The missionaries were the true heroes of the 1862 smallpox epidemic. The Halkomelem-speaking peoples were saved from near-certain decimation by the vaccination program and remain today one of the most populous and culturally viable Indian communities in the Pacific Northwest.

STAGE 2: SMALLPOX ON THE NORTH COAST

Stage 2 of the British Columbia smallpox epidemic began in May 1862, when the first Northerners were evicted from their camp outside Victoria. The refugees canoed through the Inland Passage and up the coast as far as the Stikine River in southeast Alaska. In 1862 the North Coast was relatively unsettled, populated almost entirely by Native Americans. In the entire region, almost without exception, there was no vaccine or previous vaccination, and the virulent 1862 strain of smallpox was allowed to spread virtually without impediment. The Native peoples of North Coastal British Columbia, unlike those to the south, suffered appalling losses.

Eviction of the Northerners

The Tsimshian who were evicted from the encampment in early May apparently broke into more than one party. Some hurried back to their homes on the Skeena and Nass Rivers; the Fort Simpson journal recorded their arrival on 17 May (see p. 194). Other Tsimshians remained in the south: on 11 May some were still on "small islands in the Canal de Haro"; and on 19 May the *DBC* noted a camp at Port Ludlow on the Kitsap Peninsula (Washington Territory): "many of whom have died and nearly all are down with the disease."

The main body of Northerner evacuees, 25 canoes of Haidas and 1 of Stikines, were expelled from the temporary camp at Cadboro Bay on 11 May; the rest of the Stikines were kicked out of Laurel Point on 14 May. There are no surviving firsthand records of their trip north; the logs of the British gunboats *Grappler* and *Forward,* which escorted them beyond Nanaimo and Cape Mudge, say nothing. But by mid-June the Victoria newspapers began receiving harrowing reports from the north. One group of Haida, left to their own devices when the *Grappler* was called back to Victoria, attempted to land on Discovery Island. Here they were fired on by the frightened Songhees, and three were killed before the survivors managed, "by dint of hard paddling," to escape to Cadboro Bay (*DBC,* 15 June). Those Haida escorted by the *Forward* were shot at by Quuwutsun' off Salt Spring Island, who would not stop until the gunboat aimed its barrels at them (*DP,* 18 July).[11]

11. The *DP* also reported that some Tsimshian had come ashore at the coal mines on Newcastle

Beyond Nanaimo, ships reported dead and dying Indians abandoned along the shores of the Strait of Georgia:

Lo! The Poor Indian!

Capt. Shaff, of the schooner Nonpareil, informs us that the Indians recently sent North from here are dying very fast. So soon as pustules appear upon an occupant of one of the canoes, he is put ashore; a small piece of muslin, to serve as a tent, is raised over him, a small allowance of bread, fish and water doled out and he is left alone to die. Capt. S. reports seeing many such cases his trip down, and is of the opinion that all Indians not vaccinated will die this summer. (*DBC*, 14 June)

Forty out of sixty Hydahs who left Victoria for the North about one month ago, had died. The sick and dead with their canoes, blankets, guns, etc., were left along the coast. In one encampment, about twelve miles above Nanaimo, capt. Osgood [sloop *Northern Light*] counted twelve dead Indians—the bodies festering in the noonday sun. (*DBC*, 21 June)

Captain Whitford [schooner *Explorer*], while on his passage from Stickeen, to this place, counted over 100 bodies of Indians who had died from the small-pox between Kefeaux [Cape Lazo at Comox Harbour?] and Nanaimo. In some instances, attempts had been made by the survivors to burn the dead, by heaping brush over their remains and setting it on fire, but it had failed in most instances, and the fuel had burned out, leaving the blackened, half-roasted bodies to rot, and pollute the air with their overpowering exhudations. On two islands Captain Whitford saw four squaws . . . attacked with small-pox and left . . . to die with a small quantity of food and water . . . but [they] had quite unexpectedly recovered and were subsisting on berries. They were subsequently taken off by Indians. (*DBC*, 11 July)

The forced evacuation and the deaths that accompanied it were a traumatic episode that left a collective scar in the memories of the North Coast British Columbia Indians, much as the "Trail of Tears" did among the Cherokees of the southeastern United States a quarter century earlier. Traditions of the evacuation survived among northern peoples over a century later. The following excerpts are from stories told in 1968 to Susanne Hilton by Beatrice Brown and Willie Gladstone of Bella Bella.

Island near Nanaimo, where they worked for a while. But by early July, five of them had died, one Northerner woman was dead, and another nearly so (18 July).

The Smallpox

This is a story about the people. That's not too long ago, I think, when they used to go down to Victoria, right in Victoria. . . .

And there's too many of them. I don't know what the Hudson Bay people did to the Indians when they chased them out of Victoria. They had a big, really funny coat on them and they did something on the bow of the canoes and really chased them out, the Indians. That's a long time ago.

And theres a whole bunch of them in each canoe and they started off. Not very far, the first man got sick and, a little ways, another one got sick.

And after a while all the body came out in sores and they died right there. (Brown in Hilton and Gould 1973: 5)

. . . And when they feel ill, they just go ashore and just put them in a blanket, you know, like a stretcher, you know, and put them up on the beach. They just leave them there till they die.

All along the coast, the Haida people especially—especially the Haida people—down here, below Namu, there were lots of them at the place they call Koeye, Koeye River. They just put them up on the beach, you know, and they just leave them there, you know.

And they die; lots of them.

Some get over that. Some get over the smallpox. They have kind of holes in their faces you know. (Gladstone in Hilton and Gould 1973: 75)

The Epidemic in the Inland Passage

North of the Nanaimo (on Vancouver Island) and the Squamish (on the mainland coast), the epidemic advanced, attacking Northern Coast Salish peoples, Kwagyulth and Kwakwaka'wakw, Heiltsuk and Nuxalk, and the Haida of the Queen Charlotte Islands.

Northern Coast Salish (Pentlatch, Comox, Se'shalt). The northern Coast Salish peoples had already suffered from several decades of Kwagyulth (Lekwiltok) raids (Taylor and Duff 1956), and smallpox diminished them even further. In 1864 an "old Puntledge" told Robert Brown of the Vancouver Island Exploring Expedition how his people and the island Comox came to be decimated. First the Island Comox (driven south by armed Kwagyulth) moved into Pentlatch lands. "War ensued and many were killed on either side." Then the "Great Chief above became angry with the Puntledge and killed many of them by Small pox." "Thin[ned] by war and pestilence," the Pentlatch and two other remnant groups (Eeksen and Qualicom) united with the Comox. In 1864, only 76 of the composite group remained (Brown 1864).

Although eyewitness records are also lacking for the mainland Comox and Se'shalt, circumstantial evidence suggests that they were hard hit as well. In 1860, Oblate priests "were driven away" when they attempted to missionize Se'shalt; but in 1862 a mission was opened and a rapid and near-complete process of acculturation followed. By 1868, all remnant Se'shalt were grouped together at the mission, and Oblate Father Pierre-Paul Durieu introduced his draconian "système": led by the priest, an all-Indian governmental and judicial system was adopted, dancing and potlatching were prohibited, new houses were built and gardens planted, and the Indians converted to Catholicism (Lemert 1954). Northern Coast Salish peoples, previously impervious to such drastic change, were now broken by smallpox and accepted it readily. The process was analogous to the post-1836 experience of Father Veniaminov among the Tlingit (chapter 5) and strikingly similar to what happened at the same time among Reverend William Duncan's Metlakatla Tsimshian (see below).

Kwakiutlan Peoples. The beginning of the epidemic among the southern-most of the Kwakiutlan peoples, the Kwagyulth (Lekwiltok) tribe of Discovery Passage, was attributed to infected goods stolen from Haida refugees:

This late powerful and war-like tribe, residing for centuries near Cape Mudge, on the west [*sic*] coast of this island, are dying from small pox in scores. The way the disease first spread among them is this: For many years they have been at war with the Hydahs, and espying one day recently a canoe containing four or five of their ancient enemies passing the encampment, they put out and murdered the occupants, and took possession of all their traps. The plunder thus obtained was divided among the thieves, and in a few days the dreadful disease broke out in the tribe. (*DBC*, 1 July)

Contemporary records of the epidemic among the Kwakwaka'wakw themselves are sparse.[12] Articles from the *DBC* provide hints of what happened. On 13 June, according to reports from the schooner *Nonpareil*: "The Indians at Forts Simpson and Rupert are dying from the small pox like rot-

12. The Fort Rupert journal is not extant for 1862, and the fort head, Hamilton Moffat, claimed that only five died, an unclear statement which probably refers to fort inmates alone (Moffat 1862).

ten sheep. Hundreds were swept away within a few days, and many bodies lay unburied." On the 21st, the captain of the *Northern Light* reported: "The ravages of small pox at Rupert had been frightful. The tribe native to that section was nearly exterminated." By 24 June one of the Oblate fathers and "Drs Wood and Kendall, of . . . H M Surveying steamer Hecate" had arrived at the fort and were "engaged in vaccinating the few survivors." Ten weeks later (at a time when many Indians may have been absent fishing) the master of H.M.S. *Plumper* described Fort Rupert:

11 September
Since our last Visit to this place [1858?] it is sadly Changed. the once imposing looking Village in all its rude uncivilized state is now nowhere to be seen. the smallpox which went all through the Indian Tribes about 3 months ago, did not [illegible] of these poor fellows, scores of them died and lay for days and weeks in the same spot unburied and uncared for untill the others through actual dread of their own lives from the fearful efflu[ent] pulled down the houses of the dead and scattered the pieces far and wide throwing the bodies in the sea to float away as they chose, of the fine Muscular [illegible] fellows that 4 years ago Numbered 400 men, now not fifty can be Mustered, & they are Mostly the Middle Aged or older Men, disease appears to have principally attacked the Young and Strong. (Gowlland 1862)

When Dr. John Helmcken visited Rupert in 1850, he estimated its population at 2,500 (1975: 300); in 1866 it was given as 400 (Compton in Galois 1994: 37). The best pre-epidemic estimate of total Kwakwaka'wakw population is William Tolmie's 1835 estimate of 8,850; in 1866 the equivalent number was 3,750 (Galois 1994: 37–38). Allowing for 10% mortality from the 1848 measles epidemic, the 53% decline was probably mostly due to smallpox (see chapter 8).

Heiltsuk (Bella Bella). Two surviving traditions describe how the epidemic arrived at Bella Bella. In 1866, Robert Brown reported that smallpox came from a canoe of Haida refugees who "whilst waiting on an Island for a favourable opportunity to cross to Q.C.I. all perished of this disease." In the early 1920s ethnographer Thomas McIlwraith was told that

a steamer arrived at Bella Bella carrying a man sick with smallpox, the first case known there. Large presents were offered to the young shaman if he would cure the sufferer. He undertook the task, and treated the patient during the night, but the man died before dawn. This was a terrible blow to the shaman's prestige, so he called in the people and made a speech. "You have seen my powers," he said. "Why do you doubt me even after this failure?" Then he committed suicide by shooting himself with a musket. (1948: 1.668)

By 10 June the "Bella Bellas" were reported to be "dying off very fast" (*DBC*, 21 June). On 26 June the traders at Fort Simpson received word "that nearly all the Mill Bank [Sound] Indians are taken off by the Small Pox" (McNeil 1859–62). And on 18 July the *DBC* said, "at Bella Bella only about 40 of the tribe was found alive; the remainder had been swept off by the smallpox."[13] Smallpox led to the abandonment of most winter villages and the consolidation of survivors in a few settlements. In the 1930s and 1940s ethnographer Ronald Olson's informants named Waxwas and K̓waɫṁa on Burke Channel, Kʷátus on Dean Channel, and Lúxʷbálís on Calvert Island as villages abandoned due to the epidemic (Olson 1955: 320–21).[14] Susanne Hilton's historical research indicates that movement of several local groups to the consolidated settlement at Bella Bella began following the smallpox epidemic. The Istaiɫxʷ abandoned Dean Channel in 1862; most of the Oyaliɫxʷ and Owitliɫxʷ joined them after 1880 when a mission was established; and the Yeo Island Kokwaiɫxʷ moved in 1891 after a fire destroyed their village. In the 1840s the Hudson's Bay Company censused 1,530 for the four Bella Bella tribes (excluding Haihais and Oweekeno; Douglas 1878); by 1899, when almost all had come together at Bella Bella, there were 319 (based on Hilton 1971). Virtually all of this decline and movement was attributable to the 1862 smallpox epidemic.

Stories relating to village abandonment were still being told at Bella Bella in the late 1980s:

I heard about this—what happened years ago, before my time—what they called smallpox, whatever it was, in those days. People used to live in Denny Island there. . . . They were dying. . . . I don't know how many deaths were there. And one old fellow, to get away from there, climbed a mountain, to go straight across to Hauyet. . . . They couldn't tell how many people had died. Some women lay down dead, and the little baby was still sucking their tits, and she'd be dead. They'd tell me that story. (Harkin 1997: 29)

13. I am grateful to Susanne (Storie) Hilton for alerting me to this source.
14. Boas's Bella Bella oral traditions (1928, 1932) that mention village abandonments (e.g., Wā'walis [ʔuwiga], Baxᵘ bakwā'lanuxᵘsĩ' wEᵋ [nuxʷənc]), epidemics (ɫkwi'ɫmēᵋ), and "the person with holes all over his face" (Wā'k·as) may incorporate memories from the 1860s.

Nuxalk (Bella Coola). Further inland from the Bella Bella, at the head of Dean and Burke Channels, Nuxalk villages were also decimated by smallpox. H. Spencer Palmer's surveying party, who were in the area in early July, were eyewitnesses:

During my stay this disease, which had only just broken out when I arrived spread so rapidly, that in a week nearly all the healthy had scattered from the lodges and gone to encamp by families in the woods, only, it is to be feared, to carry away the seeds of infection and death. . . . Numbers were dying each day; sick men and women were taken out into the woods and left with a blanket and two or three salmon to die by themselves and rot unburied; sick children were tied to trees, and naked, grey-haired medicine men, hideously painted, howled and gesticulated night and day in front of the lodges in mad efforts to stay the progress of the disease. (Palmer 1863: 7–8)

The surveying party's Colonel Frisbee made a report to Bishop Hills of

frightful ravages amongst the Indians by Small Pox. Dead & [illegible] bodies were lying about in all directions. Out of 2000 Indians he thought from what he saw not 500 could be left. He described the treatment of the sick cruel—as soon as taken ill a box is made for the patient—the tail of a salmon & fruit[?] is with a wooden bowl of water & the poor creature is set adrift in a Canoe or exposed & left without care. A child taken ill is tied to a tree & left. The Medicein men would occasionally come & blow & make a commotion but would listen to no advice. (Hills 1863: entry of 28 August 1862)

Haisla. Due north of the Nuxalk, a tradition related to Ronald Olson in the 1930s suggests that the Haisla (or at least the Kitimaat branch) of Douglas Channel escaped the epidemic:

At the time of the smallpox epidemic a certain shaman foretold what was to happen and what was happening in other villages. One day he said, "They (disease spirits) are coming up to get us now. Four canoe loads are coming up the channel." People did not believe him. "Now they are landing at our beach. Bring forth my bows and arrows." They brought them. Then he called for 'xsulih roots. He stuck the roots on the arrow points. "They are coming for us now, one is inside. Now I'll shoot." People saw the arrow fly. Just at the entrance the arrow stopped in mid-air. Thus he shot four arrows and all stayed in mid-air. Then he said the spirits were going in retreat. The arrows dropped. "Now they are in their canoes and leaving," he said. "They are going in three canoes and have left one behind." When they went to see there was only a snag which had not been there before. But the people here did not get the smallpox. (Olson 1940: 197)

Haida. In 1862 the population of the Haida plummeted, and a process of village abandonment and consolidation began (see chapter 8). No contemporary accounts from the Queen Charlottes themselves describing what happened after the refugee canoes of Haida returned to their homeland that summer have survived. The first on-site record comes from October 1863, when copper miner Francis Poole arrived at Skincuttle Inlet (on Moresby Island). If the source is to be believed, the disease had continued circulating among the Haida villages for over a year. Poole witnessed an outbreak at Skincuttle: there were several deaths, the Haida abandoned their camp, and Poole burnt it to the ground (1872: 158–59). When he returned from Victoria in December (with a passenger ill with the smallpox), the disease broke out again among the Ninstints people, and more perished (195).

A few Haida oral traditions may recall the 1862 epidemic. "Cloud-Watcher" describes a time when "there was much sickness . . . probably the smallpox" at Tanu village. Some people from Cumshewa, Skedans, and Old Kloo villages retreated to the west (inlet) shore of Louise Island, where, under the influence of the Cumshewa shaman Λ'nkustA, they remained free of disease (Swanton 1905b: 309–10). The "Story of Those-Born-at-Skedans" also includes a reference to "a time when there was sickness in the place." The disease was attributed to a "knife that shut up" (a pocketknife?) and that "belonged to Pestilence." It was tossed into the sea (86). Other "pestilence" myths noted in chapter 2 may incorporate memories of the 1862 epidemic.

Smallpox among the Tsimshian

Beginnings. The progress of the smallpox epidemic among the coastal Tsimshian people is fully documented by eyewitnesses in two daily journals: from Fort Simpson (fig. 14) (kept by William McNeil) and in the private journal of Anglican missionary William Duncan (fig. 15).

Smallpox spread rapidly from Victoria to the Fort Simpson area, brought by the first evacuees from the Northerners' Encampment, who were Tsimshian. The Northerners left Victoria on 1 May; just over two weeks later the Fort Simpson journal recorded:

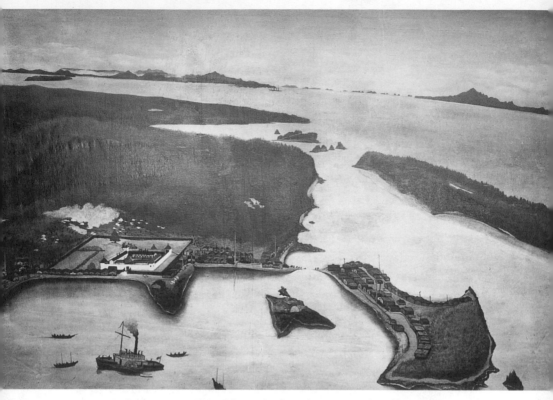

FIG. 14. In the 1920s, a Tsimshian artist drew this picture of late-nineteenth-century Fort Simpson (note the *Beaver* in the foreground). Over 500 Indians died here of smallpox in 1862. (Courtesy of Canadian Museum of Civilization, Hull, Quebec, photo no. 86130.)

17 May 1862

Four or five Canoes arrived from Victoria and report that the Small Pox was raging at that place and that some of their party died on the way here, and that some of the canoes had but two people that well enough to paddle them.

18 May 1862

A number had died on the way to this place, one Canoe was abandoned, with all that was in her. We may expect soon to have many deaths at this place, as a few *cases* have arrived. (McNeil 1859–62)

The fort authorities made no attempt to exclude these carriers from the Indian settlement or to vaccinate the locals, simple steps that might have halted the epidemic.

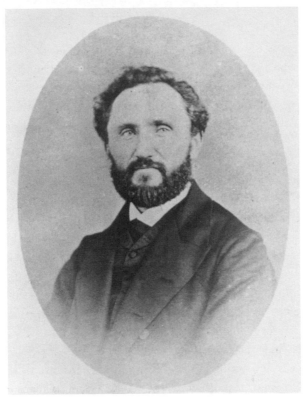

FIG. 15. Reverend William Duncan, an Anglican missionary who vaccinated Indians at Metlakatla during the 1862 smallpox epidemic, saving most of them. (Courtesy of British Columbia Archives, British Columbia Information Management Services, Victoria, photo no. A-01175.)

In accordance with the normal progression of smallpox after initial infection, the epidemic around Fort Simpson did not begin for another two weeks. In the meantime, local people were frightened. On 18 May a woman was shot for having "caused the death of one" of the evacuees (Duncan); on the 20th canoes were starting to leave "in fear of Small Pox" (McNeil). On the 24th there was "Medicine work going on all over the camp, and a piece of stick with red Medicine on it stuck on top of every house. This of course will keep the Small Pox from entering the house" (McNeil).

Red poles were indeed used as protection from smallpox; the practice is documented in both the Nisga'a tale "TsEgu'ksk^u," dated by the informant to "the first visitation of smallpox" (most likely 1836, see chapter 5), and in the Haida "Pestilence" tale "Story of the Shaman, G.A'Ndox's-Father"

(Swanton 1905b: 311–16). In the latter tale, a Haida man stole his sister from Pestilence, who had married her. "For that reason there was much sickness. . . . When many people were dying DilAgiâ' went in to dance before Pestilence. He had a long cane the surface of which was painted red. He stuck it up slantwise, stood upon it, and danced. Then he made him feel good, and the sickness ceased."

Father Duncan took advantage of the impending events to proselytize the Indians. Between 22 and 26 May he visited "all the nine tribes of the Tsimshean," telling them in their native language that the plague had been sent by the Lord as punishment for their sins, relating the "Parable of the Prodigal Son," and promising that God would "receive them back & bless them" if they repented of their sins and "came to Jesus."

On 25 May the fort journal began recording smallpox cases; two days later Duncan, with six canoes and 50 people, set off for Metlakatla, about 15 miles south, which he had selected as the site of his new Christian community. All those who left for Metlakatla were free of smallpox.

June. The epidemic began in force at the fort in the first week of June. More Tsimshian were preparing to depart: on 3 June Duncan recorded that "the old Chief Noeshlakkalnoosh & nearly all the Keitlahn [Gitlan] tribe are on their way to us." On 6 June: "the Keitlahn tribe . . . number about 200 souls. . . . They have locked up their houses at Fort Simpson bringing little or nothing with them but food & few necessary things. Small pox is still doing its deadly work I hear of about 10 or 12 deaths. . . . We number now about 300 souls."

During the third week of June the epidemic peaked at the fort. On 21 June the disease was "raging" (McNeil); on the 23d it was "doing a dreadful work" (Duncan). The Indians "lit quite a number of fires all along the beach, to drive away the Sickness" (McNeil); five of Duncan's Indian parishioners who remained at the fort were now dead. "Blessed be the Lord of all Mercy—we here are still spared" (Duncan).

Again Duncan took the epidemic as an opportunity to drive home his Christian message of punishment, repentance, and delivery:

> 25 June
> After noon I assembled them & addressed them on
> The Cause of Suffering & plague
> Sin of resisting the Voice

> The Purpose God has in mind
>
> To bring us to Repentence
>
> Plague is one instrument
>
> How long will God thus afflict
>
> The plague in Egypt—First child slain.
>
> God's people delivered upon showing a sign of their faith.
>
> The Confidence of God's People.
>
> XCI Psalm during the visitation of Plague
>
> I suppose about 150 souls attended.

When he was finished, three canoes set off for the fort to retrieve relatives. When they returned the next day, however, Duncan was forced to insist that the new arrivals be quarantined "a little distance from" Metlakatla "for a few days" before they were admitted.

July–September. By 26 June word of the epidemic had spread, and canoes of Nisga'a, Tlingit, and Haida, previously regular visitors to the fort, stopped coming. A flotilla of 13 refugee Haida canoes from Victoria appeared at the beginning of July, however, and on the fourth some were reported "camped on Finlayson's Island . . . dying daily." Fear was now general, and more canoes of Tsimshian abandoned the Fort Simpson area: "several" on 1 July and "a number" on 3 July, "for Woods Canal, bag and baggage." The settlement outside the fort was now nearly deserted.

Some Tsimshian fled to Metlakatla, requesting entry. These included refugees from tribes on the Skeena River with news "that many were dead & others sick up the river." The notorious chief of the Gispakloats, Legaik, arrived at noon on 3 July and was among "about 200 [who] assembled for prayers" in the evening. "Several" refugees from the Keetandol (Gitandau) tribe were camped "about 1/4 of a mile" from Metlakatla, hoping to be admitted. Duncan would not let them in, however, as there was smallpox among them, two Metlakatlans had shown symptoms of the disease, and a corpse of one of the Haida refugees was festering untended outside the settlement. On 6 July two Metlakatlans were sent outside to bury abandoned corpses; they were given precautions by Duncan and told to wait two days before returning. An aggrieved family of Gitandau was denied admission until after a five-day waiting period.

The next day, none too soon, there was good news. The missionary was called to the fort to collect "many things" that had been sent to him on the

Labouchere from church authorities in Victoria. These "things" included a supply of vaccine obtained from Dr. Helmcken, with instructions on how to administer it: "You can use a needle or pen-knife for making the punctures" (Cridge 1862). When Duncan arrived back at Metlakatla on 11 July: "Three had been taken sick" and "left alone to die in the bush." Although the "relatives grieved sorely," they were too frightened to attend the ill. Cases like this appeared sporadically at Metlakatla throughout July. All who became ill were isolated.[15]

Duncan began vaccinating that evening and continued doing so throughout the next two months. On 10 September he summarized:

I have vaccinated as fast as I could get matter to go on with. I think I must have done about 200 or 300 & some of them two or three times before the matter took. I have little confidence in the result to many—as the pock produced seemed to bear few symptoms of a proper Cow pock. Perhaps it was the matter passing through diseased persons or being decomposed or from my ignorance in the performance.

On 8 August "some canoes of Killentsahs [Gilutsau] arrived. The plague (in spite of their magic feathers & bark) has reached them & they are now poor creatures driven here." By this time there were 400 Indians at Metlakatla.

At Fort Simpson, without any vaccine, the epidemic was beginning to play itself out. On 25 July McNeil said two or three were dying daily, though the mortality was uneven: one-third of the "Ispotelots" (Gispakloats—Legaik's tribe) were dead, but none of the "Kil-O-Chars" (Gilutsau) (26 July). The fort journal mentions only a few cases of the disease after mid-August, nearly three months after its introduction. McNeil (1862) estimated that "at least 500 of our Indians have died" from smallpox, a number passed on to and

---

15. Duncan tracked the progress of a girl who showed signs of the disease on 18 July: she was immediately "removed from the camp" and isolated "with only a few leaves on the branch of a tree for her tent & her old grandmother to attend her." The missionary visited her on the 21st and left "medicine, rice," and instructions to pray daily. When he returned two days later: "Poor Athlthnol had bid her grandmother leave her as she felt she would die. She had also crept farther into the brush & laid down under a tree—thinking perhaps she will come to bury her when she dies. I stood on the rocky beach & called aloud—after some time the poor girl responded with a deadly hoarse voice & the grandmother made her appearance from a little distance. The poor old creature said she was very much afraid & so had got away. She then shouted for the poor girl to come. She obliged & sat where I could see her. She was spitting continually blood & pus & also blood had come from her nose. Her face was a sad sight. How sudden a change in a few days. I pointed her again to God & left her with the feeling that I should see her again no more." The next day "Poor Ahthlthnol is dead & left to be eaten by the wolves. No body dares bury her."

repeated by other Hudson's Bay Company officials. But the master of the gun-boat H.M.S. *Devastation,* on 27 September, put the total at 700 (Cooper 1862); and John Gowlland of H.M.S. *Plumper,* on 18 September, put it at 600.[16]

In September there was a brief resurgence of the disease at Metlakatla. On the 10th a distressed Duncan recorded seven cases: all were isolated, anguished families were broken apart, and by the end of the month all had died. Some of the deceased had been baptized, including Stephen Ryan, whom Duncan eulogized in a 6 March letter, and a repentant "Quthray, the cannibal chief, renamed Philip Atkinson" (1869: 94).[17] The missionary counted these two among his successes. The crafty Legaik, who took refuge at Metlakatla only when the epidemic began and then fled precipitously when new cases began to appear, had also asked to be baptized but appeared to have been motivated by "fears caused by the plague."[18] Duncan recognized that the epidemic, more than anything else, had driven most of his flock to the safety of Metlakatla and convinced them to accept conversion and ultimately reject their traditional ways.

In succeeding years, Duncan's draconian methods brought about the nearly complete acculturation of the Metlakatla Tsimshian. In addition to adopt-ing Christianity, the Metlakatlans gave up dancing, potlatching, and their social and class system, and accepted new houses and gardens, schooling in English, an elected government, and a communally run sawmill and salmon factory (Barnett 1942). The similarity to the "système Durieu" among the post-small-pox Se'shalt has been noted above.

Spread of Smallpox beyond Fort Simpson

For almost 6 weeks after the first refugee boats from Victoria appeared, and for a full month after the first case of smallpox was recorded at the fort, canoes

16. "[T]hey threatened that if Sickness had not brought them so low, they would have towed the Devastation on the beach 'and made a bonfire of her.' . . . Smallpox has made dreadful havoc amongst these Savages: 600 of them out of 2000 have already died; and even now it is raging in the Camp; numbers of their houses we see shut up and *marked,* they are full of the unburied dead in every stage of decomposition and who can help it? What can be done? if the companys men in the fort offered to bury them the Indians would not allow it and they are afraid to do so themselves" (Gowlland 1862).

17. Of Quthray, Duncan said: "Oh the dreadful and revolting things which I have witnessed him do!"

18. On Duncan and Legaik, see "When Legaix tried to murder Mr. Duncan" in Barbeau and Beynon 1987: 2.206–8.

of neighboring Indians—Nisga'a, Haida, and Tlingit—continued to arrive regularly at the fort to trade. Between 14 and 24 May well over 50 canoes came from the Nass River with eulachon grease; Nisga'a boats continued to arrive until 24 June. Haida canoes, containing "Skidegates," "Kigarnies," and "Massetts," appeared at the fort through 26 June, and Tlingit (Tongass and Stikine) canoes were named in the fort journal through 16 June. There is no doubt that many of these traders became infected with smallpox at Simpson and carried it back with them to their home villages.

The agents who carried smallpox to southeast Alaska, however, were probably refugee Stikine canoes from the Northerners' Encampment. The hegira of the refugee Stikines can be pieced together from several sources. They were evicted on 11 and 14 May from camps outside Victoria, and some were apparently escorted by the gunboat H.M.S. *Topaze* all the way to their homes in Alaska.[19] At the same time, Whites from Victoria were sailing north to the newly discovered Stikine goldfields. On 17 June at Fort Simpson the "Sloop John Thornton arrived with 35 passengers" for the Stikine goldfields, "from Victoria 20 days passage." Along with the sloop were "a Whale Boat and two Canoes," which must have held Indians, for on the 19th, at Metlakatla, "Some white men landed . . . & informed us that 25 of the Stikeen Indians, with whom they were in company on the way to the Stickeen River, had died between here & Victoria." In the first week of July, a Stikine-bound canoe carrying both Whites and Indians was fired at by Indians off Bella Bella when it attempted to "put ashore" sick Stikines; two Whites were killed (*DBC*, 23 July).

There are no extant records from Stikine itself during July and August, when the epidemic must have been spreading. But on 6 September, when H.M.S. *Devastation* passed by Point Highfield (Wrangell), they "found very few Indians at the village . . . the smallpox having decimated the tribe and was at that time raging among them" (Cooper 1862). The epidemic proceeded north into the Alexander Archipelago, but apparently only into places where the Russian vaccination program had not penetrated. These included Henya Tlingit lands on northern Prince of Wales Island, as noted some years later by ethnographer George T. Emmons:

19. In a letter dated 13 July at Victoria, Horace Talbot, master of the *Topaze,* stated he had just returned from escorting "Northern Indians . . . afflicted with the smallpox . . . 600 miles north. Not a very pleasant duty . . . but I . . . had some capital fishing."

In 1888, when I was passing through the seaward channels of Prince of Wales Island, I stopped at Tche-qwan [Shakan] on a small island about twelve miles above Tuxekan. It was a veritable city of the dead from which the survivors fled en masse after a visitation of small pox. The houses with their interior carvings and totem poles still stood intact, left to weather and decay, but passing Canoes avoided that shore, while the occupants propitiated the evil spirits with an offering of tobacco or food. (Emmons 1991: 58–59)

8 / North Coast Population History, 1774–1889

In this chapter, "North Coast" refers to the three "Northern Matrilineal" peoples (Haida; Tlingit; and Tsimshian, including the Nisg̱a'a, Git̲x̲san, and Tsimshian proper) and the several ethnic groups who traded at the Hudson's Bay Company's Fort McLoughlin (Sabassas, or "Southern Tsimshian"; Haisla; Heiltsuk, or Bella Bella; Nuxalk, or Bella Coola; and Oweekeno) (map 11). Between the early 1830s and mid-1840s, preceding and following the 1836–37 North Coast smallpox epidemic, the Hudson's Bay Company (HBC) censused virtually all these peoples (Douglas 1878).[1] The censuses, reproduced in tables 7–14 at the back of the book, are gold mines of demographic data. By themselves, they reveal a great deal of information about the varying population structures of the North Coast peoples, particularly in such sensitive indices as sex ratio and age-class composition; in comparison with earlier and later estimates and censuses, they show quite clearly the demographic effects of the 1836–37 and 1862 smallpox epidemics. Analyses of

---

1. The source is the manuscript "Census of the Indian Population on the N.W. Coast . . . ", a compendium of HBC censuses taken at different times and copied by Hubert Howe Bancroft's researcher Ivan Petrov from former Chief Factor James Douglas's "Private Papers." The original is in the Bancroft Library at the University of California, Berkeley; a microfilm copy is available in Microforms, University of Washington Libraries, Seattle. There are two printed versions of the censuses: a fairly reliable duplicate in the appendix to Paul Kane's 1859 version of *Wanderings of an Artist among the Indians of North America* and a garbled copy in Schoolcraft

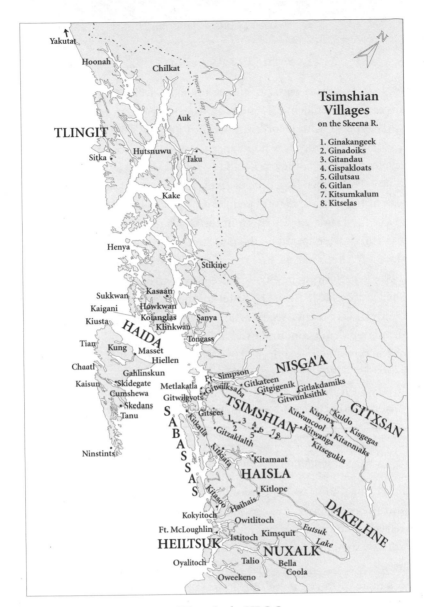

MAP 11. North Coast: Names and Places in the HBC Censuses

censuses of the Haida, Tlingit, Tsimshian, and Fort McLoughlin peoples constitute the bulk of this chapter.

1851: vol. 5. The original censuses were apparently never forwarded to the HBC headquarters, as their archives do not contain them. My figures are based mostly on the Douglas copy, cross-checked against Kane.

NORTHERN MATRILINEAL AREA

The major "disease events" of the Northern Matrilineal area include three major smallpox epidemics—in the 1770s (chapter 2), 1836 (chapter 5), and 1862 (chapter 7), with recorded mortalities ranging from one-third to two-thirds of the contemporary populations—as well as a possible fourth, minor smallpox outbreak in the 1790s and two recorded measles epidemics in 1848 and 1868, with much lower death rates. There is some variation in specific disease histories: while all three peoples experienced smallpox in the late 1700s, evidence for Haida participation in the 1836 outbreak is limited, and most island Tlingit were spared by the 1862 smallpox epidemic. There were similar local variations in exposure to minor infectious diseases.

Specific patterns of population decline vary from group to group corresponding closely to local disease histories. The island Tlingit, who experienced two early disease events, seem to have declined the least; Tsimshian peoples, with three epidemics one and two generations apart, decreased in number at a median rate; and the Haida, and to a lesser extent mainland Tlingit, severely affected by the 1862 epidemic, experienced a demographic and cultural shock so great that it threatened their continued existence as viable sociocultural entities.

Population Decline from Virgin-Soil Smallpox

There are, of course, no population statistics from the time prior to the first appearance of smallpox, and very few and crude estimates from the era immediately following it. So we do not know the true mortality from virgin-soil Northwest smallpox and can only approximate it, using a few suggestive indices.

A sample of 20 virgin-soil smallpox outbreaks from the epidemiological literature suggests an average mortality of 30% (Dixon 1962: 325). Recorded mortalities from virgin-soil epidemics of *Variola major* among American Indians, however, are uniformly much higher (e.g., Stearn and Stearn 1945; Dobyns 1966: 441). And the few surviving references to mortality due to late-1700s smallpox recorded from Northwest Indian informants also indicate sizable mortalities: "He told me that the distemper carried off great numbers of the inhabitants" (Portlock in 1787, on the Tlingit). "According to Saigakakh . . . there were only one or two persons left in each family" (Khlebnikov in 1829, on the Tlingit). "[B]y Kowe's accounts, the small Pox swept off two thirds of the people scarcely any that were affected survived" (Bishop in 1795, on the Haida). "[T]he small-pox made great ravages among them . . . it almost destroyed their country" (Green in 1829, on the North Coast). And for more southerly peoples: "So great was the mortality . . . it was impossible for the survivors to bury the dead" (Curtis in ca. 1910, on the Kwakwaka'wakw); "several villages were completely wiped out, while all suffered losses" (Suttles in 1954, on the Straits Salish); and "they all died . . . the Clatsops inform us that this disorder raged in their towns and distroyed their nation" (Clark in 1805, on the Chinookans).[2]

A second line of evidence on virgin-soil smallpox mortality comes from the several references to "abandoned villages" in the writings of early visitors to the coast. Though village sites could be "abandoned" for several reasons (most notably seasonal migration), the pronounced clustering of references to vacated settlements in the late 1700s suggests that the abandonment resulted from a singular, preceding historical event. The early explorers, to their credit, approached this problem with great caution, allowing for all possible hypotheses.[3] The earliest of these passages comes from the 1788 manuscript journal of James Colnett and refers to Kildidt Sound on the British Columbia coast:[4]

15 August 1788
Around where we lay were remains of numbers of dwellings & many corps laying in Boxes; the decay of Both Habitations & Coffins, was nearly equal, & the time of quitting this place must have been when the mortality happend. This desertion might be accounted for several ways, first after a Battle and defeated [*sic*], or a severe winter & perish'd by Famine, by the fish quitting the Ground. . . .[5]

Colnett's hypothesized reasons for the "mortality" are, ethnographically speaking, sound. A failure of fish runs and consequent winter famine are possible given the fluctuating nature of Northwest resource availability and are

2. For bibliographic citations, see chapter 2.
3. As did contemporary historian Robin Fisher (1977: 21–22).
4. Location determined by Canadian geographer Robert Galois (pers. comm., September 1996). Galois, who is annotating Colnett's journal, points out that the explorer made a similar observation at Nootka Sound, where he added yet a fourth reason for site abandonment: hygiene.
5. From the Vancouver expedition (1792), Archibald Menzies made a similar observation concerning the lands around the Strait of Georgia: "[B]ut if they might judge from the deserted

recorded frequently in the mythology (see appendix 1). Warfare is another possibility, particularly on the North Coast, where pitched battles with many deaths are well established for the late prehistoric and early contact periods.[6] But Colnett does not consider disease mortality.

Two of the more explicit accounts of abandoned villages date to the 1792 Vancouver expedition survey of the waters between Vancouver Island and the mainland, at Point Discovery (Clallam; Vancouver 1798: 1.229) and on Homfray Channel (Comox; Puget 1792: entry of 28 June).[7] In the 1793 and 1794 seasons, expedition members made similar observations on the North Coast, in Tsimshian (Puget 1793) and Tlingit (Johnstone in Vancouver 1798: 3.289) lands.

19 September 1793 (Tsimshian)
From Restoration Bay [mouth of Burke Channel] to Salmon Bay [mouth of the Nass] in the Inland parts are few Inhabitants at least our Boats found that Country nearly deserted. . . . if we may judge from the Numerous Villages which bound this & many other parts of the Inland Navigation & which now are left to decay, it is to be supposed that it was once the principal Retreat of the NW Americans.

August 1794, Kupreanof Island area (Tlingit)
[T]his branch about a mile wide stretched about five miles in an eastwardly direction . . . the remains of no less than eight deserted villages were seen; some of them were more decayed than the others. . . . In the vicinity of these ruins were many sepulchres or tombs. . . . of different sizes, and some of them contained more bodies than the others; in the largest there were not more than four or five. . . . Many of these sacred monuments seemed to have been erected a great length of time.

Similar passages describing deserted villages may be found in the 1793 journals of Johnstone (in Puget 1793: entry of 27 July, on the Skeena Tsimshian), Menzies, and Puget (11 August; on the Clarence Strait Tlingit).

———

Villages they met in this excursion, the Country appeard to be formerly much more numerously inhabited than at present, tho they could form no conjecture or opinion on the cause of this apparent depopulation which had not an equal chance of proving fallacious from their circumscribed knowledge of the manners & modes of living of the inhabitants" (1923: 63).

6. The definitive treatment of North Coast warfare is Ferguson 1984. See also Sapir and Swadesh 1939; Barbeau and Beynon 1987: vol. 2. MacDonald 1989 examines the archeological record on Tsimshian warfare.

7. Both accounts are reproduced in their entirety in Boyd 1994b: 31–32.

In isolation, these passages may be taken to support several hypotheses other than disease, including warfare, famine, seasonal movement, or various combinations thereof. Considered together, however, they suggest what archeologists term a "horizon," or abrupt change in settlement patterns. In 1982, archeologist Ann Ramenofsky hypothesized that several settlement horizons in post-1500 Native America might be the result of epidemic depopulation. Tested in three regions of North America, she found strong support for the theory.[8] Her hypothesis has also been tested in the Northwest in the middle Columbia Basin, with suggestive results (Campbell 1989), and in southwestern Oregon, where a late-1700s settlement pattern shift coincides nicely with the time frame for the first recorded appearance of smallpox (Draper 1989). Later historic Northwest settlement horizons resulting from epidemic depopulation occurred after 1862 on the North Coast and after 1830 on the lower Columbia and are described later in this chapter and in chapter 9. Comparative evidence therefore suggests that the late-1700s cluster of references to abandoned villages also represents a settlement horizon, resulting from depopulation caused by the virgin-soil smallpox experience of the 1770s.

The Earliest Population Estimates, 1774–1830

Throughout the early contact period in most of the North Coast, there were no land-based, permanent trading establishments, and most contacts with record-keeping Euro-Americans were transitory. Most estimates of Indian populations from this period were based on crude projection methods and usually covered only a segment of total tribal populations. Commonly used methods included "canoe projection," which extrapolated populations from the number and capacity of observed canoes; house and lodge counts, which assumed a standard number of occupants per structure; and warrior counts, which when multiplied by a standard number reflecting family size and number of dependents (4 is the average: see Cook 1976b: 5–6) yielded a total figure.[9] All extant estimates have been entered in tables 7–14. The most realistic estimate from the late 1700s for North Coast peoples was made for the Haida by

8. Ramenofsky's 1982 University of Washington Ph.D. dissertation, "Disease and the Archaeology of Population Collapse: Native American Responses to European Contact," was published in 1987 as *Vectors of Death: The Archaeology of European Contact.*

9. See the discussion in Boyd 1985: 190–95.

American captain William Sturgis. In 1799, he "suppose[d] . . . nearly upon 3,000 fighting men" (1978: 41), and "for the whole Kigarnee tribe . . . some 1,800 to 2,000 souls" (1978: 99). Using the standard multiplier of 4, the estimate of 3,000 warriors suggests a total population of 12,000. In the Tlingit area, the most reliable early estimate was made 5 years after the establishment of Sitka, in 1804. Urey Lisiansky estimated of those "who call themselves Colloshes . . . about ten thousand" (1814: 242).[10]

Population Estimates from 1831 to 1859

Starting in 1831, the HBC began to extend its operations northward from Fort Langley on the lower Fraser, in hopes of wresting the coastal Indian trade from the Americans. Fort Simpson was established in Tsimshian territory in 1831 and Fort McLoughlin in the land of the Heiltsuk in 1833. Two more forts, at the mouths of the Stikine and Taku Rivers, in Tlingit territory, were in operation for a few years in the early 1840s (Canada 1974: 79). The 1836 North Coast smallpox epidemic claimed, according to the Whites, one-third of the affected population. Censuses of the Haida, Tlingit, and Tsimshian were taken during the first decade of the HBC presence in the north: the Haida count apparently preceding the epidemic, the other two following it. In addition, there are two nearly contemporaneous estimates of total Haida numbers and two presmallpox estimates of Tlingit population.

Haida: Total Numbers. Three extant Haida estimates or censuses appear to have been made in the early or mid-1830s: the Hudson's Bay census (in Douglas 1878), the Reverend Samuel Parker's estimate (from 1835, in 1936: 124), and Father Ivan Veniaminov's estimate (1837, in 1981: 103); see table 7. Dating the HBC census is difficult, but most likely it was conducted sometime between 1831 and 1835.[11] The HBC total, reproduced in table 8, is 8,428.

---

10. Other tribal estimates may still survive, in manuscript, in New England archives. Albert Gallatin, for instance, had access to "the manuscript journal of Capt. William Bryant kept on that coast during the years 1820–27 embracing vocabularies of several dialects . . . [and] enumerates twenty tribes" (1836: 302).

11. Like many of the censuses in the Douglas compendium, the Haida count is undated. From its internal structure, however, the Haida census obviously represents a pre-epidemic population. If Haida were indeed affected by the 1836 smallpox epidemic, the census must predate that year, as well as postdate the establishment of the first North Coast HBC fort, which was in 1831. A likely year is 1835, when William Tolmie conducted a census of the villages in the vicinity of Fort McLoughlin (see below).

Parker's numbers were 10,692 Haida (8,600 on "Queen Charlotte's island" and 2,092 at "Kygany Harbour"), 2,264 more than the HBC census of the same groups.[12] Father Veniaminov's estimate was made in conjunction with his 1837 survey of Tlingit villages. Veniaminov did not visit the Haida area but allowed 1,350 Kaigani and 8,000 Queen Charlotte Islanders, for a total of 9,350 Haida speakers (1981: 103). His total is intermediate between Parker's and the HBC's. For the sake of the present discussion, I am using a figure of 9,490, the average of the three enumerations in the historical literature, as the closest approximation of total Haida population in the early 1800s.

Haida: Population Structure. From a demographic standpoint, the Haida census is a singular and provocative document. Alone among contemporary North Coast censuses, it records a population seemingly unaffected by the 1836 smallpox epidemic. And it indicates a population which was very large, in both total numbers and density, and which may have been increasing or had an inherent ability to do so.

The Haida are an extreme example of the "maritime hunter-gatherer" type (Yesner 1980: 729–31). Haida settlement seems to have been exclusively coastal. According to the maps compiled by Swanton (1905a) all villages were situated on saltwater. Haida subsistence also had more of a maritime orientation than did other Northwest economies: halibut, shellfish, and sea mammals, all saltwater creatures, were more important for Haida than were anadromous fishes such as salmon (Langdon 1979). The impression given by later researchers (Poole 1872; Norton 1981) is that terrestrial resources, mostly vegetal, were abundant within a short distance of village sites. The Haida very seldom hunted land animals. The subsistence base seems both diverse and concentrated; as a consequence, the Haida were more sedentary than most Northwest Coast peoples. Like other maritime hunter-gatherers, Haida society was characterized by "territoriality, resource competition, and warfare." (Yesner 1980: 731).

Demographically, two important maritime hunter-gatherer characteris-

12. There are two possible explanations for this discrepancy. The first, tentatively accepted here, is that Parker's Haida figure is drawn from a precensus HBC estimate of Haida strength and is excessive. (As with Parker's Tlingit figure, the Haida number—10,692—is divisible by 4, the assumed number of dependents per man.) The original HBC source document has apparently not survived. A second possible explanation is that the Parker number includes slaves, while the HBC census excludes them: 21% (the difference between the two) is indeed a likely percentage for slaves. The HBC Haida census is unique in not listing slaves as a separate category. But it seems more probable that they are simply included in the total of the HBC count.

tics are high population densities and low dependency ratios. Using statistics from Kroeber (1939: 135, 170) applied to a population of 9,490, Haida population density in the mid-1830s was 92 per square kilometer, or 7.9 per shoreline mile. The latter figure, given Haida settlement and subsistence patterns, is the more meaningful of the two. Dependency ratios are the proportion of economically productive to nonproductive members of the society. Nonproducers are generally considered to include children and elderly.

Because both old people and children are able to engage in activities such as shellfish collecting, and because they have lower caloric requirements, they are virtually able to support themselves in coastal zones and do not act as a sump for the population's resources. . . . Therefore, in any maritime society in which shellfish or other invertebrates are an important resource, dependency ratios tend to be lower, population pyramids broader, life expectancies higher, and potential for population increase consequently greater. (Yesner 1980: 730)

A "potential for population increase" is suggested by the high (48%) percentage of children in the 1830s census. The Haida seem to have been equally prolific in earlier times as well: in 1791, at Cloak Bay (northwest tip of Graham Island), Surgeon Roblet of the Marchand expedition observed, "If we are to judge of the fecundity of the women by the number of children which we reckoned in the habitations, it is astonishing; it always exceeded that of the women and men united" (Fleurieu 1801: 1.454). Sometime before the beginning of the historic period, Haida from the northwest tip of Graham Island colonized the southern portion of Prince of Wales Island. According to the tradition collected by John Swanton (1905b: 88–90), they defeated the Tlingit inhabitants of the area in a territorial war, killing many and forcing others to flee. Swanton believed this war and migration were the result of population pressure in the Queen Charlottes: "It would appear that the people were increasing in numbers, and that this [northwest] corner of the island was becoming overpopulated."

Once established in Tlingit territory, Haida population apparently continued to increase, pushing Tlingit to the north. It has been argued that Haida society was adapted to take advantage of an abundant halibut resource, whereas Tlingit society was patterned to make maximum use of a limited salmon resource (Langdon 1979). In regions where halibut was naturally more abundant than salmon, Haida had a competitive edge. A second factor influencing Haida fertility, added to the population equation in the early 1800s, was the early and relatively complete adoption of the white potato into Haida economy. Potato culture favors increased sedentism while simultaneously adding a needed source of carbohydrates and a potential weaning food to a high-protein seafood diet. All these factors would tend to decrease birth spacing and hence enhance fertility.[13] In 1829, an American visitor noted: "Some years since, a trader left a few English potatoes at Queen Charlotte's island, and instructed the natives in the cultivation of them. This is doubtless a benefit to the Indians, but not less so to the traders themselves. For years, at very little expense, they have been able to furnish their vessels with most excellent potatoes" (Green 1915: 51 n). By 1835 Haida at Skidegate grew "a considerable quantity of potatoes," which they traded in September at an annual "potato fair" on the Tsimshian peninsula near the mouth of the Nass (Work 1945b: 55; Scouler in Brink 1974: 35).

Most Northwest Coast peoples, in common with hunter-gatherers elsewhere, are assumed to have had stationary populations, with total numbers capped by environmental restrictions and minimal capacity for natural increase. The Haida, with a high percentage of children and historical evidence for fecundity, may have been an exception to this rule. Among all the historic population estimates of Northwest Indians in the first century of contact, there is virtually no evidence for population rebound following epidemics. Again, the Haida (at least before 1836) may have been an exception. The 1830s census, with its high percentage of Haida children, may represent a population that, circa 61 years after an initial experience with smallpox, was well on its way to recovery. Computer simulations of population rebound following smallpox epidemics among peoples with modest natural annual rates of increase suggest that population recovery should be well under way by this time (Thornton, Miller, and Warren 1991: 35).[14] Although a few other Northwest peoples (judging from high percentages of children—e.g., Coast Salish) may have had a *capacity* for relatively rapid recovery, in all other cases

13. On the history and implications of the adoption of the potato on the Northwest Coast, see Suttles 1951.

14. Specifics elude us, however. Thornton, Miller, and Warren's (1991) simulations show full recovery 75 years after an epidemic with 40% mortality for populations with 0.5% annual growth rates. We do not know these parameters for the Haida. The loss from 1770s smallpox, though here set conservatively at one-third, may have been considerably greater than that (in 1795 the Haida informant Kowe placed it at two-thirds), and though we may assume some population increase given the population structure in the mid-1830s, the actual rate is unknown.

the sequential, back-to-back nature of disease outbreaks during the first 100 years of contact effectively stalled any incipient rebound.

Tlingit: Pre-epidemic Estimates. Estimates for Tlingit populations of the early 1830s come from Russian Orthodox priest Ivan Veniaminov and HBC official James Douglas (table 9). Veniaminov's rough figure, "10,000 . . . Koloshi living . . . from Kaigan to Yakutat" (1981: 19) (which should be adjusted to 8,000, excluding the non-Tlingit Kaigani), appears to duplicate Lisiansky's identical figure from 1804. Douglas's estimate comes from an undated manuscript held by the Royal British Columbia Archives. It lists "No. of Fighting Men" for sixteen Tlingit "tribes." The grand total of men is 2,940 (or 11,760 people using Cook's multiplier of 4). The source and dating of this estimate are problematical, but all lines of ethnohistorical evidence suggest a collection date of 1834–35.[15] Pre-epidemic Tlingit population is here set at 9,880, the average of the two contemporary (Lisiansky/Veniaminov and Douglas) ethnohistorical estimates.

Tlingit: Post-epidemic Statistics. Two sets of figures from the decade after the 1836 smallpox epidemic give some idea of the demographic effect of that disease event on the Tlingit. The first set of figures were collected by Father Veniaminov during an 1837 survey of Tlingit villages (Veniaminov 1981) conducted immediately after the smallpox epidemic. The figures are rounded and obviously not the result of actual head counts. Veniaminov's numbers for some groups are unusually low; he seems to have excluded inhabited villages not actually visited by him.

The HBC census (table 10), though undated, must have been taken between the years 1842 and 1845.[16] From all indications it is quite reliable. This is apparent from both cross-checking and the internal population structure.

15. The document is titled "Statistics of the Northwest Coast of America." The strongest clue to its dating is the presence on the list of estimates of Indian numbers at Fort McLoughlin that are known to have been made in 1835. Second, though there was no HBC presence in Tlingit territory before 1840, in 1834 the HBC sent an exploratory expedition to the mouth of the Stikine (Fisher 1977: 32), a likely time for the collection of statistics on local Indian numbers. Finally, the Douglas estimates were used, with slight adjustments, by the HBC until 1842, a year after the establishment of Forts Stikine and Taku, when a formal census was undertaken. HBC Governor George Simpson, who visited the new forts in 1842, used the pre-epidemic warrior counts to project tributary populations for the two posts (Simpson 1847: 1.124, 127). The Douglas statistics were also apparently the source of Samuel Parker's 1837 estimate.

16. In 1841, as previously noted, HBC officials were still using pre-epidemic estimates; the copy reproduced in Paul Kane's appendix bears the date 1846. The Hudson's Bay Archives preserves a detailed clan-by-clan census of the Stikine Tlingit, dated 1845 (Rae 1845), which is clearly

There are a few omissions, however, which should be noted. Neither the Yakutat nor the Sitka—both of whom were within the Russian sphere of influence—were enumerated, and it seems likely that the Chilkat were again the victims of an undercount. Allowing for these omissions,[17] there were probably about 7,255 Tlingit speakers following the 1836 smallpox epidemic.

My reconstructed populations for Tlingit are 9,880 pre-epidemic and 7,255 post-epidemic, indicating a loss of about 2,625, or 27%, from the 1836 smallpox outbreak. A comparison of tribal numbers in the 1835 estimate and 1842 census suggests that mortalities were concentrated among peoples in the outlying regions (Chilkat and Henya, Auk, Kake, and Stikine). In contrast, the disease seems to have had minimal total impact on the Tlingit closest to Sitka. This difference may be due in part to varying Russian vaccination efforts (see chapter 5). Total Tlingit mortality from the 1836 epidemic, as we will see, was probably low in comparison with peoples to the south.

Tlingit: Population Structure. The 1842 HBC census is the most comprehensive document on Tlingit population extant for the period prior to the U.S. census of 1890. It includes age, sex, and slave statistics for all Tlingit *kwan* (tribes) except the Sitka and Yakutat. Although the census is not representative of a truly aboriginal population, it preserves interesting statistics on population structure, specifically sex ratios. The total sex ratio for the (non-slave) Tlingit population is 123 (males per 100 females),[18] indicating a shortage of females. The adult sex ratio is 129; that for children is 110. Significant losses of females apparently occurred in this population at more than one point in the aging process.

Skewed sex ratios indicate that some outside factor is influencing the relative numbers of males and females: among children, cross-culturally significant factors include differential care and preferential infanticide; among adults, sex differences in mortality associated with childbirth and warfare. Severe environmental conditions (a bad winter) may lead to differential care and survival of boys versus girls; smallpox epidemics disproportionately affect

---

an update of the Stikine count in the complete HBC census. All these clues have led me to select the year 1842 as the probable date of the census.

17. Add 436 Yakutat and 214 Chilkat (both figures from the 1890 census) and 829 Sitka (the average of the 1837 estimate and 1869 and 1890 censuses) to the HBC 1842 total.

18. Sex ratios are determined by dividing the number of males by the number of females and multiplying by 100. The normal sex ratio at birth "varies between 108 and 107 males per 100 females" (Howell 1973: 251); by adulthood, due to the usual greater mortality among male children, it has normally evened out.

pregnant and lactating women (Dixon 1962: 325). Preferential female infanticide is noted in the earliest ethnohistorical literature.[19] Early explorers also noted a "scarcity of women, whose number appears not to be in proportion to that of the men" (Fleurieu 1801: 1.370). The 19-point increase in sex ratio between child and adult populations (110 to 129) points to a continuing loss of females into adulthood. Female puberty confinement and childbirth were difficult among the Tlingit (Knapp and Childe 1896: 73–75, 86; Krause 1956: 151–53); in addition, it may be that there was some extra mortality of pregnant and lactating women during the 1836 smallpox epidemic.[20]

The Tlingit census preserves enough detail on the slave population that we can calculate a sex ratio for them as well. Tlingit slave sex ratio is 88 out of a total sample of 630 (or 11% of the total population). The normal North Coast pattern of slave raiding, as described for the Sitka Tlingit in 1799, explains how this skewed ratio came about. "All men prisoners taken in battle are despatched without mercy—the females they save for wives and mistresses, the children in turn get to [be] one of the tribe" (Sturgis 1978: 36). An addition of alien females to the Tlingit population improved the total sex ratio (from 123 to 118) and undoubtedly helped compensate for a lack of female labor in the workforce. There may, indeed, have been a cultural correlation among Tlingit between high sex ratios and raiding for women (DiVale and Harris 1976).[21] Following this line of reasoning, excess female mortality during epidemics may have accentuated the propensity for raiding.

19. E.g., from July 1791 at Yakutat: "The surrender of a female infant is not strange in a country where the rearing brings the mother not only great care and fatigue but also a great deprivation of conjugal pleasure, where the small number of people fitted for war and fishing gives the male a value infinitely greater than the other half of our species" (Malaspina 1934: 210).

20. It is also probable that at least some of the extra 29 males for every 100 females in the 1842 census were seasonal visitors from non-Tlingit populations. Two of the largest adult sex ratios (230 and 137) occur among *kwan* (Chilkat and Stikine) situated on salmon-run rivers. The upstream portions of both drainage systems were occupied by Athapascan peoples, who maintained close socioeconomic ties with their Tlingit neighbors and were the probable source population for the hypothesized visitors. Non-Indian enumerators, as elsewhere on the coast, assumedly were not aware of the ethnicity of non-Tlingit visitors and counted them among Tlingit men.

21. DiVale and Harris (1976) hypothesize a causal relationship between female infanticide, high sex ratios, and warfare among hunting-gathering societies. But female infanticide was certainly not the only explanation for the abnormal Tlingit sex ratio. Female infanticide appears to have occurred infrequently in many North Coast populations, and most of the region's *total* sex ratios are normal, providing no demographic impetus for raiding for females. Only one other coastal population for which adequate figures exist (Kitkatla Sabassas) offers any pos-

Tsimshian: Population Statistics. Population figures for Tsimshian peoples in the first half of the 1800s are very limited (table 11). For the pre-epidemic period there is only the 1829 "5,500 speakers of the Nass language" from a report of a cruising ship (Green 1915: 39), which certainly includes only the more accessible coastal Tsimshian. The HBC's Fort Simpson census probably dates from 1842, the same time as the Tlingit census.[22] The HBC census (table 12) includes two of the four Tsimshian-speaking groups: Nisga'a and Tsimshian proper, with total numbers of 1,615 and 2,826, respectively. A second detailed census for the Fort Simpson Tsimshian, taken in 1858, resulted in numbers nearly identical to those reported 16 years earlier. The Reverend William Duncan stated: "I have been inside 140 houses. In all I counted 2,156 souls." Allowing for those not present, the total was raised to 2,352; including lineage members married and resident elsewhere, it was 2,567 (Duncan 1869: 25–26). The inland Gitxsan were not formally enumerated until 1889, and the south coast Sabassas (the nineteenth-century name for the Kitkatla, Kitkiata, and Kitasoo) were counted in the Fort McLoughlin census and will be considered later.

Tsimshian mortality from the 1836 epidemic is known from a very specific statement by the Fort Simpson head, John Work, who maintained that smallpox "carried off nearly one-third of the Chimsyans, the tribe who inhabit about Fort Simpson" (1838). Assuming Work's observations were accurate, we may extrapolate a pre-epidemic figure: 2,423 Nisga'a and 4,239 Tsimshian proper in the early 1830s. Tsimshian and Nisga'a mortality from the 1836 epidemic would therefore approximate 2,221 (6,662 − 4,441). Haida deaths, assuming the same one-third loss figure, would be 3,163. The estimated mortality for the Tlingit is 2,625 (9,880 − 7,255, or 27%). The subtotal for the Fort Simpson District (Tlingit, Haida, Nisga'a, and Tsimshian; Gitxsan excluded and perhaps spared from this outbreak) is 8,009 deaths in 1836.

---

sible support for the DiVale-Harris hypothesis. There are, in addition, numerous other reasons, documented and hypothetical, behind Northwest warfare (see Ferguson 1984). In addition, by the historical period (the time of this census), Tlingit were resorting to other means to obtain slaves: "Though under the Russian rule wars among the Tlingit tribes became of rare occurrence, the number of slaves did not diminish. The supply was kept up by barter with the more southern tribes, and at that time a majority of the slaves belonged to the Flathead Indians of the British Possessions" (Petrov in Averkieva 1971: 330).

22. It also was printed in Kane's appendix, with the date 1846, so must refer to the period prior to that time. A marginal note indicates that it was taken after the abandonment of Fort McLoughlin, which occurred in 1842.

Tsimshian: Population Structure. The population structure of the 2,826 Coast Tsimshian recorded in the 1842 Fort Simpson census is remarkable for its "flatness." The sex ratio is normal (104), percentage of children is medium (38%), and there seem to be no significant variations, geographic or otherwise, among constituent groups. The reason for this undistinguished pattern is probably to be found in the recent history of this people. By 1842 all the Coast Tsimshian "tribes" had apparently moved from their aboriginal villages on the Skeena and coast to their historic locations in the vicinity of Fort Simpson on the Tsimshian Peninsula (Dorsey 1897: 281). Any significant local environmental influences on the various tribes had apparently already been ironed out by 1842.

Nisga'a (Nass River Tsimshian) population figures from the 1842 Fort Simpson census were collected from four villages, totaling 1,615 persons. Two characteristics of the population structure are notable. First, the adult sex ratio is skewed in favor of men, at 124. The bulk of this difference (over 100 men) is recorded for Gitkateen village, located at the mouth of the Nass, and is probably attributable to the presence of seasonal "visitors," following the mainland Tlingit model, at the Nass fishery. Likely source populations for these alien men are multiple: the village was the regional headquarters for an important spring run of eulachon and the terminus of a "grease trail" from the interior (Garfield 1951: 10). A second pattern in the Nisga'a figures is a sharp difference (29% vs. 45%) in the percentage of children between the two villages above the canyon of the Nass (Gitwunksithk and Gitlakdamiks) and those nearer the river's mouth (Gitkateen and Gitgigenik). Part of this difference may be due to the relatively small size of the sample or to differential exposure to the 1836 smallpox epidemic. On the other hand, it may be a reflection of differences in the resource base and economic well-being of the coastal and interior villages. These two patterns, apparent in the Nisga'a census but absent in the Coast Tsimshian figures, may preserve normal North Coast patterns uninfluenced by movement to trading posts.

Post-1862 Demography

In 1862 smallpox again broke out on the North Coast. This time it skipped the island Tlingit (perhaps due in part to the vaccination program undertaken by the Russians after the 1836 epidemic) but took a heavy toll among the mainland Tlingit and Tsimshian, and decimated the Haida.

Haida. The approximate population of the Haida prior to 1836 was 9,490; following the 1836 epidemic, it may have been one-third less, or 6,327; in 1882 it was near 1,658 (O'Reilly 1883; Chittenden 1884; Petrov 1884), a cumulative drop of 83%. The post-1862 statistics for the Haida are particularly interesting, for they show quite clearly the process of village abandonment and amalgamation that had occurred many times earlier on the North Coast in response to epidemic depopulation. In the mid–nineteenth century there were between 11 (Poole 1872: 309) and 13 (Douglas 1878) major inhabited villages of Queen Charlotte Haida; surveys of the Queen Charlottes made in 1882–83 showed that 8 villages were still occupied. By 1890 there were only 3, and by the turn of the century only the modern settlements of Skidegate and Masset remained. The Kaigani villages survived a bit longer. Of the five listed by Petrov in 1880, four were still in existence when the mission town of Hydaburg was established in 1911 (Brink 1974: 226; see map 12).

The abandoned settlements ranged in size from 12 to 150 inhabitants (Chittenden 1884: 23–24); in pre-epidemic times the range (excluding Masset) had been from 120 to 738 (average, 331). There seems to have been a threshhold of viability for independent villages, probably determined by a combination of factors, including availability of marriage partners (MacCluer and Dyke 1976), subsistence-related task groups (Smith 1981), and minimum group levels for other cooperative endeavors.

Finding a potential marriage partner of approximately the right age and kin status (the Haida practiced clan exogamy with preferential mother's brother's daughter marriage) would be extremely difficult under the new conditions of depopulated and scattered communities. An early missionary commented on the problem of lack of women: "The situation was so serious that the young men appealed for his help in seeking wives among the Tsimshian" (in Brink 1974: 66). There are indications, but no documentary proof, that there was a draining off of eligible females to White settlements such as Victoria, which exacerbated the situation. A partial solution to the lack of eligible women would have been an amalgamation into settlements where the age-sex distribution was broad enough that mates would be available for most individuals. A relaxation of marriage restrictions would also help. It is regrettable that we have only gross numbers for late-nineteenth-century Haida population. Census figures could be converted into sex ratios that would give us more specific information on available mates; determining the percentage of children would be a clue to the fer-

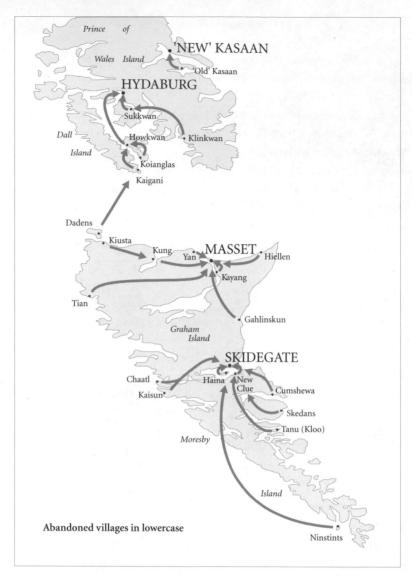

MAP 12. Haida Village Abandonment and Consolidation

tility of the population. In relation to the latter factor, an early Indian agent noted, "I was particularly struck, when visiting the several villages, by the small number of children" (O'Reilly 1883: 17). This, of course, represents a complete turnaround from the situation reported by Charles Fleurieu 90 years earlier (p. 210).

The three government-sponsored parties that visited the Queen Charlottes in 1882–84 (British Columbia Reserve Commission: O'Reilly; British Columbia

Haida Village Populations

Village	1830s[a]	1880–83[b]	1915–20[c]
Ninstints	308	30	
Tanu	545	150	
Skedans	439	12	
Cumshewa	286	60	
Kaisun	329		
Chaatl	561	108	
Skidegate	738	100	238
Gahlinskun	120		
Hiellen	280		
Tian	196		
Kung	122		
Kiusta	296		
Masset (Kayang-Uttewas-Yan)	2,473	350	350
Kaigani	234		
Koianglas	148	62[d]	
Howkwan	458	287[d]	335[e]
Klinkwan	417	125[d]	
Sukkwan	229	141[d]	
Kasaan	249	173	126
Total	8,428	1,598	1,049

[a] See Douglas 1878. Village spellings are from MacDonald 1983.

[b] See Chittenden 1884 for the Queen Charlotte villages; Petrov 1884 for the Kaigani villages.

[c] Skidegate and Masset (1915) from van den Brink 1974: 109; Hydaburg (1916–17) from Vaughan 1984: 186; New Kasaan from the 1920 U.S. census, p. 681.

[d] Survivors from these villages congregated at Hydaburg.

[e] Population of Hydaburg.

Commission of Land and Works: Chittenden; Smithsonian Institution: Swan and Deans) all traveled to and remarked upon the number of deserted villages and omnipresent mortuary structures (fig. 16). The following statements are reminiscent of those made both by the first explorers on the North Coast 90 years earlier and by emigrants to the lower Columbia in the 1830s and 1840s (chapter 9):

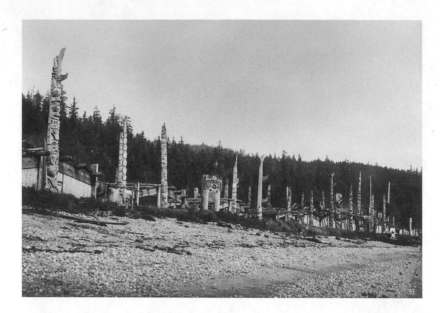

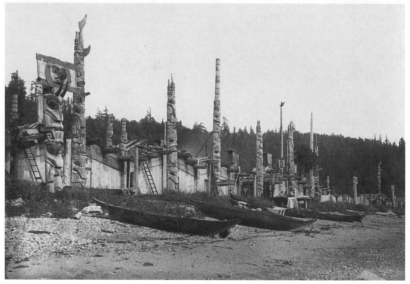

FIG. 16. Two photographs of Skidegate village taken by George Dawson on 26 July 1878, 16 years after a smallpox epidemic had devastated the Haida. They show a "forest of mortuary and memorial poles" (Cole and Lockner 1993: pl. 10), ubiquitous in Queen Charlotte Islands Indian villages of the 1870s. (Courtesy of National Archives of Canada, Ottawa, negative nos. PA-037755 and PA-037756.)

From the number and size of their houses now occupied, and ruins, from fifty to seventy in each village, their burial grounds and houses filled with the dead, these islands must have contained at least ten times their present population. (Chittenden 1884: 264)

6 September 1883

Kloo . . . [contained] 29 houses old and new, 13 totemic columns, 31 mortuary columns, 11 Posts with carved animals, and boxes on top of each containing remains of some deceased person. There are also 15 small houses containing remains of the dead. In fact the village presents more of the appearance of a cemetery than the abode of the living as the mortuary emblems outnumber the heraldic columns, and houses of the present inhabitants. (Swan 1883)

The villages described in these two quotations were totally abandoned within a few years of the observations.

Both observers also noted that village cemeteries were filled to overflowing. Haida were renowned for their totem poles, most of which were associated with death. Of the various functional types of totem poles, those used in house construction (portal poles and house fronts) appear to have a considerable antiquity, but detached poles definitely became more popular during the nineteenth century. Mortuary poles (associated with actual burials) are cited infrequently in the early-contact-period literature; memorial (commemorative) poles, however, are arguably nineteenth-century innovations. Tsimshian ethnographer Marius Barbeau suggested that the fashion for detached totem poles originated among the Nisga'a between 1840 and 1860 and became popular among the other North Coast peoples only after the latter date. Technological changes (the adoption of steel tools) and economic forces (fur trade enrichment) are reasons given for the late-nineteenth-century florescence of totem pole carving (Barbeau 1950; Duff 1964a).

No one has yet pointed out demographic changes that may have been just as important in explaining the historic florescence of totem pole art. There were heavy mortalities from smallpox in the totem pole area in both 1836 and 1862. Epidemic mortality definitely underlay the increase in size and number of Indian cemeteries on the lower Columbia in the 1830s (chapter 9). Historical shifts in material culture, fur trade enrichment, and demographic decline all contributed to an increase in the frequency, size, and intensity of nineteenth-century Kwakwaka'wakw potlatching (Codere 1950). I suspect all three factors were important in the contemporaneous rise of North Coast totem pole art. If a meaningful sample of North Coast totems could be accurately dated, it seems likely that their times of construction would cluster in two periods, 1836–46 and 1862–72. This is a hypothesis that, it seems to me, merits testing.

Tlingit. Tlingit population statistics for the 50 years after 1842 (table 9) are consistently poor.[23] The U.S. census of 1890, however, contains a detailed record of Tlingit population by both local group and village. There were 4,583 Tlingit speakers in 1890, compared to a probable 7,255 speakers 48 years earlier. This decline of 37% is attributable to three disease events: the measles outbreaks of 1848 and 1868 and the smallpox epidemic of 1862, as well as mortality associated with the bombardment of the Stikine village at Wrangell by the U.S. Navy in 1869. Mortality from the measles outbreaks was not great: probably no more than 10% of the affected populations in the 1848 visitation and a lesser proportion (due to acquired immunities) in the second. There were 508 Stikine enumerated at Wrangell in 1869 (Colyer 1870b: 11) just prior to the bombing. In 1890 Wrangell's Indian population was 228 and that of the Stikine tribe only 27 more. Casualties from this incident were not reported to be large; the statistics suggest otherwise. There is no evidence in the 1890 census that may be interpreted as dispersion from Wrangell to adjacent areas.

The remainder of the Tlingit population decline (something over 1,800 souls) was probably the result of mortality from the 1862 smallpox epidemic. In accordance with the historical record of the spread of the disease (chapter 7), most deaths seem to have been among the southern mainland (Tongass, Sanya, Stikine, Taku) and central islands (Kake, Hutsnuwu) tribes. Mortality among these peoples was probably about one-half. The figures for other Tlingit tribes in the 1842 and 1890 censuses show very little change.

Tsimshian. All of the Tsimshian peoples (Nisg̱a'a, Tsimshian proper, Git-x̱san, and Sabassas) were visited by the smallpox epidemic of 1862. Before and after population figures exist for all these groups. Four sets of figures are important: the 1842 Fort Simpson census (for the Nisg̱a'a and Tsimshian proper); William Duncan's 1858 Tsimshian proper census (which corroborates the HBC count); ethnologist George Dorsey's memory culture estimates (obtained from Indian informants in the 1890s) for all groups (most of which refer to the

23. Erman's 1861 numbers are high and out of line with their 1842 and 1890 counterparts and are therefore suspect; the Amory, Haleck, and Mahoney figures from the 1860s (with the exception of censuses of Stikine and Sitka) resulted from mere "eyeballing," and Petrov's 1881–82 "census" was in fact farmed out to a "special agent," about whom we know nothing, and whose numbers were then checked against church registers by Petrov.

pre-1862 period); and the 1889 censuses of the newly organized Northwest Coast and Babine–Upper Skeena River Indian Agencies of British Columbia. The only demographic patterns that can be discerned from these various statistics are losses, mostly attributable to the 1848 and 1868 measles outbreaks and the 1862 smallpox epidemic.

The Fort Simpson Tsimshian show 2,495 in 1842 and 2,352 in 1858, a difference close to the mortality of 250 reported by James Douglas for the 1848 measles outbreak (Bowsfield 1979: 22). The bulk of the 638 (27%) loss between 1858 and 1889 is attributable to the smallpox epidemic. The Reverend William Duncan, speaking from firsthand knowledge, stated that 500 had died at Fort Simpson alone in 1862–63 (diary entry, 6 March 1863). Total losses for the Tsimshian proper (Fort Simpson, Metlakatla, and Skeena River villages) between 1842 and 1889 were just over one-third.

The 1842 HBC census for the Nisga'a and Dorsey's memory count (1897: 278–80) (which probably refers to the period 1849–62) are nearly identical (1,615 and 1,530, respectively). In 1882 there were 877 Nisga'a; the circa 46% decline was probably due largely to smallpox and measles. The 1889 census, taken approximately one year after a dysentery epidemic (dating uncertain) on the Nass (Beynon n.d.: MSS 53 and 84), returned only 805; the 72, or 8%, difference being perhaps attributable to that disease event. Dorsey's memory culture population for the interior Gitxsan is 1,875. In 1889 the Indian Agency census returned 1,462.

Population decline for all three northern Tsimshian peoples in the mid-1800s is here set at 33%. This figure is close to the decline recorded for the Tlingit (37%) in the same time period but vastly different from that of the Haida (83%). The Tlingit and Tsimshian populations, on the whole, were able to absorb sequential epidemic losses while maintaining their sociocultural integrity. For the Tsimshian, in particular, there has been minimal change in the total number or identity of settlements between 1842 and the present. Population losses were great enough to affect the viability of local groups in only a few cases. The 1990 populations for both Tlingit and Tsimshian are close to what they were in 1838.

FORT MCLOUGHLIN DISTRICT

The Hudson's Bay Company's Fort McLoughlin, established in 1833 at the head of Milbanke Sound on the central British Columbia coast, dealt with the Sabassas ("Southern Tsimshian") villages (Kitkatla,[24] Kitkiata, and Kitasoo), the Haisla, Heiltsuk (Haihais, Istitoch, and Bella Bella) Oweekeno, and Nuxalk. The fort was abandoned in 1842. For the decade between 1835 and 1845 there are three very good sets of population statistics; one preceding, two following, the 1836 smallpox epidemic (table 13). The first is an 1835 estimate of Indian population in the entire district; the other two are censuses, dating from 1838 (Heiltsuk) and 1842 (other peoples), respectively (table 14). A summary count and later estimate by HBC officials are extant from the next decade. The 1889 census provides information which allows us to compute losses from the 1862 smallpox epidemic.

1835–1859 Statistics

The 1835 estimate was made by HBC official William Tolmie after his assignment to the fort in that year.[25] Comparison of the 1835 estimate with the 1838–42 censuses reveals some interesting patterns. The inland groups show a much greater decline in numbers than the coastal groups do. Most of this difference is undoubtedly attributable to a very real difference in smallpox mortality and the geographic extent of the epidemic.[26] From historical data presented in chapter 5 we know that smallpox did not reach Fort McLoughlin itself, though it raged at Fort Simpson. The similarity in numbers of the people nearest the fort, the Bella Bella, seems to support this historical record.

A comparison of before and after numbers for the various Fort McLoughlin peoples reveals the following. For the Kitkatla (northernmost Sabassas) there is an increase of 108 persons (15% of the 1842 total). This appears to be the beginning of a trend of Sabassas migration to the village on Porcher Island. The likely source of the migrants was Kitkiata; the stimulus, proximity to Fort

---

24. Kitkatla village traded at Fort Simpson, but its numbers are included here.

25. It exists in two parts: figures for the Bella Bella (Milbanke Heiltsuk) are in Tolmie's published diary (1963: 319); the remainder are in James Douglas's aforementioned (1878) compendium of Northwest population statistics (see n. 1, above). The Bella Bella count includes number of houses, men, and total population. The others consist of counts(?) of warriors, with total populations projected by using a multiplier of (usually) 4.2. Although this seems an unusually large multiplier I have retained it here.

26. Part of this variation is illusory, however, as the Nuxalk were certainly undercounted in the 1838 census (Talio and upriver Nuxalk villages omitted). I have corrected for this problem by replacing the 1838 Nuxalk figure (509) with a more realistic estimate (950), also made by William Tolmie, in 1856.

Simpson. If the 17% total loss for Sabassas which shows between the 1835 and 1838–42 enumerations is real, it most likely is attributable to depopulation in the southernmost Sabassas village of Kitasoo, which shows the greatest difference in numbers. Kitasoo was close to the two northernmost Heiltsuk groups, Haihais and Istitoch (see map 11), which show losses in the range of one-quarter to one-third. The population figures for the coastal groups of the Fort McLoughlin District, therefore, suggest that smallpox penetrated to the seacoast only in the vicinity of Princess Royal Island, while it missed the islands to the north and south.

The interior groups, Haisla and Nuxalk, show loss figures of 50% and 51%, respectively. The southern distribution of affected groups implies that the epidemic spread south, via Indian trails along the spine of the Coast Range. Jenness records that the Dakelhne(?) of the Eutsuk Lake area, just east of the divide, were "destroyed" by this epidemic (1943: 475). The western Dakelhne, Haisla, and Nuxalk were, like the Kitasoo, Haihais, and Istitoch on the coast, apparently too far from the HBC fort at Milbanke Sound to benefit from the stopgap measures that seem to have been initiated there (see chapter 5). Other than the Eutsuk Lake people, the greatest mortality apparently occurred in the densely and continuously populated Bella Coola River valley.

Central British Columbia Coast Population Structures. In a population sense, the region including the Kitkiata and Kitasoo Sabassas, Haisla, Heiltsuk, Nuxalk (censused from Fort McLoughlin in 1842; Douglas 1878), and Dakelhne (censused from Fort Alexandria in 1827 and 1839; McGillivray in Rich 1947; Anderson 1857) was a single interaction zone. The salient demographic characteristic of the region is a distinctive variation in population structure and resultant pattern of interaction between coastal and interior peoples:

	Sex Ratio			Point	Total (Nonslave)
	Total	Child	Adult	Difference	Population
South Dakelhne, 1827	122	161	97	+64	502
North Dakelhne, 1839	117	119	116	+3	941
Haisla, 1842	113	132	108	+24	369
Nuxalk	105	101	108	−7	509
Kitkiata and Kitasoo	95	92	96	−4	251
Istitoch and Oweekeno	108	83	122	−39	483
Bella Bella	95	72	103	−31	1,206

Some of these groups are very small, and it is possible that the Bella Bella census undercounted boys. But these potential drawbacks probably do not invalidate the overall pattern. The Dakelhne were an exclusively inland people; the Haisla and Nuxalk resided along rivers and at the heads of long coastal fjords; the southern Sabassas, Heiltsuk, and Oweekeno were exclusively coastal, saltwater peoples. The Dakelhne and Haisla have high child sex ratios (csrs), which suggests differential care of children by sex and perhaps preferential female infanticide; the coastal groups' csrs are low normal. The adult sex ratios of both interior and coastal peoples, however, are near normal. There seems to have been some population exchange between the interior and coastal groups.

One means of correcting a sexual imbalance among adults would be raiding for females by those groups lacking them. Although this seems to have been a pattern among the Tlingit and Kitkatla Sabassas, the extant ethnographic literature from the central British Columbia coast suggests that more southern peoples chose a different solution. The data on the Nuxalk (McIlwraith 1948) and adjoining Alkatcho Dakelhne (Goldman 1940) reveal an interesting pattern of intermarriage consistent with imbalanced sex ratios. According to Goldman, "most marriages appear to have been between Dakelhne men and Nuxalk women" (345); McIlwraith states, "There was a good deal of intermarriage between [the Dakelhne] and the inhabitants of the upper valley" (1948: 1.18). Given a pattern of strict patrilocality, the wife would be expected to move inland, carrying her Nuxalk traditions with her. The Dakelhne man, because of the Nuxalk marital mode of gift exchange, would become economically tied to his wife's family. In historic times, with the growth of the fur trade and subsequent enrichment of Dakelhne trappers, they were better able to afford the economic obligations involved in marrying a Nuxalk woman, and the rate of intermarriage apparently increased.

Acculturation is the logical outcome of this form of intermarriage, and indeed, all ethnographers of the Dakelhne (Goldman 1940; Jenness 1943; Steward 1960) have commented upon the rapid diffusion, in the early contact period, of coastal culture—in particular the "potlatch-rank complex"— to the Dakelhne. All have noted that intermarriage was a key factor in this process, but none has identified the underlying demographic constant that contributed to the desire of inland men to seek marital ties with coastal peoples. This same pattern—of intermarriage between coastal and interior groups encouraged by differing sex ratios—appears elsewhere on the North-west Coast, though with slightly different cultural ramifications.

CUMULATIVE EPIDEMIC MORTALITIES

Mortality from the 1836 Smallpox Epidemic

At this point we may summarize the data on mortality from the 1836 small-pox epidemic in the north. The adjusted figures, from Hudson's Bay population estimates and censuses, and coordinate ethnohistorical data are given in the following table.

	Pre-epidemic Population	*Post-epidemic Population*	*Numerical Loss*	*Percentage Loss*
Tlingit	9,880	7,255	2,625	27
Nisga'a	2,423	1,615	808	33
Tsimshian	4,239	2,826	1,413	33
Haida[a]	9,490	6,327	3,163	33[a]
Haisla	825	409	416	50
North Heiltsuk[b]	875	579	296	34
Nuxalk	1,940	1,056[c]	884	46
Total	29,672	20,067	9,605[d]	32

[a] Evidence for inclusion of Haida is limited. The HBC's figure of one-third mortality from the Fort Simpson area has been extended to the Queen Charlottes.

[b] Includes the Sabassas Tsimshian Kitasoo and the Heiltsuk Haihais and Istitoch.

[c] Tolmie's 1856 estimate has been increased to allow for 10% measles mortality in 1848.

[d] Including statistics for the remainder of the peoples of Alaska's Pacific coast (Chugach, Tanaina, Koniag, and Aleut) from Fedorova 1973: 276–77 adds nearly 3,500 more deaths.

The common wisdom among HBC officials was that the 1836 epidemic claimed one-third of the population of the North Coast (McLoughlin in Rich 1941: 271; Simpson 1847: 1.123). The 1868 U.S. government report *Message on Russian America* stated, "In 1838 ten thousand persons on the coast are reported to have fallen victims to this disease" (159). The contemporary estimates of the demographic impact of the 1836 epidemic are in very close agreement with the population data that have survived from this period.

1860–1890 Statistics

The first complete and trustworthy census of the central British Columbia coast peoples after 1842 is the 1889 Northwest Coast Indian Agency census.[27] The figures show a decline of 64%—from circa 4,212 following the 1836 epidemic to 1,507 in 1889. The decrease was mostly a result of measles and smallpox mortality, though lack of specific historical data may obscure secondary processes. As stated earlier, mortality from the 1848 measles epidemic was set by observers at 10%; the 1868 outbreak probably claimed half that figure. The Haisla, who escaped the 1862 smallpox epidemic, declined only 11% (from 409 to 364) in this half-century.

Some data from this time period indicate abandonment of several Central Coast villages whose populations had dropped beneath the threshhold of viability, and migration to centrally located Indian settlements. The evidence in this instance consists not of actual population figures from the affected villages but of ethnographic testimony collected by McIlwraith (Nuxalk) and Olson (Heiltsuk). The 23 of 45 recorded villages of the Nuxalk known to be inhabited in 1793 were reduced by about half in 1889 and were down to 3 when McIlwraith conducted his fieldwork in 1922–24 (1948: 15–16). The equally numerous villages of the Heiltsuk had diminished to 4 at the time they were censused in 1889. Survivors of 6 "village-tribes" united at the settlement at Bella Bella in the 1870s (Olson 1955: 320). A biethnic community (Haihais Heiltsuk and Kitasoo Sabassas) was formed at Klemtu.

Mortality from the 1862 Smallpox Epidemic

The bulk of the population decline was caused by the 1862 smallpox epidemic. Summary figures for this major demographic event for the entire North Coast (including Kwakwaka'wakw and Comox, not discussed here) are presented in the following table. Sources (unless otherwise indicated) are as noted in the chapter text. Loss figures for interior British Columbia peoples have not been computed.

Duff (1964b: 43) estimated that approximately 20,000 Indians died of smallpox in British Columbia during 1862–63. This reconstruction excludes Tlingit,

27. Some later HBC figures, apparently no longer extant, were used by the British explorers Warre and Vavasour for their 1845 summary statement on the Indian population of the Oregon Territory. William Tolmie's and Jonathan Amory's 1856 and 1867 figures are estimates.

	Pre-epidemic Population[a]	Post-epidemic Population[b]	Numerical Loss	Percentage Loss
Island Tlingit (Hutsnuwu and Kake)	1,088[a]	688[b]	400	37
Mainland Tlingit (Taku, Stikine, Tongass/Sanya)	2,471[a]	1,025[b,c]	1,446	59
Nisga'a	1,454[a]	923[b]	531	37
Tsimshian	2,543[a]	1,967[b]	576	23
Gitxsan	1,875	1,462	413	22
Sabassas	918	299[b]	619	67
Haida	5,694[a]	1,598	4,096	72
Nuxalk	950	398[b]	552	58
Heiltsuk	1,650[a]	506[b]	1,144	69
Kwakwaka'wakw[d]	7,965[a,e]	3,750[f]	4,215	53
Comox[d]	1,080[a,g]	847	233	22
Songhees-Saanich[d]	1,649[a]	468	1,181	72
Total	29,337	13,931	15,406	53

[a] Where appropriate, pre-1848 figures have been decreased by 10% to allow for losses from the 1848 measles epidemic.

[b] Where appropriate, post-1868 figures have been increased by 5% to allow for losses from the 1868 measles outbreak. Since most post-epidemic counts are from 1880–90 censuses, they may include nonsmallpox population decline from the years following the epidemic, hence over-stating total smallpox mortality.

[c] Includes an allowance for deaths in the 1869 Wrangell bombardment.

[d] Population history is not covered in this chapter.

[e] Source is Tolmie's 1835 estimate (1963: 317–18), revised by Galois (1994: 38).

[f] Source is Compton's 1866 estimate (Galois 1994: 36–37).

[g] 300 men (times 4) (Douglas 1931: 17).

of course, and includes interior peoples (Tsilhqot'in, Dakelhne, Stl'atl'imx, Nlaka'pamux, and western bands of Secwepemc) who were severely affected during the winter of 1862–63. My approximated loss figures suggest that Duff's 20,000 British Columbia mortality figure is very close to reality, and that in 1862 nearly 14,000 First Nations lives were lost on the British Columbia coast alone.

Conclusion

The corpus of North Coast population data, drawn from the historical literature and presented in this chapter, documents considerable depopulation
during the period 1835–90. Total population in 1835 is estimated at 33,915; in
1889–90 it was around 11,416, a decline of 66%, or about two-thirds. The bulk
of this loss, perhaps as much as 90%, was the result of mortality from two
smallpox epidemics, in 1836 and 1862. Depopulation as measured from the
aboriginal period, which terminated with the smallpox epidemic of the 1770s,
was certainly even greater.

9 / Lower Columbia Population History,
1775–1855

The "lower Columbia," as here defined, includes several ethnolinguistic groups in the lower Columbia River drainage who shared a common disease history during the first century of contact with Euro-Americans.[1] They include most Chinookan peoples, consisting of the Chinook proper (Chinook Clatsop) and four regional groupings of "Upper Chinookan"–speaking villagers: Cathlamet (Cathlamet-Wakaikam and Skilloot), "Wappato"[2] (Multnomah and other Sauvie Island area villages), Clackamas (including the villages at Willamette Falls), and Cascades (Lewis and Clark's "Shahala");[3] the Kalapuyans of the Willamette Valley (Tualatin-Yamhill and Santiam); and various smaller groups inhabiting drainages of minor lower Columbia feeder streams (those speakers of Northwest Sahaptin who are generally referred to as "Klikitat"; the northern Cascade Range segment of the Molala; the Salishan-

1. This area corresponds to the geographical core of Hajda's "Greater lower Columbia" interaction zone (1984), which is defined by a shared system of social networks and culture elements among several peoples of varying ethnicity.

2. There is no standard designation for this village cluster. Although Silverstein (1990: 534) uses the term "Multnomah" after a major village, I prefer "Wappato," the name used by Lewis and Clark.

3. I follow David French (pers. comm., 1989), but differ from vols. 7 and 14 (*Northwest Coast* and *Plateau*) of the Smithsonian's *Handbook of North American Indians* in placing the Cascades people in the Northwest Coast culture area. The furthest upstream Chinookan speakers, the White Salmon and Wasco-Wishram, whose cultural orientation was to the Plateau, are not included in the following discussion.

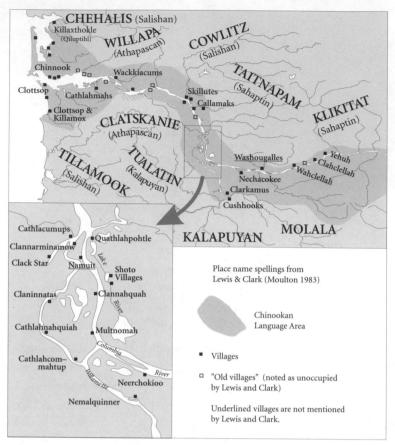

MAP 13. Chinookan Villages before 1830

speaking Cowlitz; and the Athapascan-speaking Clatskanie and Kwalhioqua). Locations of these peoples are shown on map 13.

The Indian populations of the lower Columbia suffered more from the effects of introduced diseases than those of any other subregion of the Northwest Coast culture area. The Chinookans, whose villages were situated along the banks of the Columbia, experienced epidemics of smallpox (1770s and 1801–2), an unidentified "mortality" in 1824–25 (probably smallpox, perhaps measles), malaria (1830 and later), dysentery (1844), measles (1848), and smallpox (1853).

Given this disease history, depopulation on the lower Columbia was truly fearsome. Surviving demographic data on this decline are of varying quality. There are only a few rough estimates of local groups for the initial 30 years of contact (1775–1804). Lewis and Clark's 1805–6 "Estimate of the Western Indians" is a valuable document that gives baseline total populations for most of the lower Columbia peoples. Hudson's Bay Company (HBC) statistics include early summary figures in Parker (1837, 1838, 1936) and four 1838 censuses of remnant groups. Later estimates and censuses from the 1840s and 1850s, though spotty, are sufficiently complete to clearly document the degree of depopulation following the introduction of malaria and changes in internal structures that eventually led to extinction, amalgamation, or survival of lower Columbia peoples by the late 1800s.

THE EARLIEST ESTIMATES

Although the contact period for Native Americans of the lower Columbia began with the Spanish Hezeta expedition of 1775, the earliest surviving population statistics date from the 1792 Vancouver expedition. In October of that year Lieutenant William Broughton reconnoitered the lower Columbia as far upstream as the site of modern Washougal. Off a "very large Indian village" (Quathlahpohtle) at the mouth of the Lewis River, he encountered "Twenty-three canoes carrying from three to twelve persons each," or "near two hundred" people in all (Broughton in Vancouver 1798: 2.61; Bell 1932: 143). A short distance upstream, near the Sauvie Island villages of Clannaquah and Multnomah, "an hundred and fifty natives in twenty-five canoes appeared" (62). In two days the explorers saw a total of 350 men in forty-eight canoes (7 per canoe), representing an aggregate population of 1,400 (using S. Cook's multiplier of 4), close to Lewis and Clark's April 1806 total of 1,830 for the same three villages.

LEWIS AND CLARK'S ESTIMATES

After James Douglas's compendium of HBC censuses, the second most important document in Northwest Coast demographic history is Lewis and Clark's 1805–6 "Estimate of the Western Indians" (table 15).[4] The estimate, which covered all the peoples of the Columbia River drainage, plus the Oregon and Washington coasts, was first assembled at Fort Clatsop in winter 1805–6 and revised in June 1806 on the upper Missouri (Lewis and Clark 1990: 473).

---

4. Thomas Jefferson, who conceived the expedition and appointed Meriwether Lewis to direct it, requested that the explorers gather data on a long list of ethnographic topics, among them specific information on "the names of the nations and their numbers" (letter of 20 June 1803 to Lewis, in Jackson 1978: 62).

The explorers used a combination of methods, in particular house counts and informant testimony, to arrive at their numbers. Peoples encountered on the explorers' route along the banks of the Columbia were estimated *twice*, in the autumn 1805 descent and spring 1806 ascent of the river. Numbers for those away from the river were computed after discussions with knowledge-able informants, apparently through the limited vocabulary of the Chinook Jargon. The autumn 1805 and spring 1806 versions of the estimate differ significantly in some key numbers. For Chinookan villages between Cathlamet and The Cascades rapids, the autumn estimate lists a total of 6,660; the spring equivalent is 13,740 (more than double) for the same units. For over 150 years (until 1990) only the larger, spring estimate was in print, giving an inflated impression of Chinookan populations.[5]

Seasonal Movements and Co-occupation

The substantial difference between autumn and spring Columbia river pop-ulations in the Lewis and Clark estimates appears to be a result of population movement toward the Columbia during fishing season (Boyd and Hajda 1987), a pattern that has been recognized for some time for the furthest upstream Chinookan peoples at The Dalles, the Wasco-Wishram. David French, eth-nographer of the Wasco-Wishram, discusses estimates from that area:

Spier and Sapir [in the 1930 "Wishram Ethnography"], combining data from Lewis and Clark with their own, arrive at a rough estimate of 1,000 to 1,500 for total Wishram population at the beginning of the nineteenth century. Because of ecological variability and the problem of defining the boundaries of groups, it is impossible to achieve a more accurate estimate than this. . . . [Alexander] Ross [in the 1810s] estimated that the total population at Five Mile Rapids village swelled to 3,000 during the summer fishing and trading season. (1963: 343)

Fish runs dictated this seasonal population shift. Aboriginally, the Co-lumbia River was the most productive salmon stream in the world, with five

---

5. The spring 1806 version ("Estimate of the Western Indians") appeared in the first, 1814 edition of Lewis and Clark's journals and in most reprints since that time. The autumn 1805 esti-mate ("Codex I"), a manuscript in the American Philosophical Society Library in Philadelphia, was not printed until 1990, in vol. 6 of the University of Nebraska Press's definitive edition of the Lewis and Clark journals.

salmonid (*Oncorhynchus*) species (chinook, coho, steelhead, chum, and sockeye) ascending the river between March and October. The fishing season usually began in February with an early run of the nonsalmonid eulachon (locally called "smelt," *Thaleichthys pacificus*). Chinook salmon (*O. tshawytscha*), the most favored and abundant salmonid, appeared on the river in three runs (spring, summer, and fall). Spring salmon (and eulachon too) are fat and oily and ended the lower-river peoples' long winter fast from fresh foods; the salmon of the abundant fall run, with their lower oil content, preserve well and were the major source of sustenance between November and May (Franchère 1969: 11). Salmon tend to congregate at the mouths of feeder streams before beginning their ascent to spawning grounds; lower Columbia tributaries vary widely in number and regularity of runs. As a rule, upstream peoples had fewer and less reliable runs than those on the main Columbia.

Throughout the lower Columbia in the early nineteenth century, marriages and other socioeconomic ties linked winter villages of varying ethnicity in social networks that constituted a larger interaction region (Hajda 1984). Seasonal movement and co-use and co-occupation of resource areas and villages seems to have been the norm throughout the region. Chinookan peoples moved seasonally from Willapa Bay and Seaside to the river's mouth, laterally along the Columbia between Gray's Bay and the Cowlitz, and from The Cascades rapids to the "Wappato Valley," while centrally located Wappato (Multnomah) villagers probably moved relatively little.[6]

More important, however, non-Chinookan peoples from winter villages located at some distance from the Columbia removed to the river and mixed with Chinookan populations during fishing season. These interior peoples were known to early-nineteenth-century observers as basically hunters and gatherers of roots and berries.[7] Seasonal visitors to The Dalles fishery (see above) were mostly (but not exclusively) neighboring Columbia Sahaptin-speaking peoples. A likely reconstruction of lower-river visitors includes the following. Between The Cascades and Kalama River on the north side of the Columbia, Northwest Sahaptin-speaking Klikitats converged on the Columbia

6. Documentation for these various movements is available for (1) the river mouth Chinook-Clatsop (Minor 1983; Kennedy 1824–25), (2) Cathlamet-Wakaikam and Skilloot (Minor 1983: 197–98; Lewis and Clark 1990: 201; Stuart 1935: 30), (3) Cascades (Lewis and Clark 1991: 40, 57, 99), and (4) Wappato (Dunnell, Chatters, and Salo 1973; Saleeby and Pettigrew 1983).

7. E.g., Henry 1992: 641, 657, 684, 715, on Clatskanie, Clackamas, Cowlitz, and Northwest Sahaptin, respectively.

during salmon season (Norton, Boyd, and Hunn 1983). In villages near the mouth of the Clackamas River and on Multnomah Channel there may have been a seasonal presence of Kalapuyan speakers. There were probably Molala on the Clackamas River and interior Athapascans seasonally at Wakaikam and Cathlamet and maybe even Clack Star and Killaxthokle villages. And Salishan-speaking peoples (Cowlitz and Lower Chehalis) were present at or near village clusters of the Skillutes and Chinook proper.[8]

With this background in fish ecology and socioeconomic relations in the aboriginal lower Columbia Valley, we can analyze Lewis and Clark's estimates. Table 15 reproduces and compares the figures for lower-river Chinookans from autumn 1805 and spring 1806 estimates. The autumn populations, tallied in November after the fishing season had ended, are low (half that of the spring 1806 populations) and probably represent only the permanently resident Chinookans. Village populations of the later estimate, from late March and early April 1806, approximately the end of the eulachon and the beginning of the spring salmon seasons, are more than double those from the autumn, and probably represent the arrival of inlanders on the riverbanks to take advantage of the fishery.

The largest differences between the autumn and spring estimates, for major villages and village clusters, are given in the following table:

Percentage Difference	Numerical Difference
Multnomah 75%	Clarkamus 1,000
Clack Star 71%	Skillutes 1,000
Quathlahpohtle 67%	Clack Star 850
Cathlacumups 66%	Multnomah 600
Cathlahnahquiah 63%	Quathlahpohtle 600

It is instructive to compare these differences with what is known about the spring fish runs. Village clusters located at or near the mouths of two of the three regular smelt-run rivers, the Cowlitz and the Lewis, show major increases in numbers in the spring estimates: an addition of 1,000 (40%) in the Skillute villages, and 1,450 (69%) in the two villages (Quathlahpohtle and Clack Star) located at and across from the mouth of the Lewis River. The "Clarkamus" villages, situated on a spring salmon river, increased in num-

8. Most early Euro-American observers did not comment on and were probably unable to recognize the presence of non-Chinookans, given the basic external cultural similarity of lower

bers by 1,000 (56%). And Multnomah village, located centrally on the Columbia bank of Sauvie Island, near the Willamette mouth and in an area favorable to both fishing and intergroup exchange, increased by 600 people, or 75%.

Reconstructed 1805 Upper Chinookan Populations

The above discussion suggests that the autumn 1805 and spring 1806 estimates represent two seasonally distinct populations. The 1805 numbers, collected in early November, are here assumed to approximate a core population of 6,660 Upper Chinookan speakers, resident at that time of the year in riverine winter villages. The 1806 numbers, apparently representative of the demographic situation in early April, are assumed to include a sizeable number of non-Chinookan-speaking seasonal visitors.

Many of the minor lower Columbia non-Chinookan peoples are not separately enumerated in either of the estimates. A note at the bottom of one of the "Codex I" (autumn 1805 estimate) pages acknowledges their presence thusly: "there are several other nations residing on the Columbia below the grand rappids and on some streams which discharge themselves into the same whose names we have learnt but have not any proper data from which to calculate their probable number; therefor omitted" (Lewis and Clark 1990: 475). The numbers for most of these unidentified peoples are probably included in the 7,080 difference between the autumn and spring Upper Chinookan village totals. Educated guesses as to their identities and approximate populations appear in column 2 of table 15.

All of the above numbers, of course, are representative of early-nineteenth-

---

Columbia peoples plus the presence of bilinguals and use of Chinook Jargon (Yvonne Hajda, pers. comm., 1984). Evidence for my reconstruction includes the following. (1) The name "Charcowah," one of the Willamette Falls villages, by its prefix, may be Kalapuyan (Yvonne Hajda, pers. comm., 1984); Kalapuyans came to Willamette Falls to trade and to fish for eels (Henry 1992: 658; Jacobs 1945: 43); the common ethnohistorical reference to Multnomah Channel Chinookan villages as Kalapuyan may indicate co-presence (e.g., Ross 1849: 236). (2) Molala were present at Oregon City by the 1840s (Allen 1848: 235). Ethnographic and ethnohistoric evidence supports several seasonal extensions of interior Athapascans to fishing areas (Krauss 1990); the confusion over the identity of Clack Star village (called by Clark, in Jackson 1978: 2.542, both "a separate people" and "a tribe of the Multnomah") suggests Athapascan/Chinookan mixing. (3) The Cowlitz village list collected by Edward Curtis from an informant born ca. 1835 includes several co-occupied Columbia River settlements (1913: 172). In the early decades of the 1800s, Chehalis speakers camped in their own midsummer fishing settlement near the mouth of the Columbia (Cox 1957: 56; Corney 1965: 144).

century populations and are probably significantly below the precontact totals, which would have been much reduced by the 1770s and 1801–2 smallpox epidemics. The ethnic mixing that seems to have been characteristic of Lewis and Clark's time may have been to a large degree a product of recent heavy depopulation in the riverine areas, which allowed upstream, inland peoples to move in. A similar phenomenon has been reported elsewhere in the Americas, for instance the lower Mississippi, where inland Chickasaw and Choctaw replaced depopulated riverine Tunica and Natchez villages (Dobyns 1983: 305–8). Ethnic replacement was certainly a pattern in the postfever (1830 and following) lower Columbia, as we shall see.

Kalapuya and Molala

Lewis and Clark's estimate of aboriginal Kalapuya (Willamette Valley) population, 2,000 persons, must be reevaluated. The Willamette drainage, in aboriginal times, was home to only two ethnolinguistic groups: Kalapuya (with a number of subdivisions) and Molala. Both versions of the "Estimate," however, name three bands of "Shoshones" resident at least part of the year on the "Multnomah" (Willamette) River. "Shoshone" appears to have been a common contemporary designation for Indians of a generalized interior culture, regardless of ethnic affiliation (e.g., Stuart 1935: 48). The smallest of these groups, the "Shobarboobeer" band "high up . . . on the SW Side of the Multnomah," cannot be certainly identified.[9] The second largest of the Multnomah "Shoshone" groups (3,000 in number), described as "resideing in winter and fall on the Multnomah . . . and in spring and summer . . . at the falls of the Towarnehiooks [Deschutes River] for the purpose of fishing for the Salmon" (Lewis and Clark 1990: 480) is probably the Molala (Ray 1938: 391); some Columbia Sahaptin (*tayx*) may be included (Eugene Hunn, pers. comm.). The other 6,000 Multnomah "Shoshones," apparently resident on the Willamette year-round, can only be Kalapuya (Zenk 1976: 9). In addition, on linguistic grounds, I am assigning the 200 residents of Charcowah village at Willamette Falls to the Kalapuya.[10] The sum total of the various Kalapuyan groups in the Lewis and Clark estimates is, therefore, 8,200. It

---

9. An educated guess is the Kalapuyan Yoncalla of the Umpqua River Valley.

10. An additional 850 Kalapuyans may also be included among the salmon season visitors to Chinookan villages at Willamette Falls and along Multnomah Channel (see table 15). More

should be emphasized that the Lewis and Clark Kalapuya estimates were not based on firsthand observation but obtained from Chinookan-speaking informants, probably through the limited medium of Chinook Jargon. Nevertheless, 8,200 is a ballpark figure for 1805–6 and much more compatible with the late-1820s HBC estimate of 7,785–8,780 Kalapuyans than the 2,000 that a literal reading of Lewis and Clark provides.[11]

1811–1830 ESTIMATES

Despite the continuous presence of Euro-Americans on the lower Columbia between 1811 and 1830, there are few contemporary records on Indian populations. Only three deserve mention: Astorian Robert Stuart's 1812 tally of numbers of warriors (in Stuart 1935), the total population figures preserved in the 1824–25 Fort George report (in Kennedy 1824–25), and Samuel Parker's Kalapuyan estimates for the late 1820s (in Parker 1838, 1936). All three estimates are reproduced in table 16.

Estimates of the Astorians and Nor'westers

Stuart's numbers, for the most part, seem to have been based upon firsthand observation during the height of the summer salmon season (late June to July) of 1812. (Both the 1805 and 1824–25 estimates date from the colder half of the year.) Multiplied by Cook's 4, most of his warrior counts yield totals that are consistent with the earlier and later estimates, with differences that may be explained as due to seasonal population variations.

For the downstream peoples, Stuart's summer totals (1,976 Chinook and Clatsop; 640 Cathlamet and Wakaikam) nearly double the earlier winter estimates; the difference may well be due to seasonally resident outsiders (Chehalis and Tillamook Salish; Kwalhioqua and Clatskanie Athapascans). His tallies for four Wappato Valley villages are even more instructive when compared with Lewis and Clark, as follows:

---

likely, however, these duplicate part of the population included in Lewis and Clark's "Callahpoewah Nation."

11. Anthropologist James Mooney, whose aboriginal population estimates (1928) were the standard for over 50 years, used Lewis and Clark's 2,000 to project an aboriginal (presmallpox) total of only 3,000 Kalapuyans.

Village	Lewis and Clark		Stuart (×4)
	November	*April*	*July*
Callamaks	200	200	480
Quathlahpohtle	300	900	720
Clannarminamow	280	280	280
Multnomah	200	800	520[a]
	980	2,180	2,000

[a] Two versions: 130 men in the traveling memorandum, 80 in the printed journal.

If this reconstruction is correct, local winter village populations may have doubled for the summer salmon fishery and increased nearly two and a quarter times for the early spring salmon and smelt runs.

For the second decade of the 1800s, Nor'wester (North West Company) Alexander Ross supplied an estimate of warrior strength for the area around the mouth of the Columbia (1849: 87): "All the Indian tribes inhabiting the country about the mouth of the Columbia, and for a few hundred miles round, may be classed in the following manner: 1. Chinooks;—2. Clatsops;—3. Cathlamux;—4. Wakicums;—5. Wacalamus;—6. Cattleputles;—7. Clatscanias;—8. Killimux;—9. Moltnomas; and,—10. Chickeles; amounting collectively to about 2,000 warriors." Using Cook's multiplier of 4 on Ross's warrior count yields an aggregate population of 8,000. The total for the equivalent units in Lewis and Clark's autumn 1805 estimate is 8,610.

A third estimate from the period of North West Company dominance on the lower Columbia was made by Reverend Jedediah Morse (1822: 368–72), who compiled statistics from Lewis and Clark and various fur traders for his *Report to the Secretary of War*. One new statistic was 2,400 for the "Cowlitsick," who "Dwell in 3 villages on . . . the Cowlitsick, 200 yards wide, rapid, boatable 190 miles" (1822: 368).

Hudson's Bay Company Estimates of the 1820s

In 1821 the North West Company withdrew from the Northwest Coast, and its stations were taken over by the Hudson's Bay Company. During the winter of 1824–25 an unidentified infectious disease spread throughout the Columbia River valley (chapter 2). The Fort George report (Kennedy 1824–

25),[12] which contains a partial estimate of lower Columbia populations, was apparently written shortly after this disease event. The numbers, judging by their similarities to the Lewis and Clark autumn 1805 estimate, appear to fairly accurately represent winter village populations from the mouth of the Columbia to the vicinity of Oak Point. Between Quathlahpohtle and The Cascades, only five villages along the main branch of the Columbia are listed. Their numbers seem unusually small, even for a midwinter count; it could be that they reflect population loss from the 1824–25 "mortality."[13]

A second estimate from the 1820s appears in the 1826–27 Fort Vancouver report written by Chief Factor John McLoughlin. It states, "on the Columbia alone in the Salmon-Season I am of the opinion from the Dalles to the Sea the Number of men is about two thousand" (in Rich 1947: 236). Using Cook's multiplier of 4, this implies an aggregate lower Columbia population of over 8,000. This number is also significantly lower than Lewis and Clark's spring 1806 total and may also indicate some population loss from the 1824–25 disease event.

A final estimate for the pre-fever-and-ague period is Samuel Parker's total for the Kalapuyan-speaking peoples. Acquired by Parker in 1835–36 from HBC sources, it seems to be a summary of an actual census carried out shortly before the introduction of malaria to the valley. Parker printed the estimate in two versions: the earlier—7,785—refers to "bands scattered . . . on both sides of the Willamette" (1837: 349); the second—8,780—is for "seventeen different tribes upon the Willamette River and its branches" (1838: 258). The higher number could (1) include Chinookan or bi-ethnic villages downstream from Willamette Falls and on Multnomah Channel; (2) include the southernmost band of Kalapuyans, the Yoncalla (who lived in the Umpqua River drainage and were not "resident on the Willamette"); or (3) be no more than a printer's error.[14]

12. A garbled copy of the estimate was preserved in HBC Governor George Simpson's 1824 journal (1968: 170).

13. Herbert Taylor has used the Fort George estimate to reconstruct a postulated aboriginal (precontact) Chinookan population of 5,000 people (1961, 1963).

14. When Parker's estimates were first published in book form, in 1838, they were roundly criticized by various members of the Methodist mission to Oregon. The first missionaries in the Willamette Valley, who arrived in 1834, came with the expectation of finding numerous Indian souls to convert. Instead they found no more than 2,000 Indians (Kalapuyans, Klikitats, and

1837–1841 ESTIMATES:
THE DEMOGRAPHIC IMPACT OF "FEVER AND AGUE"

After 1830, malaria became established in the lower Columbia drainage, and for each summer following claimed an annual toll of the Indian population within the range of its vector, *Anopheles freeborni.* We are fortunate in having population figures, from independent sources, that give pre-epidemic populations, post-epidemic populations, and loss figures for the two ethnolinguistic groups, Chinookan and Kalapuyan, that were most strongly affected by this imported disease. In addition, there are complete HBC censuses of six Indian villages, three at the mouth of the Columbia and three in the vicinity of Fort Vancouver, which allow us to make some statements about the relative effects of endemic malaria on internal population structures and demographic processes.

The total pre-epidemic population for those Chinookans within the Northwest Coast culture area is here set at 7,760, a figure derived from Lewis and Clark. The equivalent number for the Kalapuyan peoples is 7,785, given in 1838 by Samuel Parker. Loss figures for the Willamette Valley Kalapuya and the Wappato division of Upper Chinookans are preserved in Slacum:

December 18, 1837
All these tribes speak Kallapooyah dialect, and. . . . do not exceed 1,200.[15] The ague and fever, which commenced on the Columbia in 1829 [*sic*], likewise appeared on this river at the same time. . . . It has swept off not less than 5000 to 6000 souls. . . . From the river Cowlitz to the falls of the Columbia [Cascades] "Kassenow" claims authority. His tribe, since 1829, has lost more than 2,000 souls by fever. (1972: 15–16)

Parker's figure of 7,785 Willamette Valley Kalapuya, minus 6,000, the high end of Slacum's loss range, yields 1,785 Kalapuya survivors of fever and ague in 1837. Lewis and Clark's 1805 estimate for the Wappato Chinookans, 2,210, minus Slacum's 2,000, yields a survivorship of 210. Both figures are close to

---

Molala) in the entire valley. Gustavus Hines (1850: 236) and Daniel Lee and Joseph Frost (1844: 100) dismissed the Parker figures as totally inaccurate (which indeed they were, for the 1830s), apparently not recognizing that Parker's numbers referred to the pre-epidemic period or appreciating the fact that they originated from the most knowledgeable source on Indian affairs of the time, the Hudson's Bay Company.

15. Includes some Upper Chinookan villages on Multnomah Channel and at Kalama.

(slightly above) actual 1837 populations for the two groups. Parker himself estimated that seven-eighths of the population in those areas subject to fever and ague perished; Dr. McLoughlin stated nine out of ten (Parker 1838: 178). Two other Chinookan loss estimates, further removed in time (both date from 1841) and therefore probably not as accurate, are given below.

In 1832, intermittent fever carried off more than 10,000 members of the Chinook and Flathead tribes who live along the lower stretches of the Columbia River. . . . The Upper Chinooks still number about 1,000 individuals. However, the Lower Chinooks, who a few years ago had nearly 100 huts, today do not exceed 300 persons. (Duflot de Mofras 1937: 2.174, 182)

Upper Chinook. . . . At the period of the visit of Lewis and Clark, this was the most densely populated part of the whole Columbian region, and so it continued until the fatal year 1823 [*sic*] when the ague-fever, before unknown west of the Rocky Mountains, broke out, and carried off four-fifths of the population in a single summer. . . . The region below the Cascades . . . suffered most from this scourge. The population, which before was estimated at upwards of ten thousand, does not now exceed five hundred. Between the Cascades and the Dalles, the sickness was less destructive. There still remain five or six villages, with a population of seven or eight hundred. . . .

Lower Chinook. Twenty years ago there were, below the Multnoma Island, some five or six thousand people, speaking the same, or nearly the same language. . . . They are now reduced to a tenth of their former numbers. (Hale 1846: 215)

For the Kalapuyans, there are two statements from individuals who were resident in the Willamette Valley in the 1830s. Joseph Gervais, a French Canadian who had lived in the valley since the late twenties, told an 1841 immigrant that he had "known three thousand to die in two years on the Sacramento [*sic:* probably the Santiam] and Maries River" (Williams 1921: 65). Dr. William Bailey, a Willamette settler of 1835, stated in 1841 that "at least one fourth died off yearly" (Wilkes 1925–26: 57). It might be noted that both these figures, as well as Slacum's 1837 "5,000 to 6,000" deaths, make sense in terms of an 1830 population of circa 7,785 and an 1841 survivorship of 600.

Population figures for remnant groups between 1837 and 1841 are as follows: Willamette Valley Kalapuya, 500–800 (600 mentioned twice) (Lee and Frost 1844: 100; Hines 1850: 236; Wilkes 1925–26: 296); total Willamette Valley Indian population (including, especially, intrusive Klikitats), 1,200 (Slacum

1972: 16); Chinook, circa 500[16]; Cathlamet, about 300; Wappato, 37; Clackamas, 345; Cascades, 150 (HBC 1838; Wilkes 1925–26: 296). The most likely loss figures are Wappato, 2,210 to 37, a loss of 2,173, or 98% of the premalaria total; Willamette Valley Kalapuya, 7,785 to 600, a loss of 7,185, or 92%; Cascades, 1,500 to 150, or 90%; Cathlamet cluster, 1,800 to 300, or 83%; Clackamas, 1,150 to 345, or 70%; and Chinook, 1,100 to 500, or 55%. Cumulated loss figures for all the above peoples are 15,545 to 1,932, or 88% of the total population between circa 1805 and 1840. The magnitude of this decline is, of course, shocking. The bulk of the loss would be from mortality attributable to malaria and associated secondary diseases. Some additional deaths, from the "mortality" of 1824–25, as well as mortality and fertility shifts associated with chronic tuberculosis and venereal disease (all introduced by Euro-Americans), are likely.

Both geography and seasonal movement appear to have influenced malarial mortality. The greatest population decline was among the Wappato of swampy Sauvie Island, who apparently made only short seasonal forays from their home villages (see p. ooo). Peoples occupying low-lying riverine areas (Kalapuya, Cascades), regardless of seasonal movement, also suffered heavily. Medium mortality (70%) occurred among the Clackamas, whose territories included forested mountainous regions, and whose seasonal rounds took at least a portion of them into these uplands and out of the malarial region during the summer. Such a subsistence pattern is known ethnographically and historically for the Klikitat, Molala, and Cowlitz as well. The river-mouth territory of the Chinook proper was on the periphery of the anopheline range, and their mortality was correspondingly lower.

The three remnant populations from the Fort Vancouver area who were censused by the HBC in 1838 (HBC 1838) may have owed their survival to close association with the Euro-Americans. Kiesno (or Cassino), the "chief" of the 37 people at "Cathlaçanasese Village . . . 10 Miles below Vancouver," had a long-standing, close relationship with the HBC (Jones 1972: chap. 8). Many of the "Fort Vancouver Klikitat Tribe" were semiemployed as fur trappers and traders by the Company. Some of their children were enrolled at the fort's school, and their winter village seems to have been close by, near Washougal (Beaver 1959: 58). Both of these peoples probably had access to and used the medical facilities at Fort Vancouver (Carley 1981). The "Cath-

16. To the censused population of 429, an allowance of 71 unenumerated Shoalwater (from the 1854 census) has been added.

lal-thlalah Tribe" (apparently the same as Lewis and Clark's Clahclellah) maintained a "summer village columbia Cascades winter village Banks of the columbia opposite Vancouver" (HBC 1838; see also Demers in Landerholm 1956:
89, 168).[17]

The 1838 census includes 288 Chinook in three villages between modern
Fort Columbia and Megler (Frost 1934: 58). Added to the upstream 37
"Wapato" and 130 "Cath-lal-thlalah," this sample of 455 Chinookans has some
interesting demographic patterns. There is a slave percentage of 24% and a
notable lack of girls, especially among the river-mouth Chinook. But what is
most interesting is the percentage of children in the total population. The
Chinookans average 30% (the Klikitats, by comparison, had 45%). Thirty percent children indicates a population barely able to replace itself or in slow
decline. Of the three Chinookan communities, the most robust was at The
Cascades; the remnant settlement at *gałákanasisi* was obviously moribund.
A significant frequency of venereal-caused sterility was likely among the two
lower river Chinookan populations; but most important were certainly the
effects of endemic malaria on fertility and infant survival. Malaria produces
a pernicious anemia which, in pregnant women, may "increase the incidence
of miscarriages, premature births, and stillbirths" (Bayliss-Smith 1975: 437).
As far as the children themselves are concerned: "In endemic areas, regularly
one-third to one-half or more of all infants die of malaria in the first few years
of life" (Wood 1979: 258). Although fatalities directly attributable to malaria
drop off after about age five, "periodic attacks may lower peoples' resistance
to such an extent that other diseases which they acquire may prove fatal"
(Bayliss-Smith 1975: 437). The addition of this factor alone to stable population systems that were either stationary or experiencing moderate growth
would be enough to send them into a steady decline. Existing census materials for 1830s Chinookan populations are biased in their overrepresentation
of groups marginal (river's mouth, The Cascades) to the malarial focal area.
Inclusion of censuses from other remnant populations from the lower
Cowlitz, Willamette Falls area, or Willamette Valley would certainly under-
line the deleterious effects of endemic malaria on population survival.

17. The seasonal-movement pattern of Cascades people as reported by Lewis and Clark
placed them in winter villages at The Cascades and in summer settlements in Wappato Valley.
It could be that Cascades peoples moved seasonally in *both* directions prior to 1830 (Yvonne
Hajda, pers. comm.), but it is tempting to assign this apparent *reversal* of movement to a post-
malarial development.

A Settlement "Horizon"

Physical evidence for a recent, heavy population decline was everywhere on the lower Columbia River during the late 1830s and early 1840s. Most often mentioned were the great number of abandoned villages and the crowded cemeteries of the Upper Chinookan peoples. Map 14 shows villages and cemeteries attested in the historical literature between 1831 (the second year of fever and ague) and 1855 (the beginning of the reservation period). Compared to map 13 the difference is striking. Depopulation due to disease, looked at through time, produced a significant discontinuity in settlement patterns— in archeological terms, a true "horizon."

Several observers commented on this cause and effect. George Colvocoresses, member of the 1838–41 U.S. Exploring Expedition, reported: "We saw on both banks many Indian villages, some of which were at the time without inhabitants. This last feature was attributed to the ravages of the fever and ague, and the appearance of the burying-grounds in the vicinity served to confirm the statement; they were large and thickly studded with graves" (1852: 258). Edward Belcher, leader of an 1839 British exploring expedition, reported: "In the year 1836 [1826],[18] the small-pox made great ravages; and it was followed a few years since by the ague. Consequently, Corpse Island and Coffin Mount, as well as the adjacent shores, were studded, not only with [burial] canoes, but, at the period of our visit, the skulls and skeletons were strewed about in all directions" (1843: 293). "Corpse Island" and "Coffin Mount" were "Coffin Rock" and "Mount Coffin," so named in 1792 by William Broughton of the Vancouver expedition and located at the downstream tip (Warrior Point) of Sauvie Island and the north bank of the Columbia below the mouth of the Cowlitz River.

The "canoes" that studded these two cemeteries contained corpses. "Canoe burial" was the preferred form of corpse disposal for lower Columbia peoples from Sauvie Island to the river's mouth and south along the coast to Cape Perpetua (Hajda 1984: 139–40) and was an alternate form of interment throughout most of western Washington. Burial canoes were normally raised

---

18. The bracketed date was added by early ethnologist George Gibbs, who quoted Belcher (Gibbs 1877: 200). Gibbs, who first arrived in the Northwest in 1850 and spent many years studying its Native peoples, must have known of the mid-1820s "mortality" (chapter 2). Belcher, who was on the Columbia only briefly and had also visited Alaska and California a mere four years after those two areas had experienced their own smallpox epidemics (chapter 5), probably had his dates wrong.

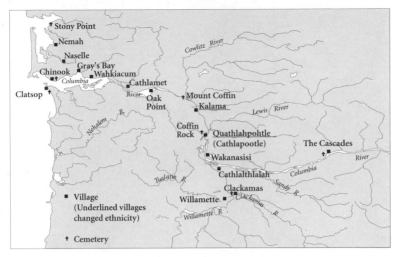

MAP 14. Chinookan Villages and Cemeteries, 1831–55

on upright planks, though they might be suspended in trees or laid on the ground. They were usually covered with boards, sometimes with a second, smaller canoe. Gender-specific grave goods were interred with the corpse, attached to the canoe's outside, or hung on poles. All were "killed" by being broken or having holes punched in them; there were holes in the canoe as well, to allow for drainage. The corpse was wrapped in mats, and dentalia might be placed in the mouth and over the eyes. Some peoples, after a few years, disinterred the bones and put them in a box or in the ground. Cemeteries appear to have been associated with village clusters, not single villages, and were generally located in isolated, difficult-of-access places such as river islands or high rocky ridges. Two paintings by Paul Kane show Coffin Rock and a Cowlitz River cemetery as they appeared in 1847 (figs. 17–18). Upstream from Sauvie Island different methods of "burial" pertained: at Multnomah village corpses were deposited on raised platforms; at Clackamas they were interred; and at The Cascades they were placed in vaults.

Specific descriptions of abandoned villages and cemeteries follow.

Sauvie Island. Writing in late 1835, the Reverend Samuel Parker stated "the Multnomah Indians . . . have become as a tribe extinct" (1838: 141). By 1835 none of the dozen villages in the "Wappato Nation" named by Lewis and Clark was permanently inhabited, and the only survivors of the 1805–6 population of 2,210 were among the 37 recorded in 1838 at Cassino's Cathlacanasese (*galákanasisi*) camp. In 1841, Dr. Silas Holmes of the Wilkes expedition recorded:

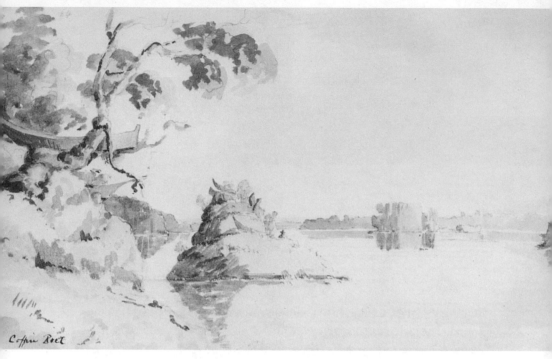

Coffin Roct

FIG. 17. *Coffin Rock*, by Paul Kane, 1847, watercolor on paper. Kane painted the cemeteries at Coffin Rock (present Warrior Point, Sauvie Island) and on the Cowlitz River shortly before they were looted and destroyed by White settlers. (Courtesy of Stark Museum of Art, Orange, Texas, accession no. 31.78/90, WWC 91.)

Dr. McLoughlin pointed out to me one morning where nine[?] large Indian villages stood a few years since, of whose inhabitants not a soul remained . . . of that tribe but a single person now remains: a man about 40 years of age, named Kasseno, whom I saw every day about the fort he was treated with great respect by the Indians who remain and who have adopted him into another tribe which is itself now nearly extinct. I have been assured that hundreds were found dead along the banks of the Columbia, whom the survivors did not attempt to bury.

Wilkes himself stated, "I am satisfied myself that the accounts given of the depopulation of this country are not exaggerated; for places were pointed out to me where dwelt whole tribes, that have been entirely swept off" (1845: 5.140). Multnomah and Cathlanaquiah villages, filled with bodies, had been burnt by order of Dr. McLoughlin in 1830; none of the other island villages is mentioned after 1830 as having inhabitants. After the Americans abandoned Fort

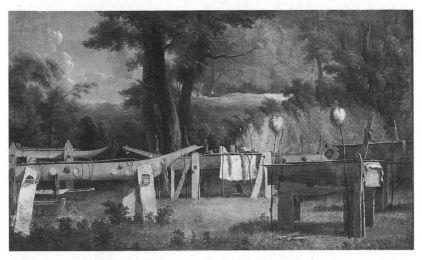

FIG. 18. *Indian Burial Place on the Cowlitz River,* by Paul Kane, 1847. Chinookan peo-
ple interred their dead in canoes raised on scaffolding. Canoe cemeteries on the lower
Columbia proliferated following the introduction of malaria in 1830. (Courtesy of the
Royal Ontario Museum, Toronto, no. 86 ETH 129, 912.1.79.)

William in autumn 1834, the island was uninhabited except for the HBC's
Laurent Sauvé and his herd of dairy cattle.

Two cemeteries are known from the southern half of Sauvie Island, at
Clannahquah on the Columbia and Cathlanahquiah on Multnomah Channel.
Both are long gone; the former washed away, the latter plowed under.
Clannahquah cemetery was apparently unique in its outlay. A reminiscence
from 1844 states:

We went into the Columbia River by the upper mouth of the Willamette, and three
or four miles down on the south [*sic:* west] bank we camped at the site of the last
Multnomah village. . . . [here] There was an extensive city of the dead, a cemetery laid
out in streets wide as the plat of the Riverview cemetery at Portland. The dead were
deposited on structures of wide split cedar boards, three or more inches thick, set
upright: sometimes three tiers of horizontal boards one above the other mortised into
and secured to the uprights by twisted inner bark of cedar. On these the dead were
laid, wrapped in cedar bark. (Minto 1895)

The cemetery at Cathlanahquiah was located on a ridge "covered with a thick
growth of oak" behind the burned village. In 1854 the site was homesteaded

by James Taylor: "Hundreds of dead Indians were placed in the branches of the oak trees, and as they fell to the ground he made it his business to gather up the bones and bury them, until today the ground is permeated with Indian skulls" (*Oregonian* 1900).[19]

Downstream Wappato Villages and Coffin Rock. All the lower Wappato villages (Clack Star, Cathlacumups, Clannarminamow, Namuit, and Quathlahpohtle) appear to have been emptied in the early 1830s, but at least one (Quathlahpohtle) was used as a seasonal campsite and may have been partially reoccupied by the early 1850s. In May 1833, William Tolmie said of this second-largest of the Wappato villages that "only its superior verdure distinguished the spot from the surrounding country" (fig. 2). But in May 1836, John Townsend treated a sick Indian girl (see chapter 4) at a settlement "on a plain below Warrior's point . . . [containing] several large lodges of Kowalitsk Indians, in all probably one hundred persons" (1978: 232). In 1854 there were 140–200 "Taitimapam" (Sahaptins) "living in the valley of the Cathlapootle [Lewis] River," though not necessarily at the former village site itself (Tappan 1854).

Coffin Rock was still intact in the late 1840s, but for reasons that will become obvious, it apparently didn't last much longer. It was an attraction, in the late forties, for anyone who was boating down the Columbia. From April 1846:

A large table-shaped rock stood near the shore, perhaps twenty feet above the water. On this there were perhaps a hundred canoes and in each was the remains of an Indian. . . . The cemetery on this rock had become literally covered. A new place of burial was selected on shore opposite Coffin Rock, where a point on the mountain sloped down to the river, and as many canoes as possible had been placed thereon, and a larger space occupied on the ground adjacent. (Tolbert 1907: 96)

One member of the party opened the largest canoe and, discovering "a number of brass rings . . . ear ornaments" and other jewelry, "removed all these

19. Upstream on the Columbia, in territory used by both Wappato and Cascades peoples, there is evidence for a second cemetery, which may have been used until the 1830s. This burial site was located behind Lewis and Clark's Nechacokee village and just to the west of Blue Lake (presently in the suburbs of northeast Portland). It is now known only from a few articles from 1939 and 1940 in the *Oregon Journal* newspaper. While excavating the land for a flood-control dike and pipeline, 1939 excavations uncovered 17 skulls and leg bones; in 1940 bulldozers turned up "hundreds of yellowed bones, most of them broken and collapsing into earth at a touch." The landowner recalled that when he first plowed the land in 1905, "Indian arrowheads, mortars, pestles and other implements" turned up "repeatedly, but all were given away" (White 1940).

ornaments, appropriating everything to himself" (97). In late 1847 painter Paul Kane stopped at the site and executed the painting that is reproduced in figure 18. Shortly following his visit, there is an account of a second group of curio hunters, who visited both Coffin Rock and Mount Coffin, appropriating at the latter cemetery "40 ankle and wrist ornaments," "66 finger rings," and a "great number of beads . . . from a canoe in which the wife of a chief had been deposited . . . equivalent to about $329" (Thornton 1849: 281).

"Skillutes" and Mount Coffin. After 1831 the only occupied village of Lewis and Clark's "Skillute Nation" was at Oak Point; the villages around the mouth of the Cowlitz itself were apparently used only seasonally by Salishan peoples from up the river. When the Cowlitz mouth sites were visited by missionaries in the 1840s, they were called "camps," and the sources note that the inhabitants were suffering from "fever and ague" (Landerholm 1956: 144; Waller 1844).

Mount Coffin was located on the north bank of the Columbia between the mouth of the Cowlitz and Oak Point and was apparently the cemetery of the Skillutes. It was separated from the mainland by a marshy area, had an oak grove atop, and along the riverside was a broken rocky face where most of the burial canoes were placed. Mount Coffin was visited by many early explorers, but the best description of the burials themselves was made by John Scouler, who visited the cemetery in 1825 in hopes of obtaining a flattened Chinookan skull for phrenological study (1905: 279–80). George Gibbs commented on the increased use of Mount Coffin between the years 1792 and 1841: the cemetery "would appear not to have been very ancient. Mr. Broughton . . . makes mention only of *several* canoes at this place. And Lewis and Clark, who noticed the mount, do not speak of them at all; but at the time of Captain Wilkes' expedition, it is conjectured that there were at least 3,000" (1877: 200).[20]

The last eyewitness account of the cemetery was made on 25 August 1841 by Charles Wilkes himself:

In the evening we reached Mount Coffin, at the mouth of the Cowlitz. This mount afforded a favorable point for astronomical observations, being 710 feet high, and quite

---

20. Gibbs was writing after the fact, and his source for 3,000 burial canoes is not known. Although Mount Coffin was very large, 3,000 seems like an excessive number. Paul Kane, also writing after the fact (in 1847), said there had been "two or three hundred" (1971: 98).

isolated. The canoes used by the Indians as coffins are seen upon it in every direction, in all stages of decay. They are supported between trees, at the height of 4 or 5 feet above the ground, & about them are hung utensils that had belonged to the deceased, or that had been offered as tokens of respect.

I remained the whole day on the top of this mount, & obtained a full set of observations; the weather being remarkably clear & beautiful. Here my boat's crew carelessly omitted to extinguish the fire they had used for cooking our dinner & as we were pulling off to the brig, I regretted to see that the fire had spread & was enveloping the whole mount; but there was no help for it. The fire continued to rage throughout the night, until all was burnt. (1845: 5.121)

Mount Coffin no longer exists; it was quarried away for gravel in the 1930s.

Little is known about conditions upstream on the Cowlitz: the population estimated at 2,400 in 1820 had dropped by 90% in the 1840s; of the more than 20 village names given to Edward Curtis in the early 1900s, none is recorded in the historical literature after 1830 (the sole documented settlement was at Cowlitz Farm); and the cemetery painted by Paul Kane in 1847 has not been located. In early September 1841 HBC governor George Simpson said:

When I descended the Cowlitz in 1828, there was a large population along its banks; but since then the intermittent fever . . . had left but few to mourn for those that fell. During the whole of our day's course till we came upon a small camp in the evening the shores were silent and solitary, the deserted villages forming melancholy monuments of the generation that had passed away. (1847: 1.107)

Willamette Falls. Depopulation was not nearly as fierce upstream on the Willamette at the Falls. Two villages remained—at *wálamt* (West Linn) and Clackamas (Gladstone)—both severely depleted. When first visited by Catholic missionaries in May 1841: "Above and below the falls are seen the sites of large villages which the fevers of 1830 entirely depopulated. . . . the village of the falls consists of four or five lodges. . . . about forty souls" (Demers in Landerholm 1956: 80, 83). As for Clackamas:

The village is situated on the left bank of the river. . . . On the right bank is seen the trace of a large village which the fever of 1830 caused to disappear. The one which I was visiting contained no more than fifteen lodges about 25 feet long by 20. In former times the houses were high and solidly built; but after the fever had ravaged, people expect to die any day; and that is why these poor natives say, they no longer take the trouble to build. One sees yet behind the village some traces of long lines of lodges which used to cover the terrain; the longest behind measured 157 steps in length. (84)

The cemetery at Clackamas (according to Wilkes) covered "quite a space" and was "crowded" with "a multitude of bones scattered about," proof to him that they "have been quite a large tribe in former times." The Clackamas people buried their dead, and raised a "two to six" foot plank, carved and painted and laden with grave goods, above the grave (1845: 4.368).

The Cascades. The five or more Cascades villages named before 1830 were diminished to two by the late thirties (Cathlalthlalah and Yehuh), and only Yehuh remained after 1844. Cathlalthlalah had 130 people in 1838; 150–200 were estimated at The Cascades itself in September 1841 (HBC 1838; Landerholm 1956: 90).[21] These *may* be the same population, but more likely Cathlalthlalah ceased to exist after the dysentery epidemic of 1844, when 400 Indians "in the vicinity" of Fort Vancouver died.

The Cascades burial site, a few miles downstream on the north bank, was described in detail by Lewis and Clark (1990: 358–61; 1991: 108) and Nor'wester Ross Cox (1957: //). It contained eight (nine in Cox) cedar-plank vault burials, each containing several skeletons or bodies bound in mats. Starting in 1843, the site was regularly visited by emigrants on the trail to Fort Vancouver. The first visitors described it as "a large Indian burying place, where the bones of hundreds were heaped together in pens"; eight years later there were "skulls and other bones of all sizes and ages lying scattered about, the wagon crushing them as it passed along" (Beckham 1984: 30–31). This is one of the last references to Indian cemeteries on the lower Columbia. Mentions of a canoe-burial site near Bruceport on Willapa Bay (Swan 1972: 68) postdate it, but none of the Chinookan cemeteries seem to have survived beyond the late 1850s.

TERRITORIAL ESTIMATES AND CENSUSES

The first round of treaty making in western Oregon took place during 1851, under the direction of Territorial Superintendent of Indian Affairs Anson Dart.

21. When Father Modeste Demers arrived at The Cascades on 16 September 1841, he said: "This new village which I wanted to conquer for J[esus] C[hrist] was composed of some thirty families. There were only young people in it, all the elders having been cut down by the fevers" (in Landerholm 1956: 88). People suffered from fever throughout Demers's 12-day visit. On his

Many of the peoples Dart or his agents treated with were censused; several were counted again in 1854.[22] Comparing these figures with those from 1838 and 1841 reveals continued population decline. Changes for the five major Chinookan groups are estimated as follows: Chinook, 500 to 238, a loss of 262, or 52%; Cathlamet, 300 to 60, a loss of 240, or 80%; Clackamas, 345 to 92, a loss of 253, or 73%; Wappato, 37 to 30, a loss of 19%; Cascades, 150 to 138, a loss of 9%. The total decline was 1,332 to 558, a loss of 774, or 58%, in 13–16 years. The continuing decline of the Chinookan populations was due to several factors: mortality from dysentery and measles in the 1840s and smallpox in 1853; depressed fertility due to venereal disease and endemic malaria; and outmarriage of women and absorption into larger neighboring groups (Chehalis, Klikitat, White). The Kalapuyan population had dropped from 600 to 560 by 1851 and to 369 by 1856 (Beckham 1990: 184), for a cumulative loss of 39%. The Kalapuya decline was probably due mostly to measles and smallpox mortality, slave raiding by Klikitat, and depressed fertility from endemic malaria and venereal diseases.

Chinookan Remnant Populations

Small remnant populations abounded on the lower Columbia in the late 1840s and early 1850s. Of the 10 "bands" of "Chinooks" near the mouth of the Columbia treated with in 1851, only 2 (Chinook proper and Tillamook) counted over 100 members. The settlement pattern of the Chinook proper around 1854 was recalled in 1902 by Chinook elder Catherine George:

At the upper end of Chinook Village at the mouth of the Chinook River were four houses. . . . A little way down from there were four more houses, and near the southeast extremity of the village, two, for a total of ten houses sheltering some 40 people. . . . At Qwatsamuts village . . . were 20 people in four houses. At the Chinook River

---

departure, he had baptized 34 children and estimated the total population at 150–200 (Landerholm 1956: 90).

22. The manuscript records of the Oregon Superintendency of Indian Affairs for 1851 include censuses of remnant Chinook (partial), Cathlamet, and Clatsop (Gibbs 1851; Shortess 1851); a total count of the Willamette Valley peoples (Spalding 1851) and censuses of Willamette Valley Klikitat and Kalapuya (partial) (Spalding 1851); and partial breakdowns of other lower Columbia groups (Dart 1852). The Washington Superintendency of Indian Affairs records include counts of north bank lower Columbia peoples (Tappan 1854); others appear in table 17.

mouth . . . lived 10 people in four houses. Further upstream at Grays Bay lived 20 Wahkiakums and Kathlamets. . . . At Nemah River was one permanent dwelling of 20 souls. . . . On the nearby Naselle River was a seven-house village of 40 people. . . . On Willapa Bay 35 Chinooks lived in two villages. . . . The total number of these Chinooks, Wahkiakums, and Kathlamets was 185 people living in thirty-seven houses. (As summarized by Ruby and Brown 1976: 216–17)

Between Cathlamet and The Cascades in 1854 the only surviving settlement that might be termed Chinookan was the village of Wakanasisi (*gałákanasisi*), or "the Fishery." In 1838 there had been 37 Indians at this location; in 1854 there were 30. William Tappan, Indian agent for southern Washington, stated that they were "a mixed race, nearly all the tribes are here represented" (1854). These included some "4 or 6" from the former Wappato village of Kalama. The name "Klikitats" frequently given to the Fishery villagers indicates their hybrid nature.

Elsewhere on the north bank of the Columbia, Tappan enumerated four bands of "Taitimapams" near the sites of former Upper Chinookan villages at the mouths of various Columbia feeder streams. There were 60 on the Cowlitz, 22 at Kalama, 140–200 on the Cathlapoodle (Lewis River), and 78 (with "Clickitat") at LaCamas Prairie east of Fort Vancouver. The Taitnapam were a Northwest Sahaptin people closely akin to the Klikitat. Tappan stated they were "of interior origin"; their historic focus was the upper Cowlitz drainage. According to Tappan, they "approached the Columbia as the lands became vacated by the Chinooks" (1854).

Demographic Patterns and Population Survival

Two very interesting demographic phenomena are apparent in the 1854 population data from the lower Columbia. Both continued aboriginal patterns, but given severely depleted local populations, neither (if they had persisted) would have been conducive to the persistence of identifiably "Chinookan" populations.

Among the river-mouth Chinook, the pattern was intermarriage with outsiders. In aboriginal times this pattern, typical of the entire Coast Salish–Chinookan continuum, created a mesh of interdependency among villages and ethnicities that was "adaptive" in a socioeconomic sense. High-ranking individuals in particular gained considerable prestige and access to economic goods through polygynous marriage with far-flung peoples: the influential Chinook chief Concomly is reputed to have had wives from the Wappato villages of Scappoose and Multnomah as well as from the non-Chinookan-speaking Willapa and Chehalis (Boyd 1976). Given patrilocal residence, Concomly's wives moved in with him, and when Concomly married off his daughters to high-prestige outsiders (usually White), they moved away from the river mouth.

In the 1851 censuses of the Clatsop and Scarborough Hill Chinook (Gibbs 1851; Shortess 1851), this pattern persisted, but with a twist. Families headed by Chinookan males all resided in Chinookan territory (17 in Gibbs's north bank census, with 19 children); additionally there is no indication of any marriages between Chinook males and White women (certainly more a reflection of White prejudices than of those of the Indians). There was significant intermarriage of Indian women with White men, however: 11 were recorded, with 36 children. The majority of these families resided apart from other Indians, and the children, one might assume, self-identified as White. For a small, distinct population surrounded and outnumbered by a growing population of culturally different migrants, such a trend could pose a threat to its existence. Among a similarly diminished group of southern California Indians in the late 1800s, this drainage of marriageable females and their reproductive capacities from Indian to White populations contributed to a continued population decline (Harvey 1967). Fortunately, among the river-mouth Chinook in the early 1850s, sex ratios were still normal, and a similar drainage had not yet occurred.[23]

The second demographic pattern, the in situ population replacement of Chinookan speakers by interior Sahaptins, likewise had its roots in pre-epidemic patterns. Chinookan families were economically bound to the productive banks of the Columbia; interior peoples were covetous of the river's resources. In the early 1800s interior peoples visited the Columbia annually; by the mid-1800s, with Chinookan depopulation, they moved downstream permanently.

As is typical of the southern Northwest Coast, rights to limited local resource areas (such as fishing stations) along the Columbia were held by local

---

23. North bank Chinook were never removed to reservations, and many stayed in their traditional territory. After the 1850s, although intermarriage and acculturation continued, a core population of Chinook persisted. Today more than 2,000 Chinook, lineally descended from the survivors of the mid-1800s, remain within the general area of their ancestors.

Chinookan families. Chinookan men, in particular, were reluctant to leave these areas and the wealth they produced, as the following quotation suggests:

14 May 1851
[T]he natives of western Oregon, so far as we have seen, without exception, are possessed of local attachments of the strongest kind. . . . The habitations of these people are, so far as regards place, not only permanent but hereditary. Divided into bands or families, now reduced in number, but retaining each their separate chiefs, occupying their own lodges in the different districts of country, having no generic name, and no ties but a common language, it has been found generally impossible to amalgamate portions of even the same people. (Gaines, Skinner, and Allen 1851)

As noted earlier in this chapter, non-Chinookan peoples inhabiting lands in the interior regions of minor tributaries of the lower Columbia did not have ready access to the salmon and other resources of the main river. During fishing season, they moved downstream to partake of the fishery. Many certainly had rights, gained by intermarriage, to fish or gather in certain areas. Others, on the model of The Dalles fishery, fished on their own or traded interior goods for riverine resources. In Lewis and Clark's time (if the interpretation of the "Estimate of Western Indians" is correct), during the fishing season local Chinookan and visiting interior populations were about equal, or in rough balance. After the "fever and ague" epidemics, the equation tipped in favor of the inlanders. Ethnographic patterns suggest how downstream replacement took place. Intermarriage persisted, and interior men may have taken advantage of the custom that allowed them to pay off the cost of a riverine wife by moving in and working for her father (Silverstein 1990: 543; cf. Boas 1894: 250). Others may simply have moved downstream to claim the property of deceased in-laws. But the largest part probably occupied empty land. By the mid-1830s most midriver Chinookan villages were already abandoned, although some were still being used as seasonal campsites by interior visitors. By the early 1850s recorded villages were mostly inhabited by Sahaptins; Chinookan survivors were few and had become a minority in their own land. The process of replacement ended with removal to reservations in 1855.[24]

24. Tappan's Cathlapootle and LaCamas Taitnapam were united with the western bands of Klikitat and removed east of the Cascade Mountains, ultimately to the Yakama reservation; most of the Kalama and Cowlitz River Taitnapam followed later.

Remnant populations like those of the lower Columbia in the early 1850s were fragile and in danger of extinction. Statistical studies (Krzywicki 1934; Livi 1949; MacCluer and Dyke 1976) suggest that endogamous populations below a total of 500 must do all that is possible to maximize their reproductive potential. Populations that encourage various forms of population control, that are characterized by wide spacing between children, that discourage large families, and that place restrictions on potential marriage (or remarriage) partners are apt to have trouble. It goes without saying that geographically fragmented populations have trouble too. Along these lines, it is instructive to compare processes in Haida versus Chinook post-epidemic populations. The Haida breakdown of internal marriage rules and readiness to group into large villages maximized the reproductive potential and persistence of the larger population unit and was adaptive. The Chinookan propensity for out-marriage and unwillingness to leave local settlements diffused the reproductive potential and geographic unity of the diminished pool of Chinookan speakers and was less conducive to sociocultural persistence.

Kalapuya Populations and Percentage of Children

The partial census of Kalapuyans taken by Agent Henry Spalding in 1851 shows, as with the Chinook, fragmented remnant populations. The aboriginal (pre-1830) pattern is not known; apparently major subdivisions corresponded to winter-village clusters, which probably in turn were grouped geographically by Willamette tributary drainage systems (Zenk 1990). In 1851 none of the eight enumerated Kalapuya bands, considered in isolation, was viable (with numbers averaging 53 persons), but all were mobile, with permeable boundaries, and should be considered a single population.

An important demographic pattern shared by Kalapuyan and several mid-nineteenth-century Chinookan populations was their abnormally small (below replacement) percentage of children. In 1851, the proportions of children among Willamette Valley Kalapuyans (14%) and among the Chinookan Cathlamet (21%) indicate declining populations (see table 18). The underlying cause was certainly endemic malaria: both populations inhabited the focal area for fever and ague. But other factors were responsible too. Even in the 1840s, Willamette Valley peoples were subject to slave raids by intrusive Klikitats, who captured children and sold them among the Columbia River peoples (e.g., Applegate 1851). Low percentages of children may also indicate a recent experience with epidemic disease. Both Kalapuyan and midriver Chinookan peoples suffered from the 1848 measles epidemic. At the mouth of the Columbia the 1853 smallpox outbreak produced a similar phenomenon: in 1851, 108 Chinook and Clatsops had 34% children; three years later a sample of 290 Chinook and Tillamook had only 61 subadults (21%) between them (Raymond 1854; Dawson 1854).

The experience of the lower Columbia peoples with successive, closely spaced epidemic visitations prompts a detailed discussion of the effects, short-range and long-range, of epidemics on the age structure of a given population. Percentage of children is the only index indicative of age structure in early-nineteenth-century Northwest Coast Indian censuses. Variations in percentage of children may relate to ecological conditions. But percentage of children also varies considerably, and in a patterned fashion, among Northwest Coast populations in relation to their recent disease history.

In the short term, the effect of any epidemic visitation is to decrease the percentage of children in a given population. There are two reasons for this phenomenon. One has to do with higher mortalities among the very young. In the case of smallpox outbreaks, three segments of the population (the very old, pregnant women, and infants) succumb in larger numbers than do others (Dixon 1962: 365). The excess mortality of children in malarial areas has been noted above. But, as described by demographer Norma McArthur in her study of the historical demography of Polynesia, more subtle influences are at work in post-epidemic times that further depress the percentage of children by impairing the normal level of fertility. McArthur claims fertility decreases because of a dramatic increase in "disrupted matings." Her reasoning is as follows:

With a mortality rate of 25%, the probability of the male partner of any mating dying would be 1/4; and the probability of the female partner dying would be the same 1/4. Matings would be disrupted by the death of either or both partners. The probability of both the male and female partners dying would be the product of the probabilities that either would die, that is 1/16. The probability that the male partner would die but not the female would be $1/4 \times 3/4$ and the probability that the male partner would survive and the female die would be $3/4 \times 1/4$. The sum of these probabilities is 7/16, which represents the likelihood of the disruption of existing matings as a result of the epidemic mortality. It also represents the extent of reduction in the number of births likely to occur in the year following the epidemic as compared with their number in the year preceding it. Although new matings would be formed subsequently, the recovery in the numbers of births each year would be gradual. (1961: 18)

Excessively low percentages of children (well below replacement) may, in fact, be taken as an index of some preceding demographic disaster, whether it be a natural event (famine, typhoon, an extremely cold winter, etc.) or an epidemic (the usual explanation in early-contact-period Northwest Indian populations).

McArthur's quotation also raises the issue of the long-term demographic effect of a single drop in the percentage of children. Under normal conditions "recovery will be gradual." Stable population theory assumes that, given a demographic disturbance, all other factors unchanged, the forces that determine the stable population structure will reassert themselves, and after a time, the fertility, mortality, and age distribution of the populations will return to their normal, predisturbance schedules. Historical demographers cite a "life time . . . perhaps 80 years . . . as soon as the whole population has been replaced" as a predictable period for a "return to normalcy" (Weiss 1975: 51; see also Howell 1973: 259). As far as *numbers* are concerned, computer simulations suggest that recovery may commence well before this time: earlier in populations where favorable ecological and social conditions combine to promote a modest annual increase; longer in stationary population systems where numbers are held in balance by ecological and social restrictions (Thornton, Miller, and Warren 1991). In the aboriginal Pacific Northwest, most population systems are assumed to have been both stable in structure and stationary in numbers. With few exceptions, recovery—both structural and numerical—should have been slow.

Local disease histories strongly influenced the natural capacity for reassertion of stable population systems and rebound in numbers. Disease-caused demographic disturbances may, of course, be rare events, or they may occur frequently. Widely spaced disturbances, such as those recorded for smallpox epidemics on the North Coast (over 60 years between the initial and second epidemic), should have allowed sufficient time for stable population systems to reassert themselves and numbers to begin to rebound. On the Central Coast, where major epidemics were more closely spaced (1770s, 1801–2, 1824–25), return to a stable demographic system and population recovery were impeded. But on the lower Columbia, given the nature of its disease history, any population recovery, systemic or numerical, was very unlikely during the pre-reservation period. Malaria, in its estival-autumnal form (appendix 2), was, in effect, a yearly epidemic that took an annual toll, concentrated among the newborn cohort. With additional mortality from less frequently occurring epidemics (influenza, dysentery, measles, smallpox) also concentrated among the young, the percentage of children was kept abnormally low, well beneath the level required for replacement and, ultimately, survival.

EPILOGUE

A final footnote to this chapter is that, following the establishment of reservations in western Oregon and Washington after 1855, many of the factors regulating population structure and size (especially regarding economic base and health care) *did* change, and after reaching nadir numbers around the turn of the century, many populations (with varying degrees of White admixture) did indeed rebound. This effect has been demonstrated in the Pacific Northwest for most Plateau populations (Boyd 1998), though the details have yet to be unraveled for the coast itself. On the lower Columbia, lineal descendants of lower Chinook today number well over 2,000 (Chinook Tribal Office, pers. comm., March 1999); there are nearly as many Cowlitz descendants; and the confederated tribes of the Grand Ronde reservation, including descendants of Kalapuyan, Clackamas, Takelma, Molala, and Clatsop peoples, have over 3,500 on their rolls (Margo Mercier, Grand Ronde Tribal Office, pers. comm., August 1996). Despite the horrendous mortalities and alarming demographic trends of the early 1800s, equally dramatic changes have occurred in the intervening century, and as of the 1990s, lower Columbia tribal populations are healthy and growing.

10 / Conclusion

Population Decline and Culture Change

In 1976, geographer William Denevan stated, "The discovery of America was followed by possibly the greatest demographic disaster in the history of the world" (1976: 7). He was, of course, referring to the effect of disease transfer on the peoples of the New World. Denevan also made a plea for more-detailed microstudies of disease and population decline in different parts of the Americas (289). Many such regional "disease and depopulation" studies have since followed.[1] This book is one such study.

Northwest Coast demographic history is summarized in table 3. Decline in the first century of contact is estimated at a minimum of 80%, or nearly 150,000 people, largely the result of mortality from introduced diseases. Estimates of total numbers and amount of decline vary in reliability dependent on date and location. "Aboriginal" (precontact) populations are difficult to determine. James Mooney's (1928) ethnohistorical estimates (table 3, column 1; 114,000 for the Northwest Coast), the standard for over 60 years, are now acknowledged as being much too low (Ubelaker 1976). The aboriginal estimates in column 2 of table 3 were calculated by working backward from the earliest reliable historical number (column 3) and compensating for preceding epidemic mortality (known or estimated). The total (183,661) is conserv-

1. A select list would include (1) for Spanish America, Cook and Borah 1971–74, Cook 1981, Reff 1991, and Jackson 1994; (2) for the Southeast, Dobyns 1983 and Smith 1987; (3) for the Plains, Ewers 1973, Ray 1974: chap. 5, 1976, Trimble 1988, and Decker 1989.

ative, as it assumes an across-the-board mortality of only one-third from the first historical smallpox visitation. A third estimate, 400,000, computed by applying a standard 20:1 "depopulation ratio" to a nadir (low-point) Northwest Coast population of 20,000 (Ubelaker 1988: 293), may be taken as the absolute high end of the range for the culture area's precontact population.[2]

The population history for North Coast and lower Columbia peoples (at least in later years) is well documented and indicates decreases of circa 66% (North Coast, 1836–80) and 90% (lower Columbia, 1805–55). Decline from the late 1700s was certainly much greater. Demographic data from other parts of the coast are not as well recorded, and population histories are not as firm. But the figures we have suggest the following—by "epidemic area"—in descending order of decline in the first hundred years: Interior Valleys, 95%; South Coast, 87%; Wakashan, 78%; Olympic, 77%; North Coast, 76%; and Inland Waters, 63%.

EPIDEMIC AREAS

Northwest Coast disease history is summarized in table 4. The various ethnolinguistic groups of the culture area have been combined into "epidemic areas," broadly defined as groups of geographically contiguous peoples who shared a common disease history (Boyd 1990: 143–47). Operatively, the concept of epidemic area arose from an attempt to summarize the complex early-contact historical epidemiology of the Northwest, plus a hypothesis of Wayne Suttles's that local disease histories might correspond to subregional social networks. As it turned out, there was indeed some correspondence when contagious diseases such as smallpox and measles were concerned, but when the vector carried, ecologically limited malaria epidemics were included, one epidemic area (Interior Valleys) turned out to be based more on environmental

---

2. The 20:1 depopulation ratio was suggested by Henry Dobyns in an important and controversial 1966 article, "Estimating Aboriginal American Population, I: An Appraisal of Techniques with a New Hemispheric Estimate." The depopulation ratio was measured from an aboriginal estimate to a nadir (historical low point) number. Dobyns examined several known and hypothesized regional American depopulation ratios and suggested that 20:1 was the most reasonable ratio to apply to the hemisphere as a whole.

The three aboriginal estimates presented here were all calculated using exclusively ethnohistorical methodologies. Auxiliary methods of population estimation, including village and house counts, density comparisons, and "carrying-capacity"/resource base evaluations, have not been attempted for Northwest Coast populations and should be encouraged.

| Group | Aboriginal Population | | | Final Post-Epidemic No.[d] |
	Mooney 1928[a]	Boyd 1996[b]	Anchor No.[c]	
NORTH COAST EPIDEMIC AREA	28,900	47,848		11,415
Tlingit	10,000	14,820	9,880	4,583
Haida	9,800	14,235[e]	9,490	1,598
Tsimshian peoples	7,000	14,645		4,492
Nisga'a		3,635	1,615	877
Gitxsan	1,500	2,813	1,875	1,462
Coast Tsimshian	5,500	6,359	2,826	1,869
Sabassas		1,838	1,225	284
Haisla	700	1,238	825	364
Nuxalk (Bella Coola)	1,400	2,910	1,940	378
WAKASHAN EPIDEMIC AREA	15,600	31,077[f]		6,895
Heiltsuk (Haihais, Bella Bella, Oweekeno)	2,000	3,027	2,018	481
Kwakwaka'wakw	4,500	13,275	8,850	2,264
Northern Coast Salish	3,100	2,400[g]	1,600	894
Nuu-chah-nulth	6,000	12,375	8,250	3,256
INLAND WATERS EPIDEMIC AREA	24,200	31,560[h]		11,603
Squamish	1,800	1,694	784	778
Halkomelem speakers	12,600	10,534	4,877	4,298
Songhees and Saanich	2,700	3,562	1,649	486
Lummi and Samish		1,974	914	660
Nooksack	1,300	1,187	412	218
Puget Salish	4,800	11,835	5,479	4,872
Twana	1,000	774	358	291
OLYMPIC EPIDEMIC AREA	4,900	9,498		2,215
Chemakum	400	260[g]	90	73
Clallam	2,000	3,208	1,485	926
Ditidaht and Makah	2,000	5,400	3,000	869
Quileute	500	630	350	347
SOUTH COAST EPIDEMIC AREA	15,700	22,800		2,966
Quinault	1,500	2,250	1,250	226
Lower Chehalis		2,340	1,300	217
Chinook and Clatsop	1,100	1,980	1,100	238
Tillamook	1,500	4,320	2,400	193
Alseans		3,060	1,700	155
Siuslawans	6,000	2,100	1,400	210
Coosans	2,000	2,250	1,500	234
Coastal Athapascans	3,600	4,500	3,000	1,493

| | Aboriginal Population | | | Final Post- |
Group	Mooney 1928[a]	Boyd 1996[b]	Anchor No.[c]	Epidemic No.[d]
INTERIOR VALLEYS EPIDEMIC AREA	24,700	40,878		2,059
Upper Chehalis		2,880	1,600	216
Cowlitz	1,000	4,320	2,400	165
Kwalhioqua and Clatskanie	1,800	2,430	1,350	21
Cathlamet, Wappato, Clackamas, Cascades	13,200	11,988[i]	6,660	300
Kalapuyans	3,000	14,760[j]	8,200	560
Takelma/Interior Athapascans	5,700	4,500[k]	3,000	797
Total	114,000	183,661		37,153

[a] Column one reproduces the estimates from Mooney 1928. Mooney collected all then-known historical estimates and censuses and, working back through time, provided a subjective estimate based on his feel for the rate of decline (see Ubelaker 1976).

[b] Revised from Boyd 1990: 136. Computation basics: An across-the-board mortality of one-third is assumed for all peoples from the first smallpox epidemic. In those cases where the anchor population postdates the epidemics of 1801–2 and 1824–25, mortalities of one-sixth are assumed (to take into account that segment of the population with acquired immunity). No provision for rebound is included in any estimate, given the back-to-back nature of epidemic visitations for most peoples and the absence of hard statistics documenting rebound.

[c] The earliest good historical number. Major sources include Lewis and Clark 1990: 473–92 (south coast peoples); Douglas 1878 (north and central coasts); and, for particular peoples, Tolmie 1963: 317–20 (central British Columbia coast); Galois 1994 (Kwakwaka'wakw); Jewitt 1975: 39–41 (Nootkans); Dorsey 1897 (Gitxsan); Douglas 1931. 17 and McDonald 1830 (Northern Coast Salish); Parker 1936: 123–24 (Takelma and Interior Athapascans); Morse 1822 and Gibbs 1877: 182 (Cowlitz and Upper Chehalis); and later censuses for a few smaller groups (e.g., Nooksack, Chemakum). See Boyd 1990 for particulars.

[d] The earliest good post-epidemic figures are given in this column; dates range from 1851 (Kalapuya) to 1890 (Tlingit). Most of the U.S. numbers date from the treaty-making and early reservation years of the middle to late 1850s and are found in the Records of the Oregon Superintendency of Indian Affairs, 1848–73; and Washington Superintendency of Indian Affairs, 1853–74 (microfilm copies from the National Archives). The British Columbia statistics date mostly from the 1880s and are recorded in the statistical tables of the Annual Report of the Department of Indian Affairs, in the Canadian Sessional Papers. See also relevant chapters in Suttles 1990.

[e] The length of time between the smallpox epidemic of the 1770s and the date of the Haida anchor (mid-1830s), plus historic evidence for change in the subsistence base (see text), may have allowed for some population recovery; hence, the aboriginal estimate may be too high.

[f] All the Wakashan Epidemic Area figures have been recalculated since 1990. The 1990 estimate included an allowance for the 1824–25 epidemic, but there is no evidence for that epidemic in Wakashan territory. New anchors (from Jewitt 1975; Galois 1994; Douglas 1931) have been used.

[g] Mortality from warfare preceding the anchor population date may make aboriginal estimates for Northern Coast Salish and Chemakum too low.

[h] Inland Waters population figures fluctuate considerably from one estimate or census to another, perhaps reflecting the seasonal consolidation/dispersion pattern of Coast Salish populations. Anchor populations given here, mostly assembled from the several censuses in Douglas 1878, are tentative and open to reinterpretation.

[i] Cascades added from Boyd 1990.

[j] Lewis and Clark's "Shobarboobeer" Shoshones dropped from Boyd 1990.

[k] Parker (1936: 123) gives 3,450 for the "Umbaqua" Indians, whom he sites in the area between the Kalapuya and the Sacramento Valley. Of the five named constituent groups, one is identifiable as Lower Umpqua, a Siuslawan people. The others *may* correspond to the Upper Umpqua and Takelma of the upper Umpqua and Rogue River drainages.

Epidemic Areas	1700s Historical	Other[a]	1801	1824	1830s	1836	1837–47	1848	1853	1862
NORTH COAST										
Tlingit	S	S				S	I	M		S
Haida	S	S				S?		M		S
Nisga'a						S				S
Gitxsan										S
Coast Tsimshian		S				S		M		S
Sabassas						S				S
Haisla						S				
Nuxalk (Bella Coola)						S				S
WAKASHAN										
Heiltsuk										S
Kwakwaka'wakw	S?	S								S
Northern Coast Salish										S
Nuu-chah-nulth										1875
INLAND WATERS										
Squamish	S	S								
Fraser Halkomelem	S	S	S					M		
Island Halkomelem	S			S/M						
Songhees	S		S					M		
Lummi	S	S								
Nooksack	S								S	
Puget Salish	S	S		S/M			I	M	S	
Twana	S		S							
OLYMPIC										
Chemakum									S	
Clallam			S					M	S	
Ditidaht	S	S							S	
Makah									S	
Quileute									S	
SOUTH COAST										
Quinault		S							S	
Lower Chehalis			S						S	
Chinook		S	S	S/M	F&A				S	
Tillamook	S								S	
Alseans		S?							S	
Siuslawans		S				S?				
Coosans		S				S?				
Tututni		S		S/M		S				
INTERIOR VALLEYS										
Upper Chehalis										
Cowlitz					F&A		D	M		
Clatskanie					F&A					
Upper Chinookan	S	S			F&A		D	M	S	
Kalapuyans				S/M	F&A		D	M		
Takelma					F&A	S		M	S?	

NOTE: S = smallpox, M = measles, S/M = smallpox or measles, F&A = fever and ague (malaria), I = influenza, and D = dysentery.

[a] Evidence from oral tradition, abandoned-village horizons, and/or archeology for smallpox during the first half-century after contact; not necessarily specific as to particular epidemic.

factors than social networks. Nevertheless, the concept of "epidemic area" may be useful in other culture areas, both to summarize epidemiological and demographic trends and to help isolate underlying social and environmental factors that influence the spread of disease.

Epidemic areas are shown on map 1 in the Introduction. The memberships and defining epidemiological characteristics of each, from north to south, are given below.

The North Coast epidemic area comprised the Tlingit, the Haida, the Tsimshian peoples, the Haisla, and the Nuxalk (Bella Coola), all of whom experienced three important smallpox epidemics, in the late 1700s, 1836, and 1862. Most of these peoples (Nuxalk excepted) shared a matrilineal form of kinship system, women wore labrets, and there was considerable economic exchange centered on the mouth of the Nass (Suttles 1990a: 13).

The Wakashan epidemic area included the various Heiltsuk-speaking peoples, the Kwakwaka'wakw, the Nuu-chah-nulth, and Northern Coast Salish. The only fully documented epidemic among these peoples is that of 1862 (1875 for the Nuu-chah-nulth), though it is probable that all experienced smallpox in the late 1700s as well. Oral traditions from this area mention shared intermarriage, ceremonial and potlatching networks, and a common form of head flattening (Suttles 1990a: 13).

The Inland Waters epidemic area was made up exclusively of Salishan peoples, from the Squamish on the north to the Twana on the south. All experienced the late-1700s smallpox epidemic and possibly secondary early outbreaks as well. Regional networks were first documented in the Salish area (Elmendorf 1971); Suttles has since elaborated on what he calls the "Coast Salish continuum" (1987b).

The Olympic epidemic area included all of the peoples of the Olympic Peninsula (Quileute, Makah, Clallam, and Chemakum) as well as the Ditidaht across the Strait of Juan de Fuca. All experienced smallpox (one or more times) during the first years of contact, and all suffered from the 1853 epidemic. Some of these peoples, although not otherwise recognized as a cultural region, potlatched together (Suttles 1987b). They were also the only whale hunters on the coast other than the Nuu-chah-nulth.

The South Coast epidemic area included all Pacific coast peoples from the central Washington to the southern Oregon coast: Quinault, Lower Chehalis, Chinook, Tillamook, Alseans-Siuslawans-Coosans, and Tututni coastal Athapascans. All suffered from early smallpox, in most cases probably more than once; most appear to have been marginally affected by fever and ague; and the northern two-thirds of the area experienced the 1853 smallpox epidemic. The South Coast and Interior Valleys epidemic areas are the two areas where the close correspondence between social factors and disease histories starts to break down, due to the ecologically limited malarial area. The regional network of the South Coast is well defined: Hajda's (1984) "Greater Lower Columbia," characterized especially by intermarriage and a special type of head flattening, included both coastal and interior peoples, from Quinault to Aleans, and extended inland along the Columbia as far as The Dalles.

The Interior Valleys epidemic area included Upper Chehalis, Cowlitz, lower Columbia Athapascans, Upper Chinookans, Kalapuyans, and Takelmans. The defining disease was malaria, which became endemic in the entire zone; but all members also experienced early smallpox, and most suffered from dysentery and measles as well.

The one area where neither epidemiological nor social analyses have yet identified a "region" but where there may in fact have been one is southwest Oregon. Epidemiologically, all southwest Oregon peoples experienced the 1836–37 smallpox epidemic (in its southern extension). Trade and movement between coastal and interior peoples on both the Umpqua and the Rogue Rivers, though not sufficiently documented, are likely. Future research should concentrate on this possibility.

MALARIA VERSUS SMALLPOX

For the Northwest Coast as a whole, the most interesting finding of this research has been the marked difference in population response between regions affected by epidemic infectious diseases and those where malaria became endemic. In the former areas, such as the North Coast, the disease response was more clean-cut and episodic. Epidemic diseases passed through the population at widely spaced intervals and were absent in intervening years. Heavy disease-caused mortality and disruption of population systems were temporally constricted to these relatively brief epidemic periods. In the absence of continued demographic "insults," population systems (and numbers) appear to have tended to return to preceding patterns. The North Coast population response to epidemics may be analogous, on the one hand, to pre-contact responses to severe perturbations in the resource base or to other environmental upsets. On the other hand, the periodicity of the outbreaks is similar to the epidemic experience in Europe, Japan, and elsewhere.

In most of western Oregon and southwest Washington after 1830, malaria became endemic and had a chronic debilitating effect on Indian populations. Population decline was sudden and rapid. Once established, malaria took a yearly toll concentrated among newborn and infants. Fertility appears to have been depressed due to maternal anemia. The impact of this disease on human populations was stronger, unrelenting, and more difficult to adjust to because of its complex ecology. In the short time span covered by this book, most affected populations declined to near extinction. Judging from malarial adaptations in other parts of the world, indigenous Northwest Coast cultures, left to their own devices, would have required many more years and wide-ranging cultural adjustments to develop an accommodation to the disease.

It is instructive to compare these patterns with trends elsewhere in the Americas. Nonmalarial areas seem to have experienced a higher rate of population and cultural survival. It may be that the episodic nature of the disease and depopulation experience in these zones was paralleled by a similar stop-and-go disruption and recovery trend in cultural change. Malarial areas in the New World, however, consistently experienced heavy depopulation and minimal population and cultural survival. There was not enough time to develop the multiple biological and cultural adaptations that allowed human populations to survive in such Eastern Hemisphere malarial areas as West Africa and Sardinia.

All of the disease and depopulation patterns documented for the Northwest Coast are potentially relevant to the history and ethnographically documented sociocultural status of small-scale ("hunting-gathering" or otherwise) or "peripheral" populations elsewhere in the world. At some time in their histories, new, highly virulent diseases were introduced to practically all of these peoples, with demographic and sociocultural disruption analogous to the Northwest Coast experience. Depending on the epidemiological characteristics of the introduced disease, disruption might be minor or systemwide, temporary, cyclical, or continuing. Sociocultural responses to this disruption should display a similar range of limited or systemic effects and short-term or long-lasting effects. Few, if any, epidemiologically "pristine" small-scale or peripheral societies are left in the world today; their numbers have declined dramatically in the last few centuries. Social scientists must not assume, therefore, that the cultures of early-contact-period small-scale societies accurately reflect the "aboriginal" state. This was a mistake commonly made in many of the early classic ethnographies of preliterate peoples that were influenced by the ahistorical perspective of Franz Boas, and it characterizes the bulk of pre-1945 Northwest Coast ethnographic studies. Whenever possible, researchers should collect information about early disease history and its effects and take it into account in their explanations of documented sociocultural patterns.

SUGGESTIONS FOR FUTURE RESEARCH

This book has focused on major introduced infectious diseases and a single systemic interaction—between these new diseases and Native population systems. Given the data base established in the preceding chapters, however, it is clear that a number of disease interactions with other social and cultural systems remain unexplored. Some of these topics for future research are discussed below.

Changes in Fertility

Population systems, as demographers like to say, result from the balance of two forces: death rates and birth rates. This book is a study of *one* side of the "population equation" among contact-era Northwest Coast Indians: death rates, and how they were affected by the introduction of infectious, epidemic diseases. The data assembled here make it clear that the population decline

FIG. 19 *(facing page)*. Survivors: two photographs from the end of the epidemic period in the 1870s that reflect different aspects of population decline: decreasing fertility and rising mortality. (Top) Quatsino Sound (Nuu-chah-nulth) women and children in 1874. Wilson Duff, who originally printed this photo, commented, "In a period of declining population, few children appear in such group photographs" (1964b: 43). (Bottom) Auk (Tlingit) mourners in Juneau, 1870s. Sergei Kan noted, "For the duration of the wake, the mourners were socially dead, their condition marked by immobility and curtailed social activities. . . . as well as their charcoal-covered faces" (1994: 138). (Top: Courtesy of the Royal British Columbia Museum, Victoria, negative no. PN2552. Bottom: Courtesy of Rare Books Division, The New York Public Library, Astor, Lenox, and Tilden Foundations.)

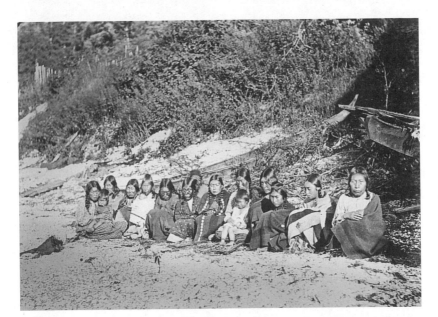

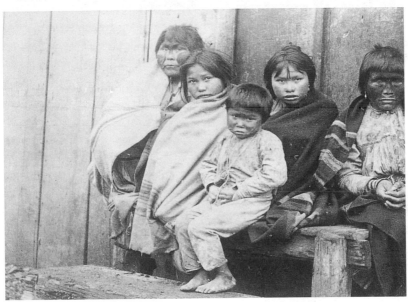

in the first century of contact was largely the result of mortality from these new diseases. But increased mortality was not the only factor: Northwest Indians' birth rates changed also.[3] The data on this problem are not nearly as forthcoming as are the data on mortality; the gross numbers of the estimates and censuses do not yield the same kind of information as, for example, the detailed birth and death registers from the Indian missions of California. The best we have at this time are clues, several of which have been mentioned in preceding pages. After epidemics, birth rates declined due to disrupted marriages; endemic malaria was accompanied by depressed fertility; and venereal diseases also negatively affected birth rates. Other factors, even more difficult to pinpoint, were at work: in the 1860s, Gilbert Sproat stated that the "principal cause" of the continued decline of the Nuu-chah-nulth peoples was the "despondency and discouragement" associated with rapid culture change (1868: 278–79). Similar arguments have been made for declining birth rates in the contact-era South Pacific (e.g., Rivers 1922). The decline in the Nuu-chah-nulth population, which (if the figures are correct) decreased from circa 8,250 people in the early 1800s to the mid-4,000s forty years later, in the absence of any recorded epidemics, may have been due to both increased mortality from chronic diseases and a marked decline in the birth rate. Fertility decline during the early contact era, its extent and causes, needs further study.

On the other hand, even though the data assembled in this book point to an unremitting across-the-board decline in population among Northwest Native peoples in the first century of contact, there may have been instances of situational, tentative rebound. This would have been most likely among North Coast peoples (Haida, Tlingit, Tsimshian), who had "breathing room" between the first recorded epidemics (perhaps 61 years), which may have allowed incipient rebound to occur. Under aboriginal conditions, most Northwest Coast populations are assumed to have been more or less stationary in numbers, backed up by a stable population system with balanced death and birth rates. Rebound assumes an inherent capacity in the population structure for births to exceed deaths. The lack of solid statistical evidence for numerical rebound among any Northwest Coast people between 1774 and 1874 argues for the preexistence of stationary population systems. But some populations

---

3. On the population equation and fertility patterns as applied to the aboriginal and contact era Native Northwest, see Boyd 1985: 415–36.

may indeed have had the capacity for rebound aboriginally, and others may have gained it after contact. The case of the Haida, discussed on pages 210–11, is instructive. Early, anecdotal accounts note the high number of children, late prehistoric population pressure may have led to wars of territorial expansion, and the high projected aboriginal population density, shared with other "outer-coastal" peoples such as the Nuu-chah-nulth, is also suggestive. The addition of cultivated potatoes to a diet lacking in carbohydrates and reliable year-round foods could conceivably have improved the general health and fat levels of females, extended the childbearing period, and reduced the interval between births, resulting in an increased fertility rate (Frisch 1977). There are analogs to this process elsewhere in the world (e.g., Lee 1972). Potato cultivation was also adopted by most Coast Salish peoples, and the relatively high percentage of children among Haida and Coast Salish populations in the HBC censuses suggests a capacity for numerical increase. Even though there is no *solid* evidence for numerical rebound of any Northwest Coast population in the century covered by this book, the topic of locally elevated contact-era birth rates is potentially significant and should be investigated further.[4]

Continuing Disease and Demographic Change

This book ends with the close of the epidemic period, with its onslaught of new diseases and unremitting population decline. The epidemic period, however, was but the first of several clear-cut stages in the postcontact disease and demographic history of Northwest Native Americans. During the reservation period (roughly the second half of the nineteenth century through World War I), a new class of diseases became prevalent while population continued a slow decline. Epidemic diseases were now largely controlled, save a few minor outbreaks among local reservation communities, and their place was taken by chronic ailments such as tuberculosis, trachoma, and the sexually transmitted diseases. Some U.S. populations experienced a brief spurt in numbers after removal to reservations, but numbers continued to drop to a population nadir after the turn of the century. Improvements in public health and health care delivery in Indian communities, particularly after

4. Robin Fisher (1996: 145) addresses the need for more study of fertility in contact-era populations.

World War I, seem to be closely tied to the population rebound that began at this time and was well under way by the last third of the twentieth century. Population rebound has been accompanied by varying degrees of intermarriage with Whites, persistence of off-reservation communities (see, e.g., Barsh 1996), and the growth of a new class of "urban Indians." With changing diets and decreased levels of physical activity following World War II, diabetes has become epidemic among Northwest Coast Indians. Many of the above patterns are shared with other North American Indians, a result of common recent historical experiences. Disease and demographic history during the reservation period has been outlined for the Plateau culture area (Boyd 1998), but no in-depth study has yet been attempted for the Northwest Coast.

Changes in Population Interrelations and Distributions

The hypothesis of differential migration and population "flow" between regions with different disease histories (urban and rural, malarial and non-malarial, highland and lowland, etc.) suggested by William McNeill (1976, 1979) and in this book might be tested elsewhere. The historic movement of upland Klikitat into depopulated malarial lowland territories of Chinookans and Kalapuyans (chapter 9) has a probable parallel along the protohistoric lower Mississippi (Dobyns 1983). Population flow as demonstrated by the Dakelhne-Nuxalk example (chapter 8) may have been operative elsewhere and earlier in the Northwest (as suggested by protohistoric downstream linguistic "flow" noted by Jacobs 1937) and might be profitably reexamined with a disease hypothesis in mind. Differential effects of disease on urban and rural and upper- and lower-class populations in Amerindian cultures and civilizations have not been studied at all. Several instances of differential mortality between semiacculturated Indians with access to White medicines and treatments and nonacculturated and distant peoples without such amenities have been noted in this book. And finally, excessive disease mortality should affect settlement patterns, influencing not only size and number but distribution (nucleated vs. dispersed, lowland vs. highland, etc.) as well. Ramenofsky (1987) suggests that such disease-caused shifts should appear in the archeological record as distinct "horizons." Preliminary tests of her thesis in the Pacific Northwest (Campbell 1989; Draper 1989) are suggestive and should be expanded.

Disease Introduction, Depopulation, and "Devolution"

In recent years some cultural anthropologists have shown an interest in what has been called cultural "devolution" or "deculturization." They have detected in some non-Western cultures experiencing significant population decline a tendency to "backtrack" or "devolve" to a point where much cumulated cultural tradition is lost, institutions break down, and social structures become simpler. These changes are adaptive in that they allow the culture to survive changed circumstances, but they run counter to the normally expected trend of cultural evolution, which is toward increasing complexity.

The case for devolution has been made most strongly in the second edition of Elman Service's *Primitive Social Organization* (1971), in his discussion of the origins of "composite bands." "The composite band lacks exogamic rules and explicit marital residence customs" (47). It "is obviously a product of the near-destruction of aboriginal bands after contact with civilization. In all cases, there is conclusive evidence of rapid depopulation by disease which resulted in the merging of previously unrelated peoples" (97). Service now believes (contrary to his position in the first edition of *Primitive Social Organization*) that certain of the simple, fluid social organizations noted among early-contact-period hunter-gatherer populations may not be typical of the "aboriginal" condition but instead be postcontact developments arising from the disruptive effects of recent contact with more-complex cultures.

A hypothesis of disease-caused "devolution" from matrilineal structures has been made for many indigenous Amazonian populations (Martin 1969; see also Murphy 1960; Henry 1964; Isaac 1977). A similar claim has been advanced for certain Subarctic Athapascan populations (Krech 1979). It should be possible to test the hypothesis of devolution for other parts of the Americas from which we have adequate knowledge of postcontact social organization, disease history, and population history.

Disease, Depopulation, and Numerically Dependent Systems

Beyond the problem of social organization itself, a few researchers have suggested that depopulation might affect the ability of a culture to maintain certain structures which require a minimum number of members of specific categories to function properly. The literature on optimal foraging theory (e.g., Smith 1981), for instance, suggests that there are minimum population levels required for the maintenance of different kinds of task groups, which in turn are necessary for carrying out certain subsistence activities. It stands to reason that depopulation which causes these task groups to fall beneath their minimum level threatens their existence and in turn affects the efficiency and/or nature of the whole group's subsistence effort. On another level, Wagley (1940, 1951) documented that age grades and feast groups, important in the ceremonial life of the Amazonian Tapirapé, decreased in numbers when depopulation cut their memberships so low that they could no longer function. As a consequence, fewer ceremonies were held, much traditional religious knowledge was lost, and the religious system became impoverished (or "simpler") in relation to the aboriginal state.

Another example of a numerically dependent aboriginal system that could no longer survive in its aboriginal state after disease-caused depopulation comes from the Northwest Coast itself. As described by Helen Codere (1950), the aboriginal potlatch system of the Kwakwaka'wakw was based upon a fixed number of individually owned statuses shared among a population that was relatively stable in number. The inheritance of each status was validated by a potlatch. When disease in the mid-1800s caused the population to decline drastically, the number of heritable statuses was unchanged, and consequently a flurry of potlatching activity was instigated by heirs apparent.

Disease, Depopulation, and Cultural Systems

Beyond specifically demographic and social effects, new diseases may interact with and cause change in other cultural systems. Two that might be profitably investigated given the Northwest Coast disease-depopulation data base are health care and religious systems.

Aboriginal treatments, health care practitioners, and explanations for disease may be strongly affected by the introduction of new diseases. Treatments that do not work may be dropped from the cultural inventory; traditional methods may be modified; new treatments and medicines from outside sources may be added. Presently, no studies deal directly with changes in the Native Northwest pharmacopoeia, despite a small literature on Indian medicines (e.g., Smith 1929). The adverse effect of one indigenous Pacific Northwest treatment—sweat bathing plus the cold-water plunge—when used to combat febrile diseases has been mentioned many times in this book. A sizable body of literature on this problem exists for the southern Northwest Coast and Plateau culture areas (Boyd 1979). Despite its documented effect on mortality, sweat bathing persists in many indigenous Northwest cultures. Sweating is still valued for its cleansing (both physical and spiritual) and "strengthening" attributes (Walker 1966), which helps explain its cultural persistence. And the febrile diseases now tend to be treated by nonindigenous methods, whereas sweating is used for minor ailments.

Disease causation in the Native Northwest was uniformly ascribed to supernatural influences: contamination, soul or spirit loss, and, in particular, witchcraft or sorcery performed by contagious and sympathetic magic or object intrusion (Drucker 1963: 159). Northwest health care practitioners (shamans) occupied the ambiguous position of being able to both cure and "cause" illness. In aboriginal times shamans might be killed in retaliation for unusual deaths; preliminary research indicates that temporal clusters of such killings and sorcery accusations occurred in parts of the Pacific Northwest during some epidemic periods (Boyd 1983). Sorcery and witchcraft accusations and "doctor-killings" are reported for other epidemic periods elsewhere in the world,[5] as well as for periods of wrenching cultural change. It has been suggested that such "epidemics" of sorcery accusations not only are symptomatic of internal cultural stresses but bring these stresses into focus, force them to be dealt with, and clear the way for possible adaptive cultural changes (Marwick 1965; Douglas 1970). In a broader sense, Northwest doctor-killings are specialized forms of scapegoating, a common cross-cultural response to epidemics and disease introduction (McGrath 1991). Several examples of scapegoating of marginalized people also appear in the preceding pages: for example, the orphan buried alive by Kalapuyans for "bringing" dysentery (p. 141) and the Makah man abandoned in the Strait of Juan de Fuca and subsequently shot for introducing smallpox (p. 168).

It is by now axiomatic that major religious changes tend to closely follow periods of wrenching cultural change (Linton 1943; Wallace 1970). In some cases epidemic diseases are major causes of this cultural upset. Cult behavior flourished during plague years in medieval Europe; the Protestant Reformation followed soon after (Langer 1964). In the Native Northwest

5. E.g., European Black Death: Langer 1964; syphilis in Europe: Andreski 1982; New Guinea Kuru: Lindenbaum 1979; Huron smallpox: Trigger 1981.

(Coast and Plateau), epidemic disease has been implicated as an important sufficient cause in the rise of many nativistic religions.[6] A major feature of Northwest Coast religion was the importance placed on trance or altered states of consciousness brought about by fasting, repetitive activities, and other forms of physical privation, both in the spirit quest and in winter ceremonies (e.g., Jilek 1982). In such instances, individuals were able to make contact with the spirit world. Indigenous prophets, aboriginally but particularly during the contact period, entered trance states, contacted the spirit world, and returned with a message. Some contact-period prophets apparently received their supernatural messages while sick with new and unusual diseases. Several examples of contact-era Native Northwest visions and prophets have been noted in this book.[7] The heightened and unexplainable mortality associated with new diseases required new explanations and methods of coping, something that the novel myths and rituals offered by Native prophets may well have supplied (Wallace 1956, 1970; Laughlin and d'Aquino 1979). Epidemics were calamitous and disturbing events, not amenable to treatment or explanation and destructive of the world as Indian peoples had known it. Missionaries were the first representatives of European religious culture to maintain continuous contact with many Native Northwest peoples. During or following major Northwest epidemics, Russian Orthodox, Anglican, and Oblate Catholic missionaries all took advantage of the fear of disease and of the disruption of epidemic times to convert their charges. In such cases, how successfully they handled the simultaneous problem of new diseases seems to have been an important factor in how completely the Christian faith was adopted by their flocks.

The Northwest Coast experience with contact-era "new diseases" was both devastating and revolutionary. Populations declined; some groups died out; the human suffering was appalling. The new diseases and associated population loss affected in one way or another virtually every aspect of Native culture, from subsistence patterns to oral literature. What happened to Northwest Coast Native peoples must not be forgotten, needs to be told, and should be a lesson to all of us who live during an era when epidemic diseases are largely a thing of the past.

6. Such as the Prophet Dance, Feather Religion, and Indian Shaker Church. See, e.g., Spier 1935; Du Bois 1938; Suttles 1957; Aberle 1959; Amoss 1982; Vibert 1995.

7. E.g., Cultee's grandfather and Tilki (p. 95); QAłax̣etł (p. 120); the Suquamish prophet (p. 156); Ləx̌i'lbid (pp. 166–67); and the disciples of Wodziwob (pp. 164–65).

Appendix 1

Northwest Coast Indigenous Ailments

In terms of health and disease, two characteristics of the Northwest Coast culture area make it different from the (mostly tropical) hunting-gathering cultures on which stage 1 of table 1 (p. 10) was based. Both relate to the high latitude and hence colder environment of the Northwest. First, during the cold half of the year (November–April), when wild foods were mostly unavailable, Northwest Coast peoples were prone to nutritional deficiencies, weight loss, and (occasionally) starvation (tables 5–6). Second, because of the colder climate, there were fewer indigenous parasites and hence infections than in tropical climates.

NUTRITIONAL PROBLEMS

Most of our information on cold-season food problems comes from the areal oral literature. Starvation runs like a leitmotif through Northwest myth texts. Several myths explicitly mention famine-induced deaths, and others note that the young and old, the poor, and those without family suffered the most.[1] Other

1. For examples of starvation in the myth texts, see the Haida "The Lost People of Yagun Inlet" (Swanton 1908: 630), Se'shalt "Tradition of a Great Snowstorm" (Hill-Tout 1978: 4.117–18), and Clackamas "They Died of Hunger" (Jacobs 1958–59: 2.458–61). Historical accounts mentioning Indian starvation include Lewis and Clark 1991: 49, Ordway 1916: 337 (on the Chinookans), and Meares 1790: 132 and Saavedra 1794: 290 (Nuu-chah-nulth). The Tsimshian "The Spider and the Widow's Daughter" (Boas 1916: 158) relates which demographic categories died.

TABLE 5. Nutritional/Dietary Ailments Known
or Hypothesized from the Northwest Coast

Condition	Characteristics
Seasonal starvation and protein poisoning	Starvation: loss of body fat and water; skin loose and thin; end-stage muscle and viscera wasting, mental derangement; cannibalism noted (Passmore and Eastwood 1986: 262–64)
	Protein poisoning: weight loss, weakness, uremic poisoning (Speth 1991: 270)
Hypervitaminosis D (vitamin D intoxication)	Excessive urination, gastrointestinal upset and vomiting, heart rhythm irregularities, weakness, mental symptoms
Scurvy (vitamin C deficiency)	Weakness, skin hemorrhages, edema, bleeding gums, anemia (Passmore and Eastwood 1986: 324–25)
Internal parasites:	
Trichinella spp.	Trichinellosis
Pinworm (Enterobius westermani)	Enterobiasis
Tapeworms	Stomachache, diarrhea, weakness
Taenia saginata	Taeniasis
Diphyllobothrium	Diphyllobothriasis
Roundworm (Anisakis simplex)	Anisakiasis: intestinal obstructions, colic, abscesses, peritonitis
Lung fluke (Paragonimus westermani)	Paragonimiasis: cough, bloody sputum
Fish fluke (Nanophyetus salmincola)[a]	Diarrhea (sometimes bloody)
Bacterial food poisoning (salmonellosis, botulism)	Salmonellosis: diarrhea and gastroenteritis (Salmonella bacteria)
	Botulism: neurological problems, paralysis (toxin from Clostridium botulinum)
Paralytic shellfish poisoning ("red tide")	Diarrhea and vomiting, heart irregularities, weakness, paralysis (20%)

[a] Flukes infected with Neorickettsia helminthoeca cause exophthalmia in fish; dogs who eat infected fish die of "salmon-poisoning disease" in western Oregon and the lower Columbia. Human infection reported in Siberia

Citations	Comments
Mythological, ceremonial, art (see references in text)	Wintertime absolute food lack or over-dependence on protein
Speth and Spielmann (1983) discuss the dangers of excessive meat consumption; Noli and Avery (1988) present the same argument for seafood	Affects young and old disproportionately Ameliorated by storage and preservation methods and by gifting and trade networks Increases susceptibility to infectious diseases
Lazenby and McCormack 1985; Chisholm, Nelson, and Schwarcz 1983	Hypothetical, winter overconsumption of seafood, particularly among children
Chinookans, 1814: spring roots "clean them of their scabs . . . and purify their blood" (Henry 1992: 703) A bleeding mouth is characteristic of possession by the South Coast *skep* spirit, manifested in winter ceremonies (Boyd 1996b: 134–37)	Hypothetical, based on ethnohistorical citations and lack of winter vitamin C sources
Fortuine 1989: 60	From bear meat
Reinhard 1990; Merbs 1992 (on neighboring regions); Schmidt and Roberts 1989 (on general characteristics)	Fecal-oral route
	From ungulates
	From fish
McKerrow, Sakanari, and Deardorff 1988	From poorly cooked salmon
	From poorly cooked crustaceans
Eastburn et al. 1987	Infected salmon
Quileute (Andrade 1931: 33–34, 154–55; Reagan 1935: 69), Quwutsun' (Hill-Tout 1978: 4.158), Clackamas (Jacobs 1958–59: 2.151)	From rancid or poorly cooked meat; possible myth references: dried fish, whale, and salmon
	Contemporary Indian botulism deaths from "salmon egg cheese" (Garvin 1989; Dolman 1964)
Tlingit (Swanton 1909: 130), Haida (Swanton 1908: 307), Kwakwa̲ka'wakw (Boas 1910: 375–77, 1935: 177), Euro-American (Fortuine 1975: 71–72)	Caused by toxin from the dinoflagellate *Gonyaulax catanella*; Indians probably avoided it in most cases

(Millemann and Knapp 1970); mythological references suggest same in lower Columbia (Adamson 1926–27; Jacobs 1945: 356–58, 1958–59: 2.548).

TABLE 6. Precontact Northwest Coast Paleopathological Conditions Identified from Bones

Ailment	Characteristics	Citations	Comments
Osteoarthritis (degenerative joint disease)	Bone malformation: eburnation, wedging, lipping; affects vertebrae (sacroiliac, thoracic, cervical) and limb joints	Noted in most Northwest Coast paleopathological studies: see esp. Cybulski 1992 (89%); Beattie 1976 (71%)	Ubiquitous among older individuals, especially women Due to mechanical stress with possible genetic predisposition
Rheumatoid arthritis	Hand (and sometimes foot) malformations	Rothschild et al. 1988; documented in Alaska (Ortner and Utermohle 1981) and Columbia Plateau (Boyd and Gregory 1995)	Prevalent among older women; autoimmune reaction to unknown infectious agent
Ankylosing spondylitis (Marie-Strümpell disease)	Fused thoracic vertebrae producing humped back	Beattie 1976 (Boundary Bay); Gofton et al. 1972 (contemporary Haida)	Prevalent among men; familial
Spondylolysis and spina bifida	Bilateral separation of neural arch in lumbar vertebrae; meninges or cord exposed	Lundy 1981 (Birch Bay); Cybulski 1992	Familial (depicted in fig. 20)
Treponematosis (probably yaws)	Lesions on extremities, particularly legs	Cybulski 1990; Rothschild and Rothschild 1996	Skin contact, mostly among children
Cancers		Cybulski and Pett 1981 (Haida and Songhees)	Rare among hunter-gatherers
Multiple myeloma	"Uniform, small" bone lesions		
Metastatic carcinoma	Round, sharp-edged lesions		
Dental diseases	High degree of attrition; abscesses common; caries rare	See esp. Hall and German 1975; Hall, Morrow, and Clarke 1986; Cybulski 1990, 1992	Clear dietary correlations; seafood and dry fish: attrition; high-carbohydrate roots (e.g., camas): caries
Cribra orbitalia (form of porotic hyperostosis)	Porosity of bones behind eyes	Cybulski 1977, 1990; Stuart-Macadam 1992	Osteological marker of iron deficiency in childhood; perhaps related to parasite overload

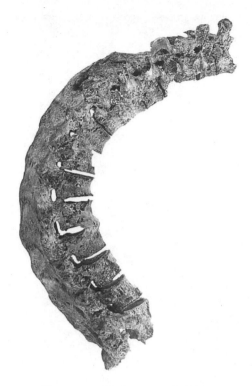

FIG. 20. Osteological problems, particularly osteoarthritis, were very common in pre-contact Indian populations. This photo shows a curved spine caused by spondylolysis, a hereditary condition, from the Boardwalk site, British Columbia. (Courtesy of Jerome Cybulski, curator of physical anthropology, Canadian Museum of Civilization, Hull, Quebec, image no. 72-16039.)

stories mention people who became too weak to move around, who were unable to stomach food when it became available, and who were reduced to skeletons.[2] Clinical starvation is characterized by mental derangement, obsession with food, and lack of concern for the welfare of others. Cannibalism is well documented during famines (Passmore and Eastwood 1986: 262–64). It is also a theme in Northwest Coast mythologies and ceremonialism. A common motif in Northwest Coast art suggests famine-related emaciation. This is the "x-ray" skeletal motif, with emphasis on the rib cage (fig. 21).

2. The Tillamook tale "Raven and Ice" has Ice becoming "mere skin and bones because he had nothing to eat" (E. Jacobs 1959: 18). The Cathlamet tale "The Spirit of Hunger" has a man wrestling with Hunger during a famine: "She was very lean; she was only skin and bones, but she was braided" (Boas 1901: 212).

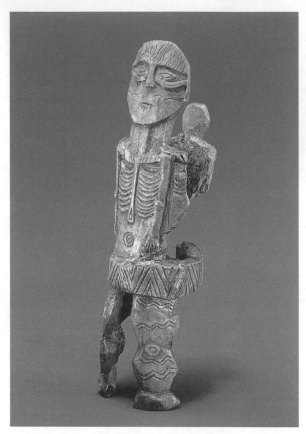

FIG. 21. Starvation is a common theme in Northwest Coast mythology and art. The "x-ray skeleton" motif pictured here, with its emphasis on the rib cage, suggests famine-related emaciation. This Chinookan elk-horn figure, from Sauvie Island, Oregon, may represent the "basket ogress." (Courtesy of the Thomas Burke Memorial Washington State Museum, Seattle, catalog no. 2-3844.)

Three reasons for starvation are mentioned in the texts: lack of a staple wild food, exhaustion of stored resources, and severe weather that made it impossible to forage. The crucial resource throughout the culture area was salmon, which (air-dried or smoked) was intended to last through the winter. But salmon runs are notoriously inconsistent, and overdependence on salmon has its own set of problems. Salmon provides plenty of protein and calcium and (like all seafood) vitamin D and unsaturated plasma essential fatty acids. It is a fair source of calories and iron and a poor source of carbohydrates and vitamin C. Shellfish, available more or less year-round, are similar nutritionally. Chemical analyses of prehistoric human bones from the

British Columbia coast indicate that 90% of protein intake came from marine sources.[3]

Overdependence on high-protein foods during the winter may, without carbohydrates or fat to help metabolize it, result in weight loss; eating protein alone for an extended period of time may result in uremic poisoning and death. It has been suggested that the seasonally high seafood diet of Northwest Coast peoples may have led to vitamin D intoxication, especially among children, and that a wintertime lack of fresh greens may have produced symptoms of scurvy. Important for the purposes of this book is the fact that people who are weak from lack of food and malnutrition are more susceptible to infectious diseases. Late winter/early spring, always a difficult time for Northwest Coast peoples, was a particularly bad time, mortality-wise, for an epidemic of introduced disease to strike.

PARASITES

Northwest Coast peoples, given their seasonal sedentism and high-seafood diet, were probably exposed to several internal parasites (listed in table 5). Some of these (particularly pinworms) may have contributed to childhood anemia. External parasites were few (relative to warmer regions) but were probably influential in the spread of the few known or likely precontact infectious diseases. Before contact, native chiggers, scabies mites, fleas, and mosquitoes, though productive of bites, are not known to have carried any important diseases. Two indigenous ticks may have caused occasional cases of tularemia and Lyme disease. And native flies and eye gnats may have helped spread conjunctivitis. But the most important indigenous disease-carrying arthropod was certainly the body louse, *Pediculus humanus* (fig. 22).

Lice are mentioned frequently in the mythology and historical texts. They infested furs, and their numbers built up in native dwellings over time.[4] One of the functions of sweat bathing (practiced everywhere but Vancouver Island) was delousing. Temperatures 4–5° C above body temperature kill lice (James and Harwood 1969: 138); sage (*Artemesia* spp.) not only imparted a

---

3. On nutritional analysis of salmon, see Hunn 1990: 177; on fatty acids, Bates et al. 1985; on shellfish, Moss 1992; on protein analysis of bones, Chisholm, Nelson, and Schwarcz 1983; and on coastal forager nutrition in general, Yesner 1987.

4. See Jacobs 1958–59: 2.394–95 for a Clackamas classification of biting insects; Fleurieu 1801: 1.328 on the hazards of trading furs; and Simpson 1968: 62 on abandonment of infested houses.

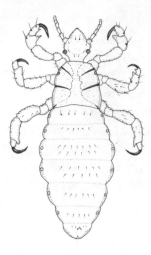

FIG. 22. *Pediculus humanus corporis,* the human body louse, causes the skin disease pediculosis. (Drawing by Shivaji Ramalingam, Dept. of Microbiology, Oregon Health Sciences University, Portland.)

fragrant odor but served as a fumigant as well (Turner 1979: 31, 177). A common myth theme has an ugly man with sores all over his body sweating several days and becoming smooth-skinned and handsome (e.g., for the Cowlitz, see Adamson 1934: 193–95; for the Skagit, see Haeberlin 1924: 433–35).

INDIGENOUS INFECTIOUS DISEASES

Lice bites cause pediculosis, a rash of red papules which, when scratched, fill with white blood cells and are apt to become infected (James and Harwood 1969: 9). Sores and scabs are mentioned frequently in the mythology. Although many conditions may be represented (such as indigenous treponematoses; see chapter 3) and exact diagnoses are not possible, the disease was probably impetigo, and the infectious agents were most likely usually varieties of the cosmopolitan *Staphylococcus* and *Streptococcus* bacteria. Impetigo is defined as a "scabby eruption," initially with "thin-walled vesicles" that rupture, leak fluid, and develop layers of "golden yellow crusts," particularly on the face (Arnold, Odom, and James 1990: 275–76). The disease spreads by physical contact and is associated with poor hygiene and crowding. It particularly affects children and, by itself, is not lethal. Impetigo lesions, however, may develop into boils, carbuncles, and abscesses.

"A scabby race of people" was how Alexander Henry described the

Chinookan people of the lower Columbia in 1814. "Their arms, legs, rumps, and bodies [were] much affected with scabs" (1992: 664). In the Clackamas myth "Coyote Went around the Land," Coyote met a man with scabs: "He saw it, horrors, his (the man's) body, something was running (oozing) from it. It was disgusting . . . that person stood up, he did something to (he scraped) his (own) body, he put (the discharge) into a pan. . . . Coyote thought . . . 'Oh oh it is nasty.' . . . He (Coyote) was disgusted and nauseated" (Jacobs 1958–59: 1.84–85). The myth theme of a scabby man who sweated and became beautiful was noted above. The Kwakwaka'wakw myth "Scab" describes a boy with "scabs all over his body" who was abandoned by his people because they feared infection. The boy scratched himself once and his "boils came off"; a second time, and from his belly emerged another boy, who was called "Scab" (Boas 1910: 39, 41). In 1889, Dr. Charles Buchanan's aged Snohomish informants described a "ss-chub-chub," a large boil with "many eyes," certainly a carbuncle.

There were also indigenous eye and ear infections. On the lower Columbia, Alexander Henry noted that "the men in general appear much affected with sore eyes. . . . Their eyes in general are also very bad, sore, and watery." Out of seven Yamhill Kalapuyans, four "had some defect in the eyes" (1992: 658). A contemporary of Henry stated, "The greater number have very sore eyes; several have only one; and we observed a few old men and women quite blind" (Cox 1957: 78). Meriwether Lewis found "soar eyes at all stages of life. . . . the loss of sight I have observed to be more common among all the nations inhabiting this river than among any people I ever observed" (Lewis and Clark 1991: 85).

Although these citations are from the Columbia River, the condition occurred all along the coast (e.g., among the Tlingit, Haida, and Nuu-chah-nulth in 1818; Roquefeuil 1823: 2.178). In 1869 an American visitor to Sitka stated "conjunctivitis and cor[n]eitis are very common owing to the constant atmosphere of smoke in their houses" (Colyer 1870a: 1024). Conjunctivitis is an inflammation of the ocular mucous membrane with exudate; the causal agents are mostly bacterial (streptococcal and staphylococcal) (Ostler 1994). Corneitis refers to complications affecting the cornea, probably keratitis (Fortuine 1989: 512). Trachoma, caused by a chlamydial infection, was epidemic among Northwest Coast Indians in the early 1900s; the above references to blindness suggest it may have occurred earlier as well.

Otitis media, an infection of the middle ear, is epidemic among contemporary Northwest Indians (Cambon, Galbraith, and Kong 1965), and it was identified paleopathologically in 10 out of a sample of 14 from Prince Rupert Harbour (Cybulski 1992: 135–36). The causal agent is (again) usually streptococcal, and symptoms include a stabbing pain, drainage of grayish pus, and, after a while, hearing loss (Sievers and Fisher 1981: 238). Ear problems and hearing loss are not mentioned, however, in either the oral traditions or early historic texts.

Appendix 2

Malaria and Smallpox:
Clinical and Epidemiological Characteristics
and Historical Epidemiology

MALARIA

Malaria is a very complex disease, in both its population interactions and clinical characteristics. The complexity comes from the three species involved in its transmission: primary host (an anopheline mosquito), parasite (a protozoan member of the genus *Plasmodium*), and secondary host (several warm-blooded species, including humans).

More than 50 species of anophelines can transmit human malaria. Though most are tropical, some are found as far as 62° north latitude (May 1961: 166–71). Breeding occurs only during warm weather and usually in warm, still water; anophelines are not common in regions with less than 30 inches of rainfall (Dutta and Dutt 1978: 74). The most important vector west of the Rockies is *A. freeborni* (fig. 23), which breeds from May to October, with a peak in September: mosquitoes, mosquito bites, and primary infections of malaria are rare between November and June. *A. freeborni* prefers "clean, sunny water" and was most common in the Northwest in the oxbow lakes and ponds along the Willamette River and in the Portland Basin (Gjullin and Eddy 1972; Aitken 1945).

The disease itself is caused by various species of the protozoan genus *Plasmodium: P. falciparum, P. malariae, P. vivax,* and *P. ovale. P. falciparum* produces the most severe disease effects in the human host and causes the highest mortality, *P. malariae* has less severe effects, and *P. vivax* and *P. ovale* usually produce a benign disease. Both severe forms were apparently present in the Northwest. Following inoculation of the host by mosquito bite, the

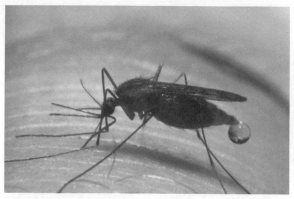

FIG. 23. *Anopheles freeborni* became the vector for the malaria-causing plasmodium parasite following the latter's introduction to the Northwest in 1830. As shown in the photograph, mosquitoes often excrete excess serum while taking a blood meal. (Courtesy of Robert K. Washino, Dept. of Entomology, University of California, Davis.)

parasite travels in the host's bloodstream to the liver, where it undergoes initial cell division. This stage corresponds to the "latency" period of the disease, with no obvious symptoms. After a variable period of time (12 days for *P. falciparum;* 30 for *P. malariae*) parasites invade red blood cells, where they multiply until the corpuscles burst; this happens simultaneously and many times in succession, producing bouts of cold shakes ("ague") and elevated fever and sweating symptomatic of the disease. The exact timing of the cycles of division in the blood cells and corresponding fits of cold and fever varies according to the parasite: daily (quotidian), every other day (tertian), every third day (quartan) (Benenson 1995: 283).

Falciparum malaria, which may invade internal organs, is the only variety that, by itself, is capable of causing death. All types of malaria, due to their blood-cell-destroying action, cause anemia in varying degrees, accompanied by a general weakening and breakdown of the body's defenses against secondary diseases. The anemia characteristic of malarial populations has been claimed by some to be a factor in cultural decline or, obversely, a retardant to development (Wood 1979). Demographically, the weakening effects of anemia are most severe among infants, and their mortality is consequently higher; fertility rates are affected by increased frequencies of miscarriages and stillbirths (Wood 1979: 258).

Following the establishment of a host-vector-parasite relationship in a given geographical area, malaria generally becomes endemic (continually present). By the late 1800s, malaria had spread from its area of origin in Africa to virtually every part of the globe where it could be supported, and "epidemics" in the recent past have resulted from sudden increases in the numbers of one of the constituent populations in already endemic areas. Malaria epidemics arising from the introduction of one or more of the three populations to a new geographic area occurred mostly in the distant past and are not well recorded.

Studies of the genus *Plasmodium* indicate that its evolutionary focus was tropical Africa (Bruce-Chwatt 1965). In his classic study Frank Livingstone (1958) reconstructed how human malaria became prevalent in the region. About 2,000 years ago two innovations prompted the cutting down of much of the forests of West Africa: iron smelting and the production of iron tools (diffused from the Nile) and yam agriculture (diffused from Southeast Asia). The opening of the forests created a new breeding environment for anopheline mosquitoes, sunlit pools. With new opportunities, both human and mosquito populations increased rapidly, and so did malaria. A period of intense natural selection followed, with consequent local increases in the sickle cell gene, which (in one of its forms) provides resistance to malaria.

Outside Africa, malaria became prevalent wherever large populations of humans, anopheline mosquitoes, and different forms of the parasite (particularly *P. falciparum*) came in close contact. Various researchers have suggested that ecological shifts promoting malarial prevalence may have been responsible for historically known periods of population and cultural decline. Such is the case for the decline of classical civilization in Sri Lanka (Nichols 1921), as a result of intensification of rice cultivation, and in Greece between ca. 550 and 450 B.C., following a period of deforestation and spread of agriculture (Jones 1909; Laderman 1975).

About the same time that it became prevalent in Greece, malaria appeared in Sardinia, where it established an intense endemic focus. Medical anthropologist Peter Brown (1980, 1981, 1983, 1986) has studied the several adaptations, both biological and cultural, that have developed in response to the requirements of living on this malarial island. As with the West African sickling gene, there has been natural selection for two genetic traits (in this case, thalassemia and favism) that provide some resistance to malaria. A complex of cultural traits—including settlement and transhumant patterns, pregnancy behaviors, and disease causation theories—has also developed to minimize malarial exposure. Both the West African and Sardinian examples show clearly what a pervasive influence endemic malaria can be and how it requires multiple adaptations, biological and cultural, for human societies to survive and persist in its presence.

Because of the relatively early spread of malaria to parts of the globe where anopheline mosquitoes are present, we know very little about the dynamics of malaria *introduction* to a given region. The last and best-recorded introduction in the Eastern Hemisphere was on the Indian Ocean island of Mauritius in the 1860s; in the Americas it was in western Oregon in the 1830s. The Mauritian example involved the introduction of an anopheline vector to an island inhabited mostly by recent immigrants from India, some of whom had chronic cases of malaria and harbored plasmodia in their blood. As in West Africa, mosquito colonization was preceded by deforestation and heavy rains, which produced innumerable breeding areas. Once the vector was introduced, the rapid breeding capacities of both mosquitoes and plasmodia took over, and a true epidemic followed. One authority describes the process: "If each starting infection produced ten others in from 20 to 30 days there would be 100 secondary cases in 50 days, 1,000 in 100 days, and so on. Since the number of carriers and the number of infected mosquitoes increase as functions of each other the multiplication of a few all-but-invisible parasites into devastating hordes can—and does—occur with a speed that will always seem miraculous however mathematically routine" (Harrison 1978: 206–7). Over 10% of the Mauritian population died, and the infection rate was many times that figure, despite a fairly good knowledge of preventive and treatment measures and the existence of the antimalarial drug quinine. The Mauritian example is most important for the rapidity of spread: it shows that true epidemics and a potential for high mortality can and do follow introduction of malaria to a new geographic area.[1]

In the last example, western Oregon in the 1830s, such an epidemic did occur (see chapter 4), and the inhabitants of the region had *none* of the adaptations—biological or cultural—found in West Africa, Sardinia, or even Mauritius. Western Oregon represents the most recent occurrence of what must have been the usual form of malarial introduction in the Americas: addition of the parasite to a preexisting mosquito-human relation. The malarial parasite seems not to have been native to the Americas.[2]

1. The Mauritian data are from a series of articles in the *Transactions of the London Epidemiological Society* for 1869 and from Harrison 1978.

2. Dunn (1965) maintains that the lack of human balanced polymorphisms (such as the sickling trait, thalassemia, and the Duffy blood group) that provide partial resistance to the disease,

An antidote to malaria was discovered in the early 1600s, in (surprisingly) South America. The bark of the cinchona tree, which grows in tropical Ecuador, contains an alkaloid, quinine, that kills the malarial parasite. Powdered cinchona bark became popular as a malarial treatment in Europe by the mid-1600s; quinine itself was not distilled and used as a medicine for another two centuries, or about the time of malaria's introduction to western Oregon (Guerra 1977).

SMALLPOX

Smallpox was normally spread by "droplet infection," usually in a sneeze, though transmission may also have occurred by physical contact with a person in the infective stage, a corpse up to three weeks after death, and, rarely, fomites (items in close contact with the patient), which could remain infective for up to a year. Once a person became infected with the *Variola* virus, the disease had to run its course; nothing could be done to arrest it and little to alleviate it.

A nonsymptomatic, noninfective incubation period of 7–18 days (average 10) followed the entry of smallpox germs into the respiratory tract. Two days of fever, headache, and body pains followed, and then a rash appeared, which proceeded through a number of well-defined stages. Initially red spots appeared on the face, hands, and feet and spread from these foci to the rest of the body. The red spots became raised lesions, which filled with liquid, like blisters. Pustules developed as white blood cells entered the lesions, and these advanced to scabs as a crust was formed. In surviving smallpox patients, the scabs fell off and deep scars (pockmarks) remained. Throughout the period when lesions were present, the patient was infective; itching and a distinct odor appeared by the pustular stage. The entire progress of the disease, from infection to recovery or death, was approximately one month (Dixon 1962; Fenner et al. 1988; Nakano and Jordan 1994; Benenson 1995).

There were two varieties of smallpox, each with differing severity of lesions and prognosis. *Variola major,* or classic smallpox, was more lethal, with a fatality rate averaging 30%. In the most severe cases, lesions became confluent (flowed together), and hemorrhaging and sloughing of skin some-

---

plus a paucity of animal malarias, argues for a post-1500 introduction of the disease to the Americas.

times occurred. "Fulminant" (rapidly progressing) cases had a very poor prognosis. *Variola minor* was much less severe, with a fatality rate of about 1%. Symptoms were not pronounced, and the disease was sometimes confused with other rash-causing diseases such as chicken pox. Clear-cut epidemics of *V. minor* did not appear before the late 1800s. Both varieties of smallpox are now extinct; the last cases were reported in 1978.

From an epidemiological standpoint, the important characteristics of smallpox were (1) its rapid and fully effective transmission, producing infection rates nearing 100% in non-immune populations; (2) its short infective period (ca. two weeks); and (3) the near 100% acquired immunity of survivors to second attacks of the disease. Smallpox typically passed through a given population very quickly and then died out for lack of susceptibles. The disease became endemic only in densely populated places such as China, India, and western Europe that had a continuous supply of susceptible newborns. In such areas smallpox developed into a mild disease of childhood, with adults largely immune. Most of the early Euro-American visitors to the Northwest Coast came from such areas.

In isolated or sparsely populated areas of the world, smallpox epidemics occurred in cycles.[3] This cyclical nature appears clearly in the recent epidemic history of western North America.

Northwest Coast	Plateau	Plains	California
ca. 1770–78	ca. 1769–80	1780–87	1780–81 (Baja)
ca. 1800–1808 (south)	ca. 1800–1808	1800–1803	
1824–25? (south)	1824–25? (south)		
		1831–32	
1836–37		1837–38	1838
1853 (south)	1853 (south)		
1862 (north)	1863 (north)		

SOURCES: Summarized from Cook 1939 (California); Taylor 1977 (the northern Plains); and this volume (Northwest Coast and Plateau).

In 1798 the Englishman Edward Jenner discovered that vaccination with the benign cowpox virus would produce immunity to smallpox infection, and

3. The lists of outbreaks and epidemics in Hirsch 1883 and Stearn and Stearn 1945 show this cyclical nature very clearly.

the technique spread rapidly across the Atlantic to the United States and Spanish colonies (Bowers 1981; Valle 1973b). One of the first Americans to use it was President Thomas Jefferson, who told Lewis and Clark to take it with them on their 1803–6 western expedition, though there is no record that they did so. Vaccine was not widely used in the Northwest until the epidemic of 1836–37 (chapter 5). In the early years, there were frequent problems with supply, viability, and improper administration of vaccine.

Appendix 3

The Unidentified "Columbia Leprosy"

Besides tuberculosis (see chapter 3), a second mycobacterial disease, leprosy, may also have been present among Northwest Coast Indians. Contemporary Euro-American observers and early-twentieth-century Native American informants consistently used the word "leprosy" to refer to a clear-cut syndrome affecting Indians on the lower Columbia and Fraser Rivers. And a mid-nineteenth-century Comox skull has been identified by a prominent paleopathologist as being clearly leprotic. But the disease has (apparently) died out, and given the historical tendency to confuse true leprosy with other destructive skin diseases such as syphilis and leishmaniasis (a tropical American disease), an accurate diagnosis is not possible.

Leprosy exists in many forms. Most produce skin lesions and not much else. The symptoms of classical (or "lepromatous") leprosy, however, are striking and well known. It is a chronic wasting disease which attacks peripheral nerve endings, producing "anesthetic lesions" and muscle wasting, especially in the face and extremities. In advanced cases, the fingers may become swollen and the hand may take on a clawed shape. The face assumes a "leonine" appearance, with thickened, sagging tissues; the nasal cartilage may be destroyed; the alveolar ridge may deteriorate and the front teeth may become loosened; blindness may arise from an inability to move the eyelids and consequent drying and ulceration of the cornea. The disease is not very contagious (like tuberculosis, it is spread by droplet infection), it takes several years for symptoms

to develop, and only a small percentage of the population appears susceptible to the most extreme forms. Leprosy is an exclusively human disease; there
is no known (natural) animal reservoir (Benenson 1995: 264–67; Plattzgraff
and Bryceson 1985).

The earliest mention of the word "leprosy" among Northwest Native
Americans is in a list of "Imported Diseases" of the Indians of the lower
Columbia, by Hudson's Bay governor George Simpson, in 1825. From the 1840s
there are two detailed descriptions from the Fort Vancouver area, by Catholic
missionary Modeste Demers and Hudson's Bay physician Dr. Forbes Barclay:

17 March 1842
The natives of the Columbia are subject to a terrible malady very similar to the leprosy of the Jews. This cruel malady is contagious, and as soon as it shows itself the
unfortunate victim is isolated without pity from his family, relatives, and friends, lodged
in a hut apart, and has no further communication with his fellow men than by voice
and from afar. They do not touch what he has used. They give him circumspectly medicines, which occasionally bring about a cure if the sickness is not obstinate and without alarming severity. A woman died of it lately in a condition difficult to describe.
Her feet, her hands, and especially her face, in complete putrefaction, shed a noisome
and unbearable odor. The malady has resisted to this day the knowledge of the doctors in the area. (Demers in Landerholm 1956: 111–12)

Libra. This is the most malignant disease which Dr. Barclay has encountered in this
part of the world. . . . the patient is first attacked with a general swelling of the solids
all over the body, and the face and hands completely disfigured—the pain is not as
severe as the swelling would make it appear. Soon after this swelling the face and legs
break out and are covered all over with putrid sores, of a flaking character, and remain
in an indolent state for a year or two, and when they scale over, they are apt to break
out on the least exposure. The appetite is generally better than when in health, notwithstanding which great and rapid emaciation takes place. . . . No internal organ appears
to be diseased, as they all perform their functions. When the patient survives the disease a few years, he is suddenly attacked with diarrhaea, which terminates in death.
The breath is always most offensive. One person in a family will sometimes have the
disease and all others enjoy good health. After death the soft parts have been observed
to drop off the bones. The treatment has been various . . . Iodine—several prepara-
tions of Mercury, [illegible], etc., have been administered, but with little or no
benefit. (Dunn 1846: 28)

The paleopathological evidence for leprosy is a Comox skull collected in 1866 with "advanced nasal spine atrophy," "maxillary alveolar process atrophy" with loose incisors, and "small, closely spaced pits" on the hard palate. All of these markers clearly indicate leprosy (Møller-Christensen and Inkster 1965). The date of collection and the fact that the skull is "mature" indicate that the individual was initially infected in the early 1800s.[1]

A final diagnostic description of leprosy comes from the medical officer of H.M.S. *Sparrowhawk* in 1869 and refers to coastal Indians of British Columbia:

Leprosy

A form of this disease allied to Lepra Guicolum occurs on the coast and is principally confined to the feet although occasionally attacking the hands. There is complete anaesthesia of the foot and palioris of the extensor muscles, the toes all contracted and the patient walks on his heel, the skin of the foot is harsh and appears of a bronze color, when attacking the hand the fingers are bent and curved like a bird claw. (Comrie 1869)

Four other references complete the ethnohistorical record on early Northwest Coast "leprosy." The 1827 Fort Alexandria report (Dakelhne, or Carrier, Indians) notes: "The Leprosy . . . transplanted from the Sea Coast" (Joseph McGillivray, in Rich 1947: 206). In 1833, at Oak Point village on the Columbia River (Chinookan/Clatskanie Athapascan), a Hudson's Bay doctor described "Yughaz the Chief (droll looking character with a square pit in the extremity of his nose capable of containing a small pea & his front of upper jaw rasped down to stumps)" (Tolmie 1963: 167). In 1841 the adolescent son of Archibald MacDonald, head of the Hudson's Bay Company's Fort Colvile, expired from the "Columbia leprosy" (Cole 1979: 201–2). In 1879 a retired Company official recalled that the half-Clatsop son of Solomon Smith "died of leprosy," one of several cases that local doctors treated with arsenic (Roberts 1962: 198–99).

Besides the lower Columbia, a second focus of leprosy accounts is the Strait of Georgia. The leprotic Comox skull and H.M.S. *Sparrowhawk* description

---

1. The Comox skull, however, should be reexamined. Jerome Cybulski, after studying a photograph of the original, ventures the opinion that its leprotic features may in fact be a result of postmortem wear (pers. comm., June 1995). The original skull is in Edinburgh, Scotland.

have been noted above; there is also a cluster of accounts in the oral literature from the lower Fraser that refer to *skom* or *qu'um* (in the Halkomelem
language), translated by the ethnographers as "leprosy." This body of oral
texts has been analyzed before, but always from a folkloristic or ethnographic
standpoint, never in the context of disease history. References to "leprosy"
in the lower Fraser stories appear in two tale types that have fairly wide dis-
tributions on the Northwest Coast. Outside the lower Fraser, references to
leprosy are replaced by more generalized references to sores, skin disease, or
the like.

The first tale type describes a "leper" married to a village woman. This man
takes off his leper skin each night to hunt, until the wife discovers the ruse,
burns the skin, and the husband becomes beautiful.[2] Variations on this theme,
with references to sores or scabs instead of leprosy, appear elsewhere on the
British Columbia coast.

The better-known tale type explains the origin of the *sxwayxwey* mask
and ceremony, which is practiced by Strait of Georgia peoples from the
Kwakwaka'wakw to the Lummi.[3] The maple mask itself is a curious con-
catenation of symbols: bulging eyes, a lolling tongue, a nose and upright "ears"
that frequently take the forms of spirit animals, and a "crest" of encircling
feathers.[4] "Owned" by certain families, it is worn in a performance associated with life rites and potlatches, and serves a ritual cleansing function (Suttles
1982).

The origin tale behind this mask and performance is uniform in outline:
A young man has a skin disease. He is unhappy and decides to drown himself in a lake. He sees loons, jumps into the water, and sinks until he lands on
the roof of the house of the lake people. He enters and sees that all and/or a

2. The Sto:lo "Myth of the Owl Husband" begins as follows: "there are only four *skumel* [pit
houses], and they are close together. There is, however, a small house on this side of the village
where a man who has the leprosy (*skom*) lives apart by himself. . . . he [a young man] comes to
the leper's dwelling, goes in and takes the man by the hair and shakes him so that his bones drop
out of his skin. The young man then dons the leper's skin and assumes the character of the leper"
(Hill-Tout 1978: 3.133). The young man's wife moves in with the "leprous" man, the villagers
scoff at and ridicule her, and the tale ends as above.

3. See Codere 1948; Duff 1952: 123–26; Lévi-Strauss 1979: chaps. 2–3, 10, 12.

4. Some of these features, incidentally, could be interpreted as referring to leprotic symptoms: bulging eyes to blindness, the lolling tongue to alveolar deterioration, and the animal nose
to a nose with deteriorated cartilage. But this is speculation, and as Wayne Suttles notes, it is dangerous to assign meanings to symbols whose full cultural content is only partially understood.

baby are lying sick with sores caused by his own saliva; he rubs saliva on them and they are cured. He arises from the water, his skin is clean, and he returns to his village, where he instructs his sister to make a basket attached to a line and throw it into the lake. She does so, and the basket is pulled out containing the *sxwayxwey* mask and rattle, which give him power and are hereafter used in the dancing performance (Codere 1948: 8–9).

The earliest version of this tale to be collected was recorded by the ethnographer Charles Hill-Tout from a Chilliwack (Sto:lo) informant around the turn of the century; it refers to *skom* (which Hill-Tout translated as "leprosy") and notes that spittle caused the spread of sores (a very logical mode of spread for leprosy).[5] But the most complete traditions were collected from two Tait Sto:lo informants, Mr. and Mrs. Robert Joe, by Marion Smith (in 1938) and Wilson Duff (in 1950). Robert Joe referred to "a disease which made [the] skin rot" and produced "sores all over and a peculiar odor" or "dark sores on the neck and face." Mrs. Joe was more explicit (in an ethnomedical sense); she referred to "*qu'm* [which] caused his skin to break and rot (the white men call it leprosy)" (Duff 1952: 123).

Wilson Duff reexamined these tales and their distribution and suggested diffusion from a center on the lower Fraser. The more complete versions cluster in this area and name villages and a lake near Union Bar as the place of action. Mrs. Joe, whose family owned the rights to the mask and performance, estimated that the events took place five generations earlier. Given her age and an average generation allowance, Duff estimated that the historical events on which the tale was grounded occurred "roughly about 1780."

5. At approximately the same time, and a short distance to the east, James Teit collected two Nlaka'pamux variants of the tale: "Origin of the *Wau'us* Mask," which called the disease *kom kome'x* and said it caused "large swellings on the body" (1912a: 272–73); and "Origin of the .*Sxo'Exo'E* Mask," which described "a loathsome disease" that caused the nose and eyes to become "swollen" (1917: 132–33).

Appendix 4

Two Local British Columbia Epidemics,
1868 and 1875

A s if the devastation caused by smallpox in 1862–63 was not enough, two
local epidemics broke out among British Columbia Indians, one in
1868 and the other in 1875. The first was a recurrence of measles among
Heiltsuk, Haisla, Tsimshian, and Tlingit; the second was a smallpox outbreak
limited to the Nuu-chah-nulth peoples of Vancouver Island, who had escaped
the 1862–63 epidemic.

THE 1868 MEASLES EPIDEMIC

Evidence for this outbreak comes from only two sources: the journal of the
German traveler Emil Teichmann, who sailed the Inland Passage from
Victoria to Sitka in the spring and summer of 1868, and U.S. government
records from the first year of occupation of southeast Alaska. Teichmann
appears to have misidentified the disease, calling it variously smallpox or scarlet fever; U.S. government medical doctors termed it measles.

Teichmann visited the Heiltsuk town of Kokai at the beginning of May,
where he observed "many" of the 200 inhabitants "suffering from smallpox
or scarlet fever, diseases which cause terrible mortality . . . since when the
fever is highest they try to get cool by plunging into the ice-cold sea, which
only too often causes death" (1963: 93). At his next stop, Fort Simpson, "our
guide advised us not to . . . go into the houses . . . on account of smallpox

and scarlet fever, which was rampant at the time" (110). At Chilkat, on 12 June 1868, American J. W. White reported: "An epidemic of measles had lately visited this people. (This disease we found at Fort Simpson in the spring, and it has since made its way through nearly every tribe up to this place.)" (1869: 7).

THE 1875 NUU-CHAH-NULTH SMALLPOX EPIDEMIC

The Nuu-chah-nulth peoples of the west coast of Vancouver Island appear, by negative evidence, to have escaped the major mid-nineteenth-century smallpox epidemics. The 1853 outbreak spread to the Pacheenaht band of Ditidaht speakers from the Makah, and the 1862 epidemic was recorded among Kwakwaka'wakw, Comox, Pentlatch, and T'Sou'ke (Sooke) peoples of Vancouver Island. Songhees and Quwutsun'–Sne-Nay-Mux^w peoples, heavily vaccinated, had few casualties. The west coast peoples, still unvaccinated, seem to have been protected only by their isolation. This state of affairs ended in mid-1875. Smallpox was recorded from four locations in Nuu-chah-nulth lands: Barkley Sound, Hesquiat Harbour, Nootka Sound, and Kyuquot Sound.

An oral tradition collected in 1964 from informant Louis Clamhouse and dated to "before 1875" recalls how smallpox first appeared at Barkley Sound on the southwest coast of Vancouver Island:

Then came a ship which entered harbour at N'aqowis, right across from Bamfield. The people went to the ship to see it, and they went aboard. . . . They looked down the hatch, the Ohiahts, and they saw that there was something wrong with many of the Whitemen, the sailors, for they were all groaning. . . . The Whitemen had smallpox sickness. I think the ship came from San Francisco. . . .

Said the Captain, "For seven days you will be well. Then you will get that sickness." . . . The Indians did not know what the sickness was; there was none like it in this country. . . . Many Ohiahts died. . . . From two thousand persons, just eighty families remained alive. . . .

Many died over the next six months. My grandfather moved to a mountain at Sarita Lake. By doing so he did not catch the smallpox sickness there. He quickly moved far away, taking along his family, his children, and by doing that he remained alive. The Americans caused them to die, the Canadian Indians, by giving them the bad sickness. All that was left alive is how many we are now. (Arima et al. 1991: 212)

In May 1975 Reverend Augustin Brabant established a Catholic Mission at Hesquiat on the central west coast. Brabant was gone for three weeks in early autumn to Victoria, and when he returned he learned that smallpox had killed "several" at Nootka Sound and that the people there were threatening to kill, in recompense, an equal number of Hesquiat. A Hesquiat woman shaman was dead of "sickness" too, and (though the account does not explicitly say so) it is likely that she may have tried, unsuccessfully, to cure the disease at Nootka Sound and that her failure was the proximate reason for the threatened revenge on her people (Brabant in Moser 1926: 39).

The Nootka attack did not materialize, however, and the epidemic at Hesquiat proceeded. What followed was reminiscent of Metlakatla 13 years previous. Brabant baptized people on the verge of death, he hired a special crew to bury bodies that most would not approach, and he vaccinated (Moser 1926: 40). Like Reverend Duncan, he detailed the personal experiences of his parishioners with the disease:

I went to see the chief's daughter, who was very low also with small-pox. She was a courageous woman and did not give up till she was quite blind and her head as black and as thick as a large iron pot. She was baptized and seemed to be in the best disposition. Her own father and another old Indian helped me bury her. The sight of the corpse was simply horrible, and as we left the shanty in which she died swarms of flies surrounded us all. (41)

A second case was Matlahaw, who had experienced a familial tragedy: both parents were dead—his father, bereaved by the loss of his wife to smallpox, had killed himself. With a warning from the villagers on Matlahaw's mental state, Brabant went to visit the man. In his lodge Matlahaw sat, gun in hand, and, trembling, requested medicine. The priest promised it and asked for the gun. But it went off, and upon receiving wounds to his hand and shoulder, Brabant fled to the village. Here he told the "loyal men of the tribe" what had happened, and armed "with axes and guns they set off to kill" Matlahaw. Not finding him, they took a canoe to the village of his sister, whom they brought back to Hesquiat, planning "to kill her in expiation of what her brother had done to me" (Moser 1926: 43–44). The priest intervened, however, and had the woman removed to the safety of a trading post at Clayoquot. Twelve days later (9 November) H.M.S. *Rocket,* with two doctors and Bishop Charles Seghers, arrived in port, and Brabant was spirited off to Victoria (46).

Bishop Seghers continued on the west coast in Brabant's stead. Although his reminiscences contain few references to disease, he recounts the number of children baptized at each port, and it is likely that he was vaccinating as well. His experience at Kyuquot, where he found an abandoned village, implies as much. Two frightened Indians related a rumor of the purpose of his mission:

23 November 1875
They had heard of our arrival but the story got mixed up. On board the schooner [*Surprise,* Capt. John Peterson] was a living man who would cut the children on the chest, and another who would rub something over the wound and it would be healed. Then the first man would begin killing the Indians, and upon the Indians trying to kill him, he would turn into stone or become a stone man. (Seghers in Moser 1926: 18)

In the 1840s a nearly complete Hudson's Bay Company census suggests a total of about 4,850 Nuu-chah-nulth (Douglas 1878, figures adjusted). The first formal British Columbia census of west coast Indians, in 1881, returned 3,256 (Guillod 1882). Although previous observers had commented on a fertility decline and the prevalence of venereal disease and tuberculosis (Sproat 1868: chap. 27), most of the approximately 33% population decline in these 40 years was probably due to the 1875 smallpox epidemic.

Population Tables

TABLE 7. Haida Population History

	1700s	1829 Green	1835—Parker Men only	1835—Parker Total	1830s HBC	1837 Veniaminov	1860 Duncan	1862–63 Poole	1867 Scott	1874 Dawson	1880–82	1883 Chittenden	1889–90 Census
QUEEN CHARLOTTE ISLANDS		3,000	2,100	8,600	6,693	8,000		5,000					
Skidegate		500			2,316					500	412[d]	810	729
Skidegate					738						317[d]	352	291
Cumshewa					286							100	198
Skedans					439						30[d]	60	
Tanu					545						25[d]	150	93
Ninstints					308						40[d]	30	
West Coast	1,700[a]				1,286			300					
Kaisun					229			100–150 men					
Chaatl					561						102[d]	108	
Tian					396								
Masset	400–500 men				3,291				300	800			
Gahlinskun					220								
Hiellen					122								
Kung					280								
Masset					2,473							350	438
Kiusta					296								
PRINCE OF WALES ISLAND													
Kaigani	1,800–2,000[b]	500–600	425	2,092	1,735	1,350			600	300	788[e]		391
Kaigani	1,000 men[c]				334								
Koianglas					148						62[e]		
Howkwan					458						28[e]		
Klinkwan					417						125[e]		
Sukkwan					229						141[e]		
Kasaan					249						173[e]		
Total	3,000 men[b]		2,525	10,692	8,428	9,350	10,000			1,600			

SOURCES: Green 1915: 39, 64, 74, 86; Parker 1936: 124; Dawson 1880: 173 and Douglas 1878 (HBC); Veniaminov 1981: 103; Duncan 1860; Poole 1872: 309; Colyer 1870a: 1005 (for the 1867 figures from Scott); Dawson 1880: 174; Chittenden 1884: 23–24. For 1889–90 census, see Canada, Dept. of Indian Affairs, 1890: 271–72 and U.S. Bureau of the Census 1893: 158.

[a] From Dixon, for 1787 (see Dixon 1789: 224). [b] From Sturgis, for 1799 (see Sturgis 1973: 41, 89). [c] Arteaga 1874: 283, southern villages only; figure extrapolated from 86 canoes seen at Cordova Bay in June 1779. [d] From O'Reilly, for 1882 (see O'Reilly 1883: 108). [e] From Petrov, for 1880 (see Petrov 1884: 32).

TABLE 8. Haida Population according
to the Mid-1830s Hudson's Bay Company Census

	Houses	Men	Women	Boys	Girls	Total
QUEEN CHARLOTTE ISLANDS[a]	430	1,736	1,742	1,576	1,639	6,693
Skidegate	158	642	620	510	544	2,316
Skidegate	48	191	182	176	189	738
Cumshewa	20	80	74	63	69	286
Skedans	30	115	121	98	105	439
Tanu (Cloo)	40	169	164	105	107	545
Ninstints (Queeah)	20	87	79	68	74	308
West Coast	63	256	269	280	281	1,086
Kaisun (Kishawin)	18	80	74	85	90	329
Chaatl (Kowwelth)	35	131	146	145	139	561
Tian (Too)	10	45	49	50	52	196
Masset	209	838	853	786	814	3,291
Gahlinskun (Aseguang)	9	34	31	27	28	120
Hiellen (Neecoon)	5	24	27	29	42	122
Kung (Nightan)	15	70	69	72	69	280
Masset[b]	160	630	650	589	604	2,473
Kiusta (Lulanna)	20	80	76	69	71	296
PRINCE OF WALES ISLAND						
Kaigani[c]	111	431	454	414	436	1,735
Kaigani (Youahnoe)	18	68	70	44	52	234
Koianglas (Quiahanless)	8	30	35	42	41	148
Howkwan (Howaguan)	27	117	121	113	107	458
Klinkwan (Clickass)	26	98	105	102	112	417
Sukkwan (Shawagan)	14	53	61	54	61	229
Kasaan (Chatcheenie)	18	65	62	59	63	249
Total	641	2,167	2,196	1,990	2,075	8,428

NOTE: Figures are based largely on Dawson 1880: 173, cross-checked against Douglas 1878. In the few instances of differences (Skidegate girls and Kiusta women), I have followed the Dawson copy.

[a] The villages are presented south to north, by geographical clusters: Skidegate = southern Graham and Moresby Islands. West Coast = Pacific Coast. Masset — northern Graham Island. Identifications by Swanton 1905a (HBC names, where significantly different, in parentheses).

[b] Masset proper contained 27 houses (528 people) according to Swanton (in Hodge 1907–10: 1.818). The HBC figure probably includes village sites on Masset Inlet as well.

[c] Southern Prince of Wales Island. Village identifications by Langdon 1979.

TABLE 9. Tlingit Population History

	1700s	1804	1829	1835—Douglas		1837	1856
			Green	Men	Total	Veniaminov	Tolmie
North						350	
Yakutat	400[a]			120	480	150	
Lituya	600					200	
Mainland				1,350	5,400	1,850	2,000
Chilkat	500[b]			600	2,400	200	250
Taku				150	600	150	250
Stikine	250[c]			600	2,400[d]	1,500	1,500
Island	3,000–4,000[f]		6,500[g]	1,290	5,160	2,150	1,570
Hoonah		500		260	1,040	250	140
Auk				100	400	200	250
Hutsnuwu				200	800	300	250
Sitka	450[h]	1,600		150	600	750	250
Kake				200	800	200	400
Kuiu				100	400	150	100
Henya				200	800	300	180
Klawak				80	320		
South				180	720	250	275
Tongass				80	320	150	220
Sanya				100	400	100	55
Total		10,000[i]		2,940	11,760	4,600	3,845

SOURCES: Green 1915: 39; Douglas 1835; Veniaminov 1981: 19; Tolmie 1856; Tikhmenev 1978: 428 (for the 1861 Erman figures); Amory 1868: 83–84; Colyer 1870a: 1004, 1017 (for the 1868 Halleck and the 1869 Mahoney figures); Petrov 1884: 31–32; U.S. Bureau of the Census 1893: 158.

[a] Malaspina 1934: 208.

[b] Number of canoes on Lynn Canal in July 1794 (Vancouver 1798: 3.256).

[c] 20 canoes counted near Cape Caamano in September 1793 (Vancouver 1798: 2.396).

[d] In 1841 (using pre-smallpox figures), Sir George Simpson estimated "600 men or 3,000 souls" as the Stikine population, and 4,000–5,000 who were "dependent on Fort Stikine for supplies." "Seven tribes," numbering "about 4,000 souls," frequented Fort Taku (1847: 1.124, 127).

[e] Both the Stikine and Sitka were censused in 1869. There were 508 at the Stikine village of Wrangell (Colyer 1870b: 11) and 1,251 at Sitka (Ludington 1871: 28).

| 1861—Erman | | | | 1867 | 1868 | 1869 | 1881–82 | 1890 |
Male	Female	Slave	Total	Amory	Halleck	Mahoney	Petrov	Census
428	435	107	970				826	436
163	168	49	380			300	626	
265	267	58	590				200	
1,371	1,373	281	3,025	2,650	3,500	5,700	1,555	1,290
728	728	160	1,616	1,200	2,000	2,500	988	812
335	337	40	712	450	500	2,000	269	223
308	308	81	697	1,000	1,000	1,200[e]	317	255
1,680	1,502	211	3,393	4,050	6,500	4,800	4,090	2,602
154	154	23	331	1,150	1,000	1,300	908	592
				700	800	750	640	279
280	280	40	600	700	1,000	1,000	666	420
715	535	94	1,344		1,200	1,000[e]	721	815
210	210	25	445	200	1,200	750	568	234
126	126	10	262	800	800		60	
195	197	19	411	500	500		587	262
							27	
210	210	31	451	400	500	800	273	255
154	154	25	333	250	500		173	
56	56	6	118	150			100	
3,689	3,520	630	7,839	7,100	10,500	11,600	6,744	4,583

[f] Langsdorf's estimate of 3,000–4,000 (1814: 1.86) probably refers to only those peoples closest to Sitka in contact with Russians.

[g] Green's estimate of "Sitka language" speakers probably excludes most mainlanders. Very similar is Samuel Parker's 1835 estimate (from the HBC) of "Hanaga and Chatham straights, Nine bands numbering 1540 men . . . 6160 [total]" (1936: 124).

[h] Dixon 1789: 186.

[i] Lisiansky's figure (1814: 151, 237, 242; repeated by Veniaminov in 1835). Excluding the non-Tlingit Kaigani, the total should be ca. 8,000.

TABLE 10. Tlingit Population according
to the circa 1842 Hudson's Bay Company Census

	Men	Women	Adult Sex Ratio	Boys	Girls
North (Yakutat and Lituya)		Not Enumerated			
Mainland	956	636	150	376	322
Chilkat	267	116	230	71	66
Taku	127	110	115	71	66
Stikine	562	410	137	234	190
Island	855	721	119	327	286
Hoonah	258	234	110	108	88
Auk	72	61	118	35	31
Hutsnuwu	274	240	114	85	76
Sitka and Kuiu		Not Enumerated			
Kake	169	106	159	70	64
Henya	82	80	103	29	27
South	180	185	97	141	157
Tongass	85	90	94	60	65
Sanya	45	50	90	39	43
"Port Stuart"[c]	50	45	111	42	49
Total	1,991	1,542	129	844	765

NOTE: This census, from James Douglas's private papers (1878), differs in several numbers from that printed in Petrov 1884: 36–37 and reprinted in de Laguna 1990: 205 (in Emmons 1991: 432). Significant differences are in number of men (Chilkat 167, Hutsnuwu 247, Kake 109) and all Stikine numbers (total 1,586).

Sex ratios are determined by dividing the number of males by the number of females and multiplying by 100.

[a] In this and the following tables, "% Children" is for the free population only (child slave numbers are not given).

Child Sex Ratio	Total Sex Ratio (Free)	% Children[a]	Slaves		Total Sex Ratio (including slaves)	Total
			No.	%		
Not Enumerated						
117	139	30	341	13	130	2,631
108	186	26	78	13	174	598
108	113	37	119	24	109	493
123	134	30	144	9	124	1,540[b]
114	117	28	274	12	115	2,463
123	114	28	94	12	108	782
113	116	33	4	2	116	203
112	114	24	81	11	112	756
Not Enumerated						
109	141	33	44	10	138	453
107	104	26	51	19	105	269
90	94	45	15	3	93	678
92	94	42	15	5	92	315
91	90	46	—	—	90	177
86	98	49	—	—	98	186
110	123	31	630	11	118	5,772

[b] The 1845 Stikine census returned a total of 1,574 (Rae 1845).

[c] Port Stewart is on the Cleveland Peninsula, in southernmost Stikine territory. De Laguna (in Emmons 1991: 432) classifies with Stikine. The closest recorded village, however, is Sanya, and the population structure (high percentage of children, no slaves, balanced sex ratio) most resembles that of Sanya (and, secondarily, Haida).

TABLE 11. Tsimshian Population History

	1829 Green	1840s HBC	Men	Women	1858—Duncan Sex Ratio	Chil- dren	% Chil- dren	Total
Nisga'a		1,615						2,500
Gitkateen		520						
Gitgigenik		429						
Gitwunksithk		381						
Gitlakdamiks		285						
Tsimshian	5,500[c]	2,826						
Fort Simpson		2,495	637	756	84	763	35	2,352[d]
Fort Simpson								
Metlakatla								
Port Essington		331						
Kitsumkalum		147						
Kitselas		184						
Gitxsan								2,500
Kitwanga								
Kitwancool								
Kitsegukla								
Kitanmaks								
Kispiox								
Kisgegas								
Kuldo								
Total								7,500

SOURCES: Green 1915: 64; Duncan 1869: 25–26; Colyer 1870a: 1005 (for the 1867 Scott figures); Dorsey 1897; O'Reilly 1883. For the censuses, see Canada, Dept. of Indian Affairs, 1890: 271–72 and U. S. Bureau of the Census 1893: 158.

[a] Dorsey's figures, based on memory culture, predate the 1888(?) dysentery epidemic and may, in some cases, precede the 1862–63 smallpox epidemic.

[b] Most of the lower Nass villagers recongregated at the mission villages of Kincolith and Lakkulzap, in 1867 and 1872, respectively.

| 1867 | 1870–80 | 1882 O'Reilly Reserve Survey | | | | | 1889 |
| | | | | | % | | |
Scott	Dorsey[a]	Men	Women	Children	Children	Total	Censuses
2,000	1,530	257	301	319	36	877	805
	350	46	59	75	42	180	} 420[b]
	630	94	109	99	33	302	
	200	37	45	47	36	129	104
	350	80	88	98	37	266	281
	1,300						1,869
1,500	850						1,714
900							762
600							952
	450						155
	150						69
400	300						86
1,900	1,875						1,462
300	250						143
400	350						195
300	250						172
	200						285
400	400						398
500	275						223
	150						46
5,800	4,705						4,136

[c] "Nass language."

[d] Duncan counted 2,156 persons but upped this to 2,352 to account for those absent at the time; including relatives married outside, the total was 2,567. In his letter of 25 October 1860, Duncan gave 2,500 as the total for each of the three Tsimshian groups: at Fort Simpson and on the Nass and Skeena Rivers.

TABLE 12. Tsimshian Population according to the circa 1842 Hudson's Bay Company Census

	Adult			Child			% Children	Slaves		Total	
	Men	Women	Sex Ratio	Boys	Girls	Sex Ratio		No.	%	Sex Ratio	Total
Nisga'a	543	438	124	314	308	102	39	12	1	114	1615
Gitkateen	182	109	167	126	103	122	44			145	520
Gitgigenik	117	111	105	97	104	93	47			100	429
Gitwunksithk	146	118	124	48	69	70	31			104	381
Gitlakdamiks	98	100	98	43	32	134	27	12	4	103	285
Tsimshian	868	848	102	529	506	105	38	75	3	104	2826
Fort Simpson	737	778	95	465	447	104	38	68	3	99	2495
Gispakloats	116	150	77	99	71	139	39	11	2	96	447
Gitlan	129	134	96	75	76	99	36	10	2	98	424
Gitsees	71	75	95	43	30	143	33	1		110	220
Ginadoiks	63	74	85	43	39	110	37	4	2	94	223
Gitwilgyots	64	73	88	41	36	114	36	18	8	98	232
Gitzaklalth	31	36	86	20	29	69	42	1	1	80	117
Gilutsau	104	85	122	50	58	86	36	5	2	110	302
Ginakangeek	87	68	128	48	62	77	42	8	3	104	273
Gitandau	54	70	77	35	43	81	39	10	5	84	212
Gitwilksaba	18	13	138	11	3	366	31			181	45
Port Essington	131	70	187	64	59	108	38	7	2	150	331
Kitsumkalum	59	23	257	35	28	125	43	2	1	182	147
Kitselas	72	47	153	29	31	94	34	5	3	130	184
Gitxsan					Not Enumerated						

TABLE 13. Fort McLoughlin District Population History

| | 1835[a] | | | 1838–42 | % Loss (Tolmie |
	Houses	Men	Total	HBC	minus HBC)
Sabassas		280	1225	1020	17
Kitkatla		150	625	733	
Kitkiata		60	250	194	
Kitasoo		70	350	93	67[b]
Haisla		198	825	409	50
Kitamaat		144	600	222	63
Kitlope		54	225	187	17
Nuxalk	67	468	1940	509[d]	51[d]
Kimsquit	10			220	
Bella Coola	53			289	
Talio	4				
Heiltsuk		664	2018[e]	1833	9
Haihais		36	150	98	35
Istitoch		90	375	281	25
Bella Bella	52	490	1293	1249	3
Owitlitoch	23	215	590	511	13
Oyalitoch	16	175	399	430	+8
Kokyitoch	13	100	304	308	+1
Oweekeno	8	48	200	205	+3
Total			6003	3771	

SOURCES: Douglas 1878 and Tolmie 1963: 319–20 (for 1835 figures); Ross 1842; Warre 1909: 61; Tolmie 1856; Amory 1868: 84; O'Reilly 1883; Canada, Dept. of Indian Affairs, 1890: 171–72.

[a] Most numbers are from Douglas 1878; house counts and Bella Bella numbers are from Tolmie.

[b] The southernmost Sabassas at Kitasoo appear to have been the only ones to suffer significant smallpox losses; the increase in numbers in the northern two villages suggests that survivors from the south fled north. This smallpox loss figure has been adjusted to include migration loss as well.

1842 Ross	1845 Warre	1856 Tolmie	1867 Amory	1882 O'Reilly	1889 Census	% Loss 1840–89
		1225	500		284	72
		700	300	220	193	74
		450	100		91	53
	1429[c]	75	100	70		100
		315			364	11
		250	200		261	(+)
		65			103	45
		950		570	378	60
		280		200	106	52
650		550		370	226	59
		120			46	62
1500	1628	910	500		481	74
			100		52	47
		140				100
		600	300	290	259	79
				230	188	56
				60	71	77
		170	100	150	170	17
					1510	64

[c] "Sabassas 5 Tribes Gardiner's Canal."

[d] The Nuxalk 1838–42 figures in Douglas 1878 are probably incomplete. To compute losses from the 1836 smallpox epidemic, Tolmie's 1856 total (950) has been used.

[e] Repeated as "2180" by Samuel Parker in 1835 (1936: 124). In 1841 Sir George Simpson gave 5,200 as the total population of the Fort McLoughlin District.

TABLE 14. Fort McLoughlin District Populations according to the Hudson's Bay Company, circa. 1838–42

	Adult			Child			Total	%	Slaves		Total
	Men	Women	Sex Ratio	Boys	Girls	Sex Ratio	Sex Ratio	Children	No.	%	
Sabassas	328	272	121	193	156	124	122	37	71	7	1020
Kitkatla	239	179	134	160	120	133	133	40	35	5	733
Kitkiata	63	66	95	20	22	91	94	25	23	12	194
Kitasoo	26	27	96	13	14	93	95	34	13	14	93
Haisla	146	135	108	50	38	132	113	24	40	10	409
Kitamaat	80	75	107	24	18	133	112	21	25	11	222
Kitlope	66	60	110	26	20	130	115	27	15	8	187
Nuxalk	160	148	108	101	100	101	105	39			509
Kimsquit	66	59	111	44	51	86	100	43			220
Bella Coola	94	89	106	57	49	116	109	37			289
Talio					Not Enumerated						
Heiltsuk	884	902					98		47	3	1833
Haihais	47	51					92				98
Istitoch	112	81	138	39	46	85	119	31	3	1	281
Bella Bella	467	454	103	119	166	72	95	24	44	3	1249[a]
Owitlitoch	252	243					104		16	3	511
Oyalitoch	223	196					114		11	4	430
Kokyitoch	111	180					62		17	4	308
Oweekeno	71	69	103	29	36	81	95	32			205
Total											3771[b]

NOTE: Compiled from three sheets (two censuses?) in Douglas 1878. Sabassas, Haisla, and Bella Bella totals from the ca. 1842 Fort Simpson (Tsimshian) census; Nuxalk and all other Heiltsuk groups from two sheets dated to 1838.

[a] Total numbers from two sheets vary by one point: 1,250 for the Bella Bella total; 1,249 as the total of three Bella Bella subgroups.

[b] Adjusted total = 4,212 (950 instead of 509 Nuxalk). See chap. 8, n. 26.

TABLE 15. Lower Columbia Peoples in Lewis and Clark's Estimates

Name	Ethnicity	Autumn 1805	Spring 1806	Differences Counts	%
Sha-ha-la Nation	Cascades Chinookan	1,500	2,800	1,300	+46
y-e-huh	(seasonal visitors:				
Clah-clel-lah	mostly Northwest				
Wah-clel-lah	Sahaptin)				
Ne-er-cho-ki-oo					
Wap-pa-to Nation	Multnomah Chinookan	2,210	5,290	3,080	+58
Ne-cha-co-kee		100	100		
Mult-no-mah	(Visitors: diverse)	200	800	600	+75
Clan-nah-quah		130	130		
Shotos	(Seasonal visitors:	180	460	280	+61
Quath-lah-poh-tle	Northwest Sahaptin)	300	900	600	+67
Cal-la-maks		200	200		
Cath-lah-cum-ups	(Seasonal visitors:	150	450	300	+66
Clack Star	Athapascan?)	350	1,200	850	+71
Clan-nar-min-a-mow		280	280		
Clan-in-na-tas	(Seasonal visitors:	100	200	100	+50
Cath-lah-nah-quiah	Kalapuyan?)	150	400	250	+63
Cath-lah-com-mah-tup		70	170	100	+59
[Clackamas] villages		1,150	2,650	1,500	+57
Ne-mal-quln-ner		100	200	100	+50
Clark-a-mus	(Visitors: Molala?)	800	1,800	1,000	+56
Cush-hooks	(Visitors: Kalapuyan?)	250	650	400	+62
[Cathlamet] villages		1,800	3,000	1,200	+40
Skil-lutes	(Visitors: Cowlitz)	1,500	2,500	1,000	+40
Wack-ki-a-cums	(Seasonal visitors:	100	200	100	+50
Cath-lah-mahs	Athapascan)	200	300	100	+33
[Upper Chinookan subtotal]		6,660	13,740	7,080	+52
[Lower Chinook]		700[a]			
Chin-nooks		400			
Clat-sops		200			
Kil-laxt-ho-kles[b]		100			
[Kalapuyan]		8,200			
Char-cow-ah		200			
Cal-lah-po-e-wahs		2,000			
Sho-sho-nes [on the Multnomah]		6,000			

SOURCE: Originals in Lewis and Clark 1990: 473–89. (See chap. 9, n. 5.) Based on chart 11 in Boyd 1985 and table 1 in Boyd and Hajda 1987.

[a] Neither version apparently includes 400 additional Chinook resident on a "river" north of Baker's Bay (Moulton 1983: map 82; Lewis and Clark 1990: 61). They should perhaps be added to the total.

[b] Probably the same as Curtis's Qĭláptĭhl, at the site of Bruceport on Willapa Bay. Perhaps seasonally co-occupied with Athapascan Kwalhioqua (Lewis and Clark 1990: 491).

TABLE 16. Lower Columbia Population History, Pre-1830

	Lewis and Clark		Stuart 1812		1820	1824–25	Late 1820s
	1805	1806	Men	×4	(Morse 1822)[a]	Kennedy	HBC
SALISH							
Quinault	1,250				1,250		
Lower Chehalis	1,300		234	936	1,360, 1,400		
Upper Chehalis		(1,350)					
Cowlitz		(1,000)[b]	250	1,000	2,400		
ATHAPASCAN							
Willapa		(100)					
Clatskanie		(1,250)			1,200	175	
CHINOOKAN[c]	7,760	14,840					
Chinook	1,100[d]				3,100	1,040	
Shoalwater	100				100		
Chinook	800		280	1,120	1,700	910	2,000 men[e]
Clatsop	200		214	856	1,300	130	
Cathlamet	1,800	3,000			3,400		
Cathlamet	200	300	94	376	600	125	
Wakaikam	100	200	66	264	400	210	
Skilloot	1,500	2,500	200	800	2,400	285	
Middle	4,860	10,740					
Wappato	2,210	5,290	440–490	1,760–1,960	5,790	655	
Clackamas	1,150	2,650	80[f]	320[f]	2,000		
Cascades	1,500	2,800			1,800, 2,800	250	
WEST KLIKITAT							
Skamania County		(1,300)					
Clark County		(880)					

MOLALA (NORTH)	3,000 (part)	(1,000)^g				8,780^h
KALAPUYAN	9,200				20,000	
North	2,200	(850)^i	300^j	1,200	1,800	
Central	6,000					
Yoncalla	1,000^k					
TILLAMOOK	2,400				2,400	
North	1,200		200	800	1,200	
South	1,200				1,200	
ALSEAN	1,700				1,700	

SOURCES: Stuart 1935: 4, 28–33, 43; Morse 1822: 368–72; Kennedy 1824–25; for late 1820s HBC counts, Rich 1947: 236 (McLoughlin) and Parker 1838: 258.

a Some names listed more than once.

b Numbers in parentheses estimated by subtracting the printed (winter) estimate from the manuscript (spring) estimate for villages downstream from Athapascan and Sahaptin bands. See table 13 for computations.

c Excludes White Salmon, Wasco, and Wishram.

d Includes 18 lodges and 400 people north of Baker's Bay (Moulton 1983: map 82; Lewis and Clark 1990c 61).

e McLoughlin's 1826 estimate of people "on the Columbia in Salmon-Season . . . from the Dalles to the Sea" is identical to Alexander Ross's 1811 "tribes . . . about the mouth of the Columbia," which excludes Upper Chinookans from The Cascades to The Dalles but includes Chehalis and Tillamook (1849: 87).

f "[O]n an Eastern branch . . . above the [Willamette] Falls . . . dwell the Cathlathlas" (Stuart 1935: 33). May possibly be Molala.

g The excess salmon season visitors on the Clackamas River may be the same as the Shoshones resident seasonally on the "Multnomah" (Willamette) and Towarnehiooks (Deschutes) Rivers.

h This is Parker's second figure (1838: 258). His earlier total was 7,785 (1936: 123). The larger number may include mixed and Chinookan villages on the Willamette downstream from Willamette Falls and on Multnomah Channel or the Kalapuyan Yoncalla of the Umpqua River valley.

i The excess salmon season visitors at Willamette Falls and on Multnomah Channel may be included in Lewis and Clark's 2,000 "Callapoewahs."

j "[T]he first nation above the [Willamette] Falls are the Cathlapooyas." Continuing "along the river . . . natives [unenumerated] are very numerous and go by the name of Shoshones" (Stuart 1935: 33).

k The "Shobarboobeer" Shoshones, 1,600 in the spring estimate, which may be a transcription error.

TABLE 17. Lower Columbia Population History, Post-1830

	1830s		1840s				1848		1851	1854–56
	Losses	Numbers	Missions	Wilkes	HBC/Warre	Meek	Thornton	Newell		
SALISH										
Quinault			700					300		158
Lower Chehalis				2,000[sic]						217
Upper Chehalis				300–350	500					216
Cowlitz					, 240	500		120		140
ATHAPASCAN	−10,000[a]								21	
Willapa				100					13	
Clatskanie				100				300	8	
CHINOOKAN										
Chinook		800	300		429	400				238
Shoalwater										71
Chinook		288		209			200	100	142	126
Clatsop				220			180	50	71	41
Cathlamet				300				, 58	60	41
Middle					800[b]			200[c]		
Wappato	−2,000[d]	37								
Willamette			40/150[e]	70/100[e]		300		20	13	30
Clackamas				275[f]	200	400	80	60	88	78
Cascades		130	150–200	150		1,000	400	130	120	138
WEST KLIKITAT										
Clark County		345			500		80		60	240
Willamette									492	

MOLALA (NORTH)	−5,000–6,000	1,200–1,500	600		200				123
KALAPUYAN		600	500,500	300				560	
North							150		
Tualatin					200		60	65	
Yamhill							90	59	
Central					500				
Santiam-Pudding								141	
Calapooya-Mary's							75	175	
Yoncalla								48	
TILLAMOOK	200 (north)	500	400,700	1,500	500	370	200	150	193
ALSEAN			600–700		600–700		200		96

SOURCES: Loss figures for the 1830s are from Duflot de Mofras 1937: 2.174; Slacum 1972: 15–16. Total numbers for the 1830s are from Slacum 1972: 15–16; Frost 1934: 58; HBC 1838. The 1840s mission figures are from Demers in Landerholm 1956: 83, 90; Hines 1850: 91, 236; Lee and Frost 1844: 308; Duflot de Mofras 1937: 2.175. The Wilkes figures can be found in Wilkes 1925–26: 296, 1845: 4.366, 5.144; Hale 1846: 204, 212, 217, 218. For the HBC/Warre figures, see Warre and Vavasour 1909: 61; Douglas 1931: 7 (Cowlitz: 60 men × 4). Figures from Meek and Thornton are in Polk 1848: 9–10. Newell's figures are in Newell 1959: 171–74. For 1851, most figures are from Dart 1852; Kalapuya numbers are from Spalding 1851; Cathlamet, Gibbs 1851; Tualatin, Gaines, Skinner, and Allen 1852; and Clatskanie, Dart 1851b. The Chinookan numbers in Dart 1852 do not correspond to those of Gibbs 1851, used in table 18. For 1854–55, see Tappan 1854; Raymond 1854; Swan 1972: 346; Beckham 1990: 184.

a Includes all Chinookans below The Cascades rapids, as well as neighboring seasonal visitors to the Columbia (Duflot de Mofras 1937: 2.174).

b Includes Cathlamet, Wappato, and Cascades.

c Includes "Kathlemit, Konick, Wakanasceces, Wakamucks, Namanamin and Namoit" (Newell 1959: 171).

d Includes Wappato only.

e Winter village versus "fishing season" numbers.

f Includes Clackamas and Willamette.

TABLE 18. Lower Columbia Post-Fever-and-Ague Population Structures

Group	Men	Women	Boys	Girls	% Children	Total	Total with Slaves	Women Married Out	Half-Blood Offspring	Total including Half Bloods
CHINOOKANS										
1838 Hudson's Bay Company Censuses										
Chinook	73	88	41	28	30	230	288			
Wappato	9	12	1	3	16	25	37			
Cascades	29	31	11	20	34	91	130			
1851 Treaty Censuses[a]										
Chinook	33	38	19	18	34	108	135	15	55	205
Chinook	17	17	9	11	36	54	73	11	36	120
Clatsop	16	21	10	7	31	54	62	4	19	85
Cathlamet	17	20	4	5	21	46	60			
Clackamas + "Tumwaters"	24	35	— 42 —		42	101				
Cascades	45	— 75 —				120				
KALAPUYANS										
Kalapuya	169	166	36	52	21	423				
"Lower"	136	133	19	24	14	312				
Yamhill	25	27	3	4	12	59				
Pudding	23	25	2	4	11	54				
Santiam (+ "Forks Santiam")	34	35	9	9	21	87				
Mary's R.	36	31	1	3	6	71				
Kalapooya	18	15	4	4	20	41				
"Upper"	23	33	17	28	41	111				
McKenzie	19	18	10	16	41	63				
Yoncalla	14	15	7	12	40	48				

SOURCES: For 1838, see Frost 1934: 58; HBC 1838. For 1851 Chinookans, see Gibbs 1851 (Chinook, Clatsop, Cathlamet); Dart 1852: 477 (Clackamas, Cascades). For 1851 Kalapuyans, see Spalding 1851. Gibbs's 1851 numbers do not correspond to those of Dart 1852, used in table 17.

[a] Both the Chinook and the Kalapuya counts are incomplete: neither the Willapa Bay peoples nor the Tualatin were censused.

References

Aberle, David

   1959   "The Prophet Dance and Reactions to White Contact." *Southwestern Journal of Anthropology* 15(1): 74–83.

Ackerknecht, Erwin

   1945   "Malaria in the Upper Mississippi Valley." *Bulletin of the History of Medicine Supplement* no. 4.

Adamson, Thelma

   1926–27   Unarranged sources of Chehalis ethnology. Box 77, Melville Jacobs Collection. Manuscripts and University Archives. University of Washington Libraries, Seattle.

   1934   *Folk-Tales of the Coast Salish.* Memoirs of the American Folk-Lore Society 27. New York.

Aitken, Thomas

   1945   "Studies on the Anopheline Complex." *University of California Publications in Entomology* 7(11): 273–364.

Alcala Galiano, Dionisio

   1991   *The Voyage of the Sutil and Mexicana, 1792.* Translated by John Kendrick. Spokane: Arthur H. Clark Co.

Alderman, Lewis

   1957   "Mission Rose Farm." *Champoeg Pioneer* 2(23): 1.

Allan, George

    1882   "Reminiscences of Fort Vancouver, Extracts from a Letter of 1832." In *Transactions of the Oregon Pioneer Association for the Year 1881,* pp. 75–80. Salem: E. M. Waite.

Allen, Miss A. J.

    1848   *Ten Years in Oregon: Travels and Adventures of Dr. E. White and Lady.* . . . Ithaca: Mack, Andrus, and Co.

Allison, M., J. Mendoza, and A. Pezzia

    1973   "Documentation of a Case of Tuberculosis in Pre-Columbian America." *American Review of Respiratory Disease* 107: 985–91.

Alvarado, Juan

    n.d.   "Historia de California." Translated by Elizabeth Buckingham. MS C-D4. Bancroft Library. University of California, Berkeley.

Alvord, Benjamin

    1884   "The Doctor-Killing Oregons." *Harper's Magazine,* January: 364–66.

Amory, Jonathan

    1868   "The Northern Indians." In *Message on Russian America,* 40th Cong., 2d sess. House Executive Doc. 177, vol. 13 (Serial no. 1339), pp. 81–84. Washington.

Amoss, Pamela

    1982   "Resurrection, Healing and 'the Shake': The Story of John and Mary Slocum." In Michael A. Williams, ed., *Charisma and Sacred Biography,* pp. 87–109. *Journal of the American Academy of Religion, Thematic Studies* 48(3–4).

Anastasio, Angelo

    1972   "The Southern Plateau: An Ecological Analysis of Intergroup Relations." *Northwest Anthropological Research Notes* 6(2): 109–229.

Anderson, Alexander

    1857   "Some Notes for Captain Prevost Ret. H.M.S. 'Satellite.'" Cathlamet, 8/25. Royal British Columbia Archives, Victoria.

Andrade, Manuel

    1931   *Quileute Texts.* Columbia University Contributions to Anthropology 12. New York.

Andreski, Stanislav

    1982   "The Syphilitic Shock: A New Explanation of the 'Great Witch Craze' of the 16th and 17th Centuries in the Light of Medicine and Psychiatry." *Encounter* 45: 7–26.

Appleby, Geraldine

 1961 *Tsawwassen Legends.* Ladner, B. C.: Dunning Press.

Applegate, Jesse

 1851 Letter of 2 June to Anson Dart. Records of the Oregon Superintendency of Indian Affairs, 1848–1873. National Archives, Washington.

Arima, Eugene, et al.

 1991 *Between Ports Alberni and Renfrew: Notes on West Coast Peoples.* Mercury Series Paper 121. Hull: Canadian Museum of Civilization.

Armelagos, George

 1991 "Human Evolution and the Evolution of Disease." *Ethnicity and Disease* 1: 21–25.

Armelagos, George, and John Dewey

 1970 "Evolutionary Response to Human Infectious Diseases." *BioScience* 20(5): 271–75.

Arnold, Harry, Richard Odom, and William James

 1990 *Andrews' Diseases of the Skin.* 8th ed. Philadelphia: W. B. Saun-ders Co.

Arteaga, Ignacio

 1874 "Voyage of the *Princesa* and the *Favorita* up the California Coast in 1779." In "Viajes en la Costa al Norte de las Californias, 1774–1790," vol. 1, pp. 267–98. Translated by George Davidson. MS in Bancroft Library, University of California, Berkeley.

Ashburn, Percy

 1947 *The Ranks of Death: A Medical History of the Conquest of the Americas.* New York: Coward-McCann.

Averkieva, Julia

 1971 "The Tlingit Indians." In Eleanor Leacock and Nancy Lurie, eds., *North American Indians in Historical Perspective,* pp. 317–42. New York: Random House.

Babbott, Frank, and John Gordon

 1954 "Modern Measles." *American Journal of the Medical Sciences* 228: 334–61.

Bailey, Margaret

 1986 *The Grains, or Passages in the Life of Ruth Rover.* Corvallis: Oregon State University Press.

Baker, Brenda, and George Armelagos

 1988 "The Origin and Antiquity of Syphilis: Paleopathological Diagnosis and Interpretation." *Current Anthropology* 29(1): 103–20.

Ball, John

1925 *Autobiography.* Grand Rapids: Dean-Hicks Co.

Bancroft, Hubert (and Ivan Petrov)

1886 *History of Alaska, 1730–1885.* San Francisco: History Co.

Barbeau, Marius

1950 *Totem Poles.* 2 vols. National Museum of Canada Bulletin 119. Ottawa.

Barbeau, Marius, and William Beynon

1987 *Tsimshian Narratives.* 2 vols. Edited by John Cove and George Mac-Donald. Mercury Series Directorate Paper no. 3. Hull: Canadian Museum of Civilization.

Barclay, Forbes

1848 Letter of 18 March. MS D. 5/21, fols. 541–42. Hudson's Bay Company Archives, Winnipeg.

Barker, Burt, ed.

1948 *Letters of Dr. John McLoughlin, 1829–32.* Portland: Binfords and Mort.

Barman, Jean

1991 *The West beyond the West: A History of British Columbia.* Toronto: University of Toronto Press.

Barnett, Homer

1942 "Applied Anthropology in 1860." *Applied Anthropology* 1(3): 19–32.

Barsh, Russell

1996 "Puget Sound Indian Demography, 1900–1920: Migration and Economic Integration." *Ethnohistory* 43(1): 65–97.

Bartlett, John

1925 "Narrative of Events. . . . " In Elliot Snow, ed., *The Sea, the Ship, and the Sailor,* pp. 287–343. Salem: Marine Research Society.

Basedow, Herbert

1932 "Diseases of the Australian Aborigines." *Journal of Tropical Medicine and Hygiene* 35: various pp.

Bates, Charles, et al.

1985 "Plasma Essential Fatty Acids in Pure and Mixed Race American Indians on a Diet Exceptionally Rich in Salmon." *Prostaglandins, Leukotrienes, and Medicine* 17: 77–84.

Bayliss-Smith, Tim

1975 "Ontong Java: Depopulation and Repopulation." In Verne Caroll, ed., *Pacific Atoll Populations,* pp. 417–83. Honolulu: University Press.

Beaglehole, John, ed.

  1967   *The Voyage of the "Resolution" and "Discovery," 1776–1780.* Vol. 3. of *The Journals of Captain James Cook.* . . . Cambridge: Cambridge University Press.

Beals, Herbert

  1989   *Juan Perez on the Northwest Coast: Six Documents of His Expedition in 1774.* Portland: Oregon Historical Society Press.

Beattie, Owen

  1976   "Skeletal Pathology of Prehistoric Human Remains from Crescent Beach." In Roy Carlson, ed., *Current Research Reports,* pp. 155–64. Department of Archaeology, Simon Fraser University, Publication no. 3. Burnaby.

Beaver, Herbert

  1959   *Reports and Letters, 1836–1838, of Herbert Beaver.* . . . Edited by Thomas Jessett. Portland: Champoeg Press.

Beaver, H.M.S.

  1863   Medical Officer's Journal. Mf. 67. Oregon Historical Society, Portland. (Original in Royal Naval Hospital, Portsmouth, England.)

Beckham, Stephen

  1984   *"This Place Is Romantic and Wild": An Historical Overview of The Cascades Area, Fort Cascades, and the Cascades Townsite, Washington Territory.* Heritage Research Associates Report no. 27. Eugene.

  1986   *Land of the Umpqua: A History of Douglas County, Oregon.* Roseburg: Douglas County Commissioners.

  1990   "History of Western Oregon since 1846." In Suttles 1990c: 180 88.

Belcher, Edward

  1843   *Narrative of a Voyage Round the World, performed in Her Majesty's Ship Sulphur, during the years 1836–1842.* . . . London: Henry Colburn.

Bell, Edward

  1792–94 Journal of a Voyage in H.M.S. *Chatham.* Special Collections. University of British Columbia Library, Vancouver.

  1932   Excerpt from Edward Bell's Journal. In J. Neilson Barry, ed., "Columbia River Exploration, 1792." *Oregon Historical Quarterly* 33: 31–42, 143–55.

Benenson, Abram, ed.

  1995   *Control of Communicable Diseases Manual.* 16th ed. Washington: American Public Health Association.

Beynon, William

n.d.   The Beynon Manuscripts. Mf. A6655. Microforms. University of Washington Libraries, Seattle. (No. 53: "The Epidemic of Excrement of Blood," informant Wm. Ksanigitgigeni. No. 84: "The Narrative of why the Tsimshians got the Epidemic of Excrement of Blood," informant John Tate.)

Biddle, Nicholas

1814   *History of the Expedition Under the Command of Captains Lewis and Clark.* . . . 2 vols. Philadelphia: Bradford and Inskeep.

Bishop, Charles

1967   *The Journal and Letters of Captain Charles Bishop on the North-west Coast of America.* Edited by Michael Roe. Hakluyt Society, vol. 81. Cambridge.

Black, Francis

1966   "Measles Endemicity in Insular Populations: Critical Community Size and Its Evolutionary Implication." *Journal of Theoretical Biology* 11: 207–11.

Blackman, Margaret

1981   *Window on the Past: The Photographic Ethnohistory of the Northern and Kaigani Haida.* National Museum of Man Mercury Series, Canadian Ethnology Service Paper no. 74. Ottawa: National Museum of Canada.

Boas, Franz

1894   *Chinook Texts.* Bureau of American Ethnology Bulletin 20. Washington.

1901   *Kathlamet Texts.* Bureau of American Ethnology Bulletin 26. Washington.

1902   *Tsimshian Texts.* Bureau of American Ethnology Bulletin 27. Washington.

1910   *Kwakiutl Tales.* Columbia University Contributions to Anthropology 2. New York.

1916   "Tsimshian Mythology, Based on Texts Recorded by Henry W. Tate." In *Thirty-first Annual Report of the Bureau of American Ethnology for the Years 1909–1910,* pp. 29–1037. Washington.

1928   *Bella Bella Texts.* Columbia University Contributions to Anthropology 5. New York.

1932   *Bella Bella Tales.* Memoirs of the American Folk-Lore Society 25. New York.

1935   *Kwakiutl Culture as Reflected in Mythology.* Memoirs of the American Folk-Lore Society 28. New York.

1975   *Indian Legends of the North Pacific Coast of America.* Translated from the 1895 German by Dietrich Bertz, for the British Columbia Indian

Language Project, Victoria. Special Collections. University of British Columbia Library, Vancouver.

Bodega y Quadra, Juan Francisco de la

1912   "Expeditions in the Years 1775 & 1779 towards the West Coast of North America." Translated by G. F. Barwick from "Anuario de la Direccion de Hidrografia, año III, 1865, Seccion Historica." Typescript. Royal British Columbia Archives, Victoria.

Bolduc, Jean-Baptiste

1979   Journal, Cowlitz, 15 February 1844. In Edward Kowrach, trans., *Mission of the Columbia,* pp. 103–21. Fairfield, Wash.: Ye Galleon Press.

Bolon, Augustus

1854   Report to Isaac I. Stevens, 30 September. Records of the Washington Superintendency of Indian Affairs, 1853–74. National Archives, Washington.

Boone, George

1941   "Boone Family Reminiscences as Told to Mrs. Dye." *Oregon Historical Quarterly* 42(3): 220–29.

Bowen, William

1975   "The Oregon Frontiersman: A Demographic View." In Thomas Vaughan, ed., *The Western Shore: Oregon Country Essays Honoring the American Revolution,* pp. 181–98. Portland: Oregon Historical Society Press.

Bowers, John

1981   "The Odyssey of Smallpox Vaccination." *Bulletin of the History of Medicine* 55: 17–33.

Bowsfield, Hartwell, ed.

1979   *Fort Victoria Letters, 1846–1851.* Winnipeg: Hudson's Bay Record Society.

Boyd, Mark

1941a   "An Historical Sketch of the Prevalence of Malaria in North America." *American Journal of Tropical Medicine* 21: 223–44.

———, ed.

1941b   *Symposium on Human Malaria.* Washington: American Association for the Advancement of Science.

Boyd, Robert

1975   "Another Look at the 'Fever and Ague' of Western Oregon." *Ethnohistory* 22(2): 135–54.

1976   "Concomly of the Chinooks: A Biography from Ethnohistorical Sources." Typescript.

1979 "Old Cures and New Diseases: The Sweatbath and Febrile Diseases in the Aboriginal Pacific Northwest." Typescript.

1983 "'Doctor-Killings' in the Aboriginal Pacific Northwest: An Index of Systemic Stress Associated with Epidemic Mortality and Rapid Culture Change." Typescript.

1985 "The Introduction of Infectious Diseases among the Indians of the Pacific Northwest, 1774–1874." Ph.D. diss., University of Washington, Seattle.

1990 "Demographic History, 1774–1874." In Suttles 1990c: 135–48.

1992a "The Columbia River as a Corridor for Disease Introduction: 'New Diseases' of the 1840s in the Pacific Northwest." Paper presented at Great River of the West Conference, Longview, Wash., November.

1992b "Population Decline from Two Epidemics on the Northwest Coast." In Verano and Ubelaker 1992: 249–55.

1994a "The Pacific Northwest Measles Epidemic of 1847–1848." *Oregon Historical Quarterly* 95(1): 6–47.

1994b "Smallpox on the Northwest Coast: The First Epidemics." *BC Studies* 101: 5–40.

1995 "Kalapuya Disease and Depopulation." In *What Price Eden? The Willamette Valley in Transition, 1812–1855,* Salem: Mission Mill Museum.

1996a "Commentary on Early Contact Period Smallpox in the Pacific Northwest." *Ethnohistory* 43(2): 307–20.

1996b *People of The Dalles: The Indians of Wascopam Mission.* Lincoln: University of Nebraska Press.

1998 "Demographic History to 1990." In William Sturtevant, ed., *Handbook of North American Indians,* vol. 14, *Plateau,* edited by Deward Walker, pp. 467–83. Washington: Smithsonian Institution Press.

Boyd, Robert, and C. Dolores Gregory

1995 "[Plateau] Health and Disease before Contact." Typescript.

Boyd, Robert, and Yvonne Hajda

1987 "Seasonal Population Movement along the Lower Columbia River: The Social and Ecological Context." *American Ethnologist* 14(2): 309–26.

Brewer, Laura

1845 Letter of 15 August, Wascopam Mission. Canse Collection. Washington State Historical Society, Tacoma.

Brink, Jacob van den

1974 *The Haida Indians: Cultural Change Mainly between 1876–1970.* Leiden: E. J. Brill.

The British Columbian (New Westminster)

1862   Articles on smallpox, 14 May ff.

Brooks, Charles

1876   "Report of Japanese Vessels Wrecked in the North Pacific Ocean, from the Earliest Records to the Present Time." *Proceedings of the California Academy of Sciences* (San Francisco) 6: 50–66.

Brown, Joseph

1878   "Settlement of Willamette Valley." Mf. 176. Oregon Historical Society, Portland. (Original in Bancroft Library, University of California, Berkeley.)

Brown, Milton

1847   "Diary. . . . " MSS 268. Oregon Historical Society, Portland.

Brown, Peter

1980   "New Considerations on the Distribution of Thalassemia, Favism, and Malaria in Sardinia." Paper presented at the 49th Meeting of the American Association of Physical Anthropologists, Niagara Falls.

1981   "Cultural Adaptations to Endemic Malaria in Sardinia." *Medical Anthropology* 5(4): 313–37.

1983   "Demographic and Socioeconomic Effects of Disease Control: The Case of Malaria Eradication in Sardinia." *Medical Anthropology* 7(2): 63–87.

1986   "Cultural and Genetic Adaptations to Malaria: Problems of Comparison." *Human Ecology* 14(3): 311–32.

Brown, Robert

1864   Journal of the V. I. Exploring Expedition. Typescript by Winnifreda Macintosh, 1968. Royal British Columbia Archives, Victoria.

1866   "The Land of the Hydahs, a Spring Journey due North." Add. MSS 794, vol. 5. Royal British Columbia Archives, Victoria.

Bruce-Chwatt, Leonard

1965   "Paleogenesis and Paleo-epidemiology of Primate Malaria." *Bulletin of the World Health Organization* 32: 363–87.

Buchanan, Charles

1889   "Some Medical Customs, Ideas, Beliefs and Practices of the Snohomish Indians of Puget Sound." *St. Louis Courier of Medicine* 21. Typescript of original. Special Collections. University of Washington Libraries, Seattle.

Buckley, Cornelius

1989   *Nicholas Point, S. J.: His Life and Northwest Indian Chronicles.* Chicago: Loyola University Press.

Buikstra, Jane, ed.

1981   *Prehistoric Tuberculosis in the Americas.* Northwestern University Archaeological Program Scientific Paper 5. Evanston.

Buikstra, Jane, and Sloan Williams

1991   "Tuberculosis in the Americas: Current Perspectives." In Donald Ortner and Arthur Aufderheide, eds., *Human Paleopathology: Current Syntheses and Future Options,* pp. 161–72. Washington: Smithsonian Institution Press.

Burnet, Frank, and David White

1972   *Natural History of Infectious Diseases.* 4th ed. New York: Cambridge University Press.

Caamaño, Jacinto

1790   Extract of the Log on the *Princesa.* Mexican Archives, History, vol. 69(1). "Official Documents Relating to Spanish and Mexican Voyages of Navigation, Exploration, and Discovery Made in North America in the Eighteenth Century." Translated by Mary Daylton. WPA project no. 2749. Seattle, 1939–40. Special Collections. University of Washington Libraries, Seattle.

Cambon, K., J. D. Galbraith, and G. Kong

1965   "Middle Ear Disease in the Indians of the Mount Currie Reservation, British Columbia." *Canadian Medical Association Journal* 93: 1301–5.

Camp, Charles

1966   *George C. Yount and His Chronicles of the West.* Denver: Old West Publishing Co.

Campa Cos, Miguel de la

1964   *A Journal of Explorations Northward along the Coast from Monterey in the Year 1775.* Translated by John Galvin. San Francisco: John Howell.

Campbell, Sarah

1989   "Postcolumbian Culture History in the Northern Columbia Plateau, A.D. 1500–1900." Ph.D. diss., University of Washington, Seattle.

Canada, Department of Indian Affairs

1880–90   *Annual Reports.* Sessional Papers. Ottawa: I. B. Taylor.

Canada, Department of Mines and Technical Surveys

1974   *National Atlas of Canada.* Ottawa: Macmillan.

Carey, Charles, ed.

1922   "The Mission Record Book of the Methodist Episcopal Church, Willamette Station, Oregon Territory." *Oregon Historical Quarterly* 23(3): 230–66.

Carley, Caroline

1979　"Historical and Archaeological Evidence of Nineteenth Century Fever Epidemics and Medicine at Hudson's Bay Company's Fort Vancouver." M.A. thesis, University of Idaho, Moscow.

1981　"Historical and Archaeological Evidence of 19th Century Fever Epidemics and Medicine at Hudson's Bay Company's Fort Vancouver." *Historical Archaeology* 15(1): 19–35.

Chance, David

1973　*Influences of the Hudson's Bay Company on the Native Cultures of the Colvile District.* Northwest Anthropological Research Notes 7(1), Memoir 2. Moscow: University of Idaho.

Chardon, Francis

1932　*Chardon's Journal at Fort Clark, 1834–1839.* Edited by Annie Abel. Pierre, S.D.

Chirouse, Casimir

1862　Letters of 6 May, 14 July, and 6 August. Oblates of Marie Immaculate. MSS 1581 (microfilm). Oregon Historical Society, Portland.

Chisholm, Brian, D. Erle Nelson, and Henry Schwarcz

1983　"Marine and Terrestrial Protein in Prehistoric Diets on the British Columbia Coast." *Current Anthropology* 24(3): 396–98.

Chittenden, Newton

1884　*Hyda Land and People: Official Report of the Exploration of the Queen Charlotte Islands for the Government of British Columbia.* Victoria.

Christiansen, Povl, et al.

1952–53　"An Epidemic of Measles in Southern Greenland, 1951." *Acta Medica Scandinavica* 144(4–5): various pp.

Clark, George, et al.

1987　"The Evolution of Mycobacterial Disease in Human Populations: A Reevaluation." *Current Anthropology* 28(1): 45–62.

Clarke, Samuel

1905　*Pioneer Days of Oregon History.* 2 vols. Portland: J. K. Gill Co.

Cleland, J. Burton

1928　"Disease amongst the Australian Aborigines." *Journal of Tropical Medicine and Hygiene* 31: various pp.

Cockburn, Aidan

1959　"The Evolution of Infectious Diseases." *International Review of Medicine* 172: 493–508.

1963   *The Evolution and Eradication of Infectious Diseases.* Baltimore: Johns Hopkins University Press.

1967   *Infectious Diseases: Their Evolution and Eradication.* Springfield: Charles C. Thomas.

1971   "Infectious Diseases in Ancient Populations." *Current Anthropology* 12(1): 45–60.

Codere, Helen

1948   "The Swai'xwe Myth of the Middle Fraser River: The Integration of Two Northwest Coast Cultural Ideas." *Journal of American Folk-Lore* 61: 1–18.

1950   *Fighting with Property: A Study of Kwakiutl Potlatching and Warfare, 1792–1930.* American Ethnological Society Monograph 18. New York.

Cole, Douglas, and David Darling

1990   "History of the Early Period." In Suttles 1990c: 119–34.

Cole, Douglas, and Bradley Lockner

1993   *To the Charlottes: George Dawson's 1878 Survey of the Queen Charlotte Islands.* Vancouver: University of British Columbia Press.

Cole, Jean

1979   *Exile in the Wilderness: The Biography of Chief Factor Archibald McDonald, 1790–1853.* Seattle: University of Washington Press.

Collins, G. W.

1866   *Report of August 15, Alsea Indian Sub-Agency.* 39th Cong., 2d sess. House Executive Doc. 1 (Serial no. 1284), pp. 84–85, Washington.

Collins, June

1949   "John Fornsby, the Personal Document of a Coast Salish Indian." In Marian Smith, ed., *Indians of the Urban Northwest,* pp. 287–341. Columbia University Contributions to Anthropology 36. New York.

Collison, William

1981   *In the Wake of the War Canoe: a stirring record of forty years' successful labour, peril, and adventure amongst the savage Indian tribes of the Pacific coast, and the piratical head-hunting Haida of the Queen Charlotte Islands, British Columbia.* 1915. Reprint edited by Charles Lillard, Victoria: Sono Nis Press.

Colnett, James

1788   Journal, *Prince of Wales,* 16 October to 7 November. Public Record Office, Adm. 55/146, Kew, Surrey, England. (Mf. A250, Microforms. University of Washington Libraries, Seattle.)

1940   *The Journal of Captain James Colnett aboard the "Argonaut" from April 26, 1789, to Nov. 3, 1791.* Toronto: Champlain Society.

Colvocoresses, George

1852   *Four Years in a Government Exploring Expedition. . . .* New York: Cornish, Lamport & Co.

Colyer, Vincent

1870a   *Alaska Report.* 41st Cong., 2d sess. House Executive Doc. 144 (Serial no. 1418). Washington.

1870b   *Wrangell, Alaska, Previous to Bombardment.* 41st Cong., 2d sess. Senate Executive Doc. 68 (Serial no. 1406). Washington.

Comrie, P.

1869   Medical Officer's Journal, H.M.S. *Sparrowhawk.* Mf. 67. Oregon Historical Society, Portland. (Also in Public Record Office, Adm. 101/178, Kew, Surrey, England. Original in Royal Naval Hospital, Portsmouth, England.)

Cook, Noble David

1981   *Demographic Collapse: Indian Peru, 1520–1620.* New York: Cambridge University Press.

Cook, Sherburne

1935   "Diseases of the Indians of Lower California in the Eighteenth Century." *California and Western Medicine* 43(6): 432–34.

1937   "The Extent and Significance of Disease among the Indians of Baja California from 1697 to 1773." *Ibero-Americana* (Berkeley) 9.

1939   "Smallpox in Spanish and Mexican California, 1770–1834." *Bulletin of the History of Medicine* 7(2): 153–91.

1955   "The Epidemic of 1830–33 in California and Oregon." *University of California Publications in American Archaeology and Ethnology* 43(3): 303–26.

1956   *The Aboriginal Population of the North Coast of California.* Anthropological Records 16(3). Berkeley and Los Angeles: University of California Press.

1976a   *The Population of the California Indians, 1769–1970.* Berkeley and Los Angeles: University of California Press.

1976b   *The Indian Population of New England in the Seventeenth Century.* University of California Publications in Anthropology 12. Berkeley.

1978   "Historical Demography." In William Sturtevant, ed., *Handbook of North American Indians,* vol. 8, *California,* edited by Robert Heizer, pp. 91–98. Washington: Smithsonian Institution Press.

Cook, Sherburne, and Woodrow Borah

1971–74   *Essays in Population History: Mexico and the Caribbean.* 2 vols. Berkeley
           and Los Angeles: University of California Press.

Cook, Warren

1973   *Flood Tide of Empire: Spain and the Pacific Northwest, 1543–1819.* New
           Haven: Yale University Press.

Cooper, Donald

1965   *Epidemic Disease in Mexico City, 1761–1813.* Austin: University of Texas
           Press.

Cooper, James

1862   Letter of 17 October. Correspondence with H.M.S. *Devastation.* MS
           F1210. Royal British Columbia Archives, Victoria.

Corney, Peter

1965   *Early Voyages in the North Pacific, 1817–18.* 1896. Reprint, Fairfield, Wash.:
           Ye Galleon Press.

Corruccini, Robert, and Samvit Kaul

1983   "The Epidemiological Transition and Anthropology of Minor Chronic
           Non-infectious Diseases." *Medical Anthropology* 7: 336–50.

Couture, Marilyn

1978   "Recent and Contemporary Foraging Practices of the Harney Valley
           Paiute." M.A. thesis, Portland State University.

Cox, Ross

1957   *The Columbia River.* 1831. Edited by Edgar and Jane Stewart. Norman:
           University of Oklahoma Press.

Coxe, William

1780   *Account of the Russian Discoveries between Asia and America.* London:
           T. Cadell.

Cridge, Edward

1862   Letter of 16 June. Microfilm. William Duncan Papers. Special Collec-
           tions. University of British Columbia Library, Vancouver.

Crosby, Alfred

1972   *The Columbian Exchange: Biological and Cultural Consequences of 1492.*
           Westport, Conn.: Greenwood.

1976   "Virgin Soil Epidemics as a Factor in the Aboriginal Depopulation of
           America." *William and Mary Quarterly* 33(2): 290–99.

1978   "God . . . Would Destroy Them, and Give Their Country to Another
           People. . . . " *American Heritage* 29(6): 39–42.

Curtis, Edward

1911   "The Chinookan Tribes." In *The North American Indian*, vol. 8, pp. 85–154, 172–83, 198–205. Norwood, Mass.: Plimpton Press.

1913   *Salishan Tribes of the Coast.* Vol. 9 of *The North American Indian.*

1915   *The Kwakiutl.* Vol. 10 of *The North American Indian.*

Cutter, Donald

1969   *The California Coast: A Bilingual Edition of Documents from the Sutro Collection.* Norman: University of Oklahoma Press.

Cybulski, Jerome

1977   "Cribra Orbitalia, a Possible Sign of Anemia in Early Historic Native Populations of the British Columbia Coast." *American Journal of Physical Anthropology* 47(1): 31–40.

1990   "Human Biology." In Suttles 1990c: 52–59.

1992   *A Greenville Burial Ground: Human Remains and Mortuary Elements in British Columbia Coast Prehistory.* Archaeological Survey of Canada Mercury Series, paper no. 146. Hull: Canadian Museum of Civilization.

1994   "Culture Change, Demographic History, and Health and Disease on the Northwest Coast." In Clark Larsen and George Milner, eds., *In the Wake of Contact: Biological Responses to Conquest,* pp. 75–85. New York: Wiley-Liss.

Cybulski, Jerome, and L. Bradley Pett

1981   "Bone Changes Suggesting Multiple Myeloma and Metastatic Carcinoma in Two Early Historic Natives of the British Columbia Coast." In Jerome Cybulski, ed., *Contributions to Physical Anthropology, 1978–1980,* pp. 176–86. Archaeological Survey of Canada Mercury Series, paper no. 106. Ottawa: National Museum of Canada.

Daily British Colonist (Victoria)

1862   Articles on smallpox, 18 March ff.

Daily Press (Victoria)

1862   Articles on smallpox, 26 March ff.

Dart, Anson

1851a   Letter of 14 May. Records of the Oregon Superintendency of Indian Affairs, 1848–73. National Archives, Washington.

1851b   "Articles of a Treaty, Made and Concluded at Tansey Point, Near Clatsop Plains [5–9 August, with ten bands]." Records of the Oregon Superintendency of Indian Affairs, 1848–73. National Archives, Washington.

1852 *Report to the Commissioner of Indian Affairs, April 19, 1851.* 32d Cong., 1st sess. House Executive Doc. 2 (Serial no. 636), pp. 472–83. Washington.

1854 Letter of 15 January to I. I. Stevens. Records of the Washington Superintendency of Indian Affairs, 1853–74. National Archives, Washington.

Dawson, George

1880 "On the Haida Indians of the Queen Charlotte Islands." In *Geological Survey of Canada: Report of Progress for 1878–79,* pp. 103–75. Montreal: Dawson Brothers.

1887 *Notes and Observations on the Qwakiool People of the northern part of Vancouver Island and adjacent coasts, made during the Summer of 1885....* Transactions of the Royal Society of Canada 11. Reprint, Fairfield, Wash.: Ye Galleon Press, 1973.

Decker, Jody

1989 " 'We Should Never Be Again the Same People': The Diffusion and Cumulative Impact of Acute Infectious Diseases Affecting the Natives of the Northern Plains of the Western Interior of Canada, 1774–1839." Ph.D. diss., York University, Toronto.

de Laguna, Frederica

1972 *Under Mount Saint Elias: The History and Culture of the Yakutat Tlingit.* 3 vols. Smithsonian Contributions to Anthropology, vol. 7. Washington.

1990 "Tlingit." In Suttles 1990c: 203–28.

de Lesseps, [Jean-Baptiste-Barthélemy, Baron]

1790 *Travels in Kamtschatka, during the years 1787 and 1788.* London: J. Johnson.

Demers, Modeste

1844 Letter of 31 August. MS in Archdiocesan Archives, Portland.

Denevan, William

1976 *The Native Population of the Americas in 1492.* Madison: University of Wisconsin Press.

De Smet, Pierre-Jean

1906 *Oregon Missions and Travels over the Rocky Mountains in 1845–46.* Edited by Reuben Thwaites. Travels in the Far Northwest, vol. 2. Cleveland: Arthur H. Clark Co.

d'Herbomez, Louis

1863 Letter of 11 December. In *Missions de la Congrégation des Missionaires Oblats de Marie Immaculée,* quatrième année, 1865, p. 308.

DiVale, William, and Marvin Harris

1976   "Population, Warfare, and the Male Supremacist Complex." *American Anthropologist* 78(3): 521–38.

Divin, Vasilii

1993   *The Great Russian Navigator A.I. Chirikov.* Translated and annotated by Raymond Fisher. Fairbanks: University of Alaska Press.

Dixon, Cyril

1962   *Smallpox.* London: J. and A. Churchill.

Dixon, George

1789   *A Voyage Round the World, but more particularly to the North-West Coast of America: performed in 1785, 1786, 1787 and 1788 in the King George and Queen Charlotte.* . . . London: George Goulding.

Dobyns, Henry

1966   "Estimating Aboriginal American Population, I: An Appraisal of Techniques with a New Hemispheric Estimate (and Comments)." *Current Anthropology* 7(4): 395–416, 425–49.

1983   *Their Number Became Thinned: Native American Population Dynamics in Eastern North America.* Knoxville: University of Tennessee Press.

1992   "Native American Trade Centers as Contagious Disease Foci." In Verano and Ubelaker 1992: 215–22.

1993   "Disease Transfer at Contact." *Annual Review of Anthropology* 22: 273–91.

Dollar, Clyde

1977   "The High Plains Smallpox Epidemic of 1837–38." *Western Historical Quarterly* 8(1): 15–38.

Dolman, C.

1964   "Botulism as a World Health Problem." In K. Lewis and K. Cassel, eds., *Botulism: Proceedings of a Symposium,* pp. 20–23. Cincinnati: U.S. Public Health Service.

Dominis, John

1827–30   Log of *Owyhee,* 21 January 1827 to 21 October 1830 (kept by the first mate). MS 16. California Historical Society, San Francisco.

Donald, Leland

1996   "Slavery and Captivity: A Comparison of Servitude on the Northwest Coast and among Interior Salish." In Don Dumond, ed., *Chin Hills to Chiloquin: Papers Honoring the Versatile Career of Theodore Stern,* pp. 75–86. University of Oregon Anthropological Paper 52. Eugene.

Dorsey, George

1897   "The Geography of the Tsimshian Indians." *American Antiquarian* 19(4): 276–82.

Douglas, David

1905   Letters of 11 October 1830, 24 October 1832, and 9 April 1833. In "Second Journey to the Northwestern Parts of the Continent of North America during the years 1829–'30–'31–'32–'33." *Oregon Historical Quarterly* 6(3): 288–309.

Douglas, James

1835   "Statistics of the Northwest Coast of America." In James Douglas Diary, MS B 40 D72.5, fols. 138–40. Royal British Columbia Archives, Victoria.

1848a   Letter of 16 March. MS D. 5/10, fols. 474, 479. Hudson's Bay Company Archives, Winnipeg.

1848b   Letter of 5 December. MS B. 223/b/38, fols. 59–60. Hudson's Bay Company Archives, Winnipeg.

1878   "Census of the Indian Population on the N.W. Coast. . . . " Transcription by Ivan Petrov. Private Papers, 2d ser. Bancroft Library. University of California, Berkeley. (Microfilm A 92. Microforms. University of Washington Libraries, Seattle.)

1931   "Douglas Expeditions, 1840–41." Edited by Herman Leader. *Oregon Historical Quarterly* 32(1): 1–22 (pt. 1).

Douglas, Mary

1970   "Introduction: Thirty Years after Witchcraft, Oracles, and Magic." In Mary Douglas, ed., *Witchcraft Confessions and Accusations,* pp. xiii–xxxviii. London: Tavistock.

Drake, Daniel

1850   *A systematic Treatise, Historical, Etiological and Practical, on the principal diseases of the interior valley of North America. . . .* Cincinnati: Winthrop B. Smith and Co.

Draper, John

1989   "A Proposed Model of Late Prehistoric Settlement Systems on the Southern Northwest Coast, Coos and Curry Counties, Oregon." Ph.D. diss., Washington State University, Pullman.

Drucker, Philip

1951   *The Northern and Central Nootkan Tribes.* Bureau of American Ethnology Bulletin 144. Washington.

1955 "Sources of Northwest Coast Culture." In *New Interpretations of Aboriginal American Culture History,* pp. 59–81. Washington: Anthropological Society of Washington.

1963 *Indians of the Northwest Coast.* Garden City: Natural History Press.

Drury, Clifford

1958 *The Diaries and Letters of Henry H. Spalding and Asa Bowen Smith Relating to the Nez Perce Mission, 1838–1842.* Glendale: Arthur H. Clark.

1973 *Marcus and Narcissa Whitman and the Opening of Old Oregon.* Vol. 2. Glendale: Arthur H. Clark.

Du Bois, Cora

1938 *The Feather Cult of the Middle Columbia.* General Series in Anthropology 7. Menasha, Wisc.: George Banta.

1939 *The 1870 Ghost Dance.* Anthropological Records 3(1). Berkeley and Los Angeles: University of California Press.

Duff, Wilson

1952 *The Upper Stalo Indians of the Fraser Valley, British Columbia.* Anthropology in British Columbia Memoir no. 1. Victoria: Provincial Museum of British Columbia.

1964a "The Contributions of Marius Barbeau to West Coast Ethnology." *Anthropologica* 6(1): 63–96.

1964b *The Indian History of British Columbia.* Vol. 1, *The Impact of the White Man.* Anthropology in British Columbia Memoir no. 5. Victoria: Provincial Museum of British Columbia.

Duflot de Mofras, Eugene

1937 *Duflot de Mofras' Travels on the Pacific Coast.* 1844. 2 vols. Translated, edited, and annotated by Marguerite Wilbur. Santa Ana: Fine Arts Press.

Dumond, Don

1996 "Poison in the Cup: The South Alaskan Smallpox Epidemic of 1835." In Don Dumond, ed., *Chin Hills to Chiloquin: Papers Honoring the Versatile Career of Theodore Stern,* pp. 117–29. University of Oregon Anthropological Paper 52. Eugene.

Duncan, William

1860 Letter of 25 October. William Duncan Papers. Mf. AW1 R2547. University of British Columbia Library, Vancouver. (Original in Metlakahtla Christian Mission, Annette Island, Alaska.)

1862   Journal. William Duncan Papers. Mf. AW1 R2547. University of British Columbia Library, Vancouver. (Original in Metlakahtla Christian Mission, Annette Island, Alaska.)

1869   *Metlahkatla: Ten Year's Work among the Tsimsheean Indians: from the Journals and Letters of William Duncan.* London: Church Missionary House.

Dunn, Frederick

1965   "On the Antiquity of Malaria in the Western Hemisphere." *Human Biology* 37(4): 385–93.

1968   "Epidemiological Factors: Health and Disease." In Richard Lee and Irven DeVore, eds., *Man the Hunter*, pp. 221–28. Chicago: Aldine.

Dunn, J. R.

1846   Journal on H.M.S. *Fisgard*. Public Record Office, Adm. 101/100.4 XC A/3930, Kew, Surrey, England.

Dunn, John

1845   *The Oregon Territory and the British North American Fur Trade.* Philadelphia: G. B. Zieber.

Dunnell, Robert, James Chatters, and Leslie Salo

1973   *Archaeological Survey of the Vancouver Lake–Lake River Area . . . Report to the U.S. Army Corps of Engineers, Portland District.* Portland: U.S. Army Corps of Engineers.

Dutta, Hiran, and Ashok Dutt

1978   "Malarial Ecology: A Global Perspective." *Social Science and Medicine* 12: 69–84.

Eastburn, Richard, et al.

1987   "Human Intestinal Infection with *Nanophyetus salmincola* from Salmonid Fishes." *American Journal of Tropical Medicine and Hygiene* 36(3): 586–91.

Edwards, Philip

1932   *The Diary of Philip Leget Edwards.* San Francisco: Grabhorn Press.

Eells, Myron

1889   "The Twana, Chemakum, and Klallam Indians of Washington Territory." In *Annual Report of the Smithsonian Institution for the Year 1887*, pp. 605–81. Washington.

Elliot, Mrs.

1927   "The Story of the Evolution of the County from a Primitive State." *Hillsboro Argus*, 15 November.

Elliott, William

1931   "Lake Lillooet Tales." *Journal of American Folk-Lore* 44: 166–81.

Ellis, William

1782   *An Authentic Narrative of a Voyage Performed by Captain Cook and Captain Clerke. . . .* 2 vols. London: G. Robinson.

Elmendorf, William

1960   *The Structure of Twana Culture.* Washington State University Research Studies 28(3), Monographic Supplement no. 2. Pullman.

1971   "Coast Salish Status Ranking and Intergroup Ties." *Southwestern Journal of Anthropology* 27(4): 353–80.

1990   "Chemakum." In Suttles 1990c: 438–40.

Emmons, George F.

1841   "Journal kept while attached to the Exploring Expedition . . . No. 3." Microfilm of WA MS 166. Western Americana Collection. Beinecke Library. Yale University, New Haven.

Emmons, George T.

1991   *The Tlingit Indians.* Edited by Frederica de Laguna. Anthropological Papers of the American Museum of Natural History, vol. 70. Seattle: University of Washington Press.

Ermatinger, Francis

1980   *Fur Trade Letters of Francis Ermatinger . . . 1818–1853.* Edited by Lois McDonald. Glendale: Arthur H. Clark.

Evans, Lucylle

1981   *Good Samaritan of the Northwest: Anthony Ravalli, S. J., 1812–1884.* Stevensville: Montana Creative Consultants.

Ewers, John

1973   "The Influence of Epidemics on the Indian Populations and Cultures of Texas." *Plains Anthropologist* 18: 104–15.

Fedorova, Svetlana

1973   *The Russian Population in Alaska and California, Late 18th Century–1867.* Translated and edited by Richard Pierce and Alton Donnelly. Kingston, Ont.: Limestone Press.

Fenner, Frank

1971   "Infectious Disease and Social Change." *Medical Journal of Australia* 1: 1143–51.

Fenner, Frank, et al.

1988   *Smallpox and Its Eradication.* Geneva: World Health Organization.

Ferguson, R. Brian

1984   "A Re-examination of the Causes of Northwest Coast Warfare." In R.
        Brian Ferguson, ed., *Warfare, Culture, and Environment*, pp. 267–328.
        Orlando: Academic Press.

Fiennes, Richard

1978   *Zoonoses and the Origins and Ecology of Human Disease.* New York:
        Academic Press.

Finlayson, Duncan

1846–50 Fort Victoria Journal. MS B. 226/a/1. Hudson's Bay Company Archives,
         Winnipeg.

Finlayson, Duncan, and John Work

1834–38 Fort Simpson Journal. MS B. 201/a/3. Hudson's Bay Company Archives,
         Winnipeg.

Fisher, Raymond

1996   "Finding America." In Stephen Haycox and Mary Mangusso, eds., *An
        Alaska Anthology: Interpreting the Past*, pp. 3–20. Seattle: University of
        Washington Press.

Fisher, Robin

1977   *Contact and Conflict: Indian-European Relations in British Columbia,
        1774–1890.* Vancouver: University of British Columbia Press.

1996   "The Northwest from the Beginning of Trade with Europeans to the
        1880s." In Bruce Trigger and Wilcomb Washburn, eds., *The Cambridge
        History of the Native Peoples of the Americas*, vol. 1, *North America*, pt.
        2, pp. 117–82. Cambridge: Cambridge University Press.

Fleurieu, Charles P. Claret, Comte de

1801   *A Voyage Round the World Performed During the Years 1790, 1791, and
        1792 by Étienne Marchand.* 2 vols. London: T. N. Longmans and O.
        Rees.

Fortuine, Robert

1975   "Paralytic Shellfish Poisoning in the North Pacific: Two Historical
        Accounts and Implications for Today." *Alaska Medicine* 17(5): 71–76.

1984a   "Communicable Disease Control in the Early History of Alaska, I:
        Smallpox." *Circumpolar Health* 84: 187–90.

1984b   "Communicable Disease Control in the Early History of Alaska, II:
        Syphilis." *Circumpolar Health* 84: 191–94.

1986   "Early Evidence of Infectious Disease among Alaskan Natives." *Alaska
        History* 2(1): 38–56.

1989 *Chills and Fever: Health and Disease in the Early History of Alaska.* Fairbanks: University of Alaska Press.

Fouquet, Leon

1862 Letter of 16 July. In *Missions de la Congrégation des Missionaires Oblats de Marie Immaculée,* troisième année, no. 2—juin 1864, pp. 161–207. Paris: Typographie Hennuyer et Fils.

Frachtenberg, Leo

1914 "Kalapuya: Ethnology." MS 1923-c. National Anthropological Archives. Smithsonian Institution, Washington.

1920 *Alsea Texts and Myths.* Bureau of American Ethnology Bulletin 67. Washington: Government Printing Office.

Franchère, Gabriel

1969 *Journal of a Voyage on the North West Coast of North America during the Years 1811, 1812, 1813, and 1814.* Edited and translated by W. Kaye Lamb and Wessie Lamb. Toronto: Champlain Society.

Fraser, Simon

1960 *The Letters and Journals of Simon Fraser, 1806–1808.* Edited by W. Kaye Lamb. Toronto: Macmillan.

French, David

1963 "Wasco-Wishram." In Edward Spicer, ed., *Perspectives in American Indian Culture Change,* pp. 337–429. Chicago: University of Chicago Press.

Friedlander, Judith

1970 "Malaria and Demography in the Lowlands of Mexico: An Ethnohistorical Approach." In Robert Spencer, ed., *Forms of Symbolic Action: Proceedings of the 1969 Annual Spring Meeting of the American Ethnological Society,* pp. 217–33.

Frisch, Rose

1977 "Nutrition, Fatness and Fertility: The Effect of Food Intake on Reproductive Ability." In W. Henry Mosley, ed., *Nutrition and Human Reproduction,* pp. 91–122. New York: Plenum Press.

Frost, Joseph

1934 "Journal, 1840–43." Edited by Nellie Pipes. *Oregon Historical Quarterly* 35: various pp.

Gaines, John, Alonzo Skinner, and Beverly Allen

1851 Letter of 8 February to Commissioner Luke Lea. Records of the Oregon Superintendency of Indian Affairs, 1848–73. National Archives, Washington.

1852   Letter of 14 May 1851. 32d Cong., 1st sess. House Executive Doc. 2 (Serial no. 636), pp. 468–72. Washington.

Gairdner, Meredith

1834   Letter of 7 November. Vol. 62, no. 82, fol. 163. Kew Gardens Herbarium Archives, Kew, Surrey, England.

Gallatin, Albert

1836   *A Synopsis of the Indian Tribes . . . in North America.* Transactions of the American Antiquarian Society, Archaeologia Americana, vol. 2. Worcester, Mass.

Galois, Robert

1994   *Kwakwa̱ka̱'wakw Settlements, 1775–1920: A Geographical Analysis and Gazetteer.* Vancouver: University of British Columbia Press.

1996   "Measles, 1847–1850: The First Modern Epidemic in British Columbia." *BC Studies* 109: 31–43.

Garfield, Viola

1951   "The Tsimshian and Their Neighbors." In *The Tsimshian: Their Arts and Music,* pp. 1–70. American Ethnological Society Publication 18. New York: J. J. Augustin.

Garrett, F. A.

n.d.   Reminiscences [of Alexander Garrett]. Typescript, with diary excerpts. MS E B G19. Royal British Columbia Archives, Victoria.

Garrett, Laurie

1994   *The Coming Plague: Newly Emerging Diseases in a World out of Balance.* New York: Farrar, Straus, and Giroux.

Garvin, Richard

1989   "Botulism and Prehistoric Populations on the Northwest Coast." *Northwest Anthropological Research Notes* 23(2): 167. (Abstract of paper presented at the 42d Annual Northwest Anthropological Conference, Spokane, 23–25 March.)

Gary, George

1923   "Diary of Rev. George Gary." Edited by Charles Carey. *Oregon Historical Quarterly* 24: various pp.

Gass, Patrick

1958   *A Journal of Voyages and Travels of a Corps of Discovery. . . .* Minneapolis: Ross and Haines.

Gibbs, George

1851   "January. Census of the Chinook tribe of Indians & Census of the

Clatsop tribe of Indians." Records of the Oregon Superintendency of Indian Affairs, 1848–73. National Archives, Washington.

1855   Report . . . to Captain Mc'Clellan, on the Indian Tribes of the Territory of Washington. In "Report of Explorations for a Route . . . from St. Paul to Puget Sound," in vol. 1 of *Reports of Explorations and Surveys . . . from the Mississippi River to the Pacific Ocean . . . 1853–54,* pp. 419–65. 33d Cong., 1st sess., House Executive Doc. 129 (Serial no. 736). Washington.

1857   "Observations on the Coast Tribes of Oregon." MS 196-a. National Anthropological Archives. Smithsonian Institution, Washington.

1877   "Tribes of Western Washington and Northwestern Oregon." *Contributions to North American Ethnology* 1(2): 157–361.

1955–56   "George Gibbs' Account of Indian Mythology in Oregon and Washington Territories." Edited by Ella Clark. *Oregon Historical Quarterly* 56(4): 293–326; 57(2): 125–67.

Gibson, James

1976   *Imperial Russia in Frontier America, 1784–1867.* New York: Oxford University Press.

1982–83   "Smallpox on the Northwest Coast, 1835–1838." *BC Studies* 56: 61–81.

1988   "The Maritime Trade of the North Pacific Coast." In William Sturtevant, ed., *Handbook of North American Indians,* vol. 4, *History of Indian-White Relations,* edited by Wilcomb Washburn, pp. 375–90. Washington: Smithsonian Institution Press.

Gjullin, Claude, and Gaines Eddy

1972   *The Mosquitoes of the Northwestern United States.* USDA Agricultural Research Technical Bulletin no. 1447. Washington.

Glushankov, Ivan

1973   "The Aleutian Expedition of Krenitsyn and Levashov." Translated by Mary Sadouski and Richard Pierce. *Alaska Journal* 3(4): 204–10.

Gofton, J. P., et al.

1972   "Sacroiliitis and Ankylosing Spondylitis in North American Indians." *Annals of Rheumatic Diseases* 31: 474–81.

Goldman, Irving

1940   "The Alkatcho Carrier of British Columbia." In Ralph Linton, ed., *Acculturation in Seven American Indian Tribes,* pp. 333–89. Gloucester, Mass.: P. Smith.

Good, John

n.d.   "The Utmost Bounds of the West: Pioneer Jottings on Forty Years of

Missionary Reminiscences of the Out West Pacific Coast, AD 1861 to AD 1900." Microfilm 650A. Royal British Columbia Archives, Victoria.

Gould, Richard

1978 "Tolowa." In William Sturtevant, ed., *Handbook of North American Indians,* vol. 8, *California,* edited by Robert Heizer, pp. 128–36. Washington: Smithsonian Institution Press.

Gowlland, John

1862 Journal of H.M.S. *Plumper.* Microfilm 447a. Royal British Columbia Archives, Victoria.

Green, Jonathan

1915 *Journal of a Tour on the NorthWest Coast of America in the Year 1829. . . .* New York: Charles F. Heartman.

Greer, Richard

1965–66 "Oahu's Ordeal—the Smallpox Epidemic of 1853." *Hawaii Historical Review* 1(2): 221–42; 2(1): 248–66.

Guerra, Francisco

1977 "The Introduction of Cinchona in the Treatment of Malaria." *Journal of Tropical Medicine and Hygiene* 80(6–7): 112–18, 135–40.

1988 "The Earliest American Epidemic: The Influenza of 1493." *Social Science History* 12(3): 305–25.

Guillod, Harry

1882 "Report on the Tribes of the West Coast of Vancouver Island." In Dominion of Canada, *Annual Report of the Department of Indian Affairs for the Year 1881,* pp. 161–65. Ottawa.

Gunther, Erna

1925 *Klallam Folk Tales.* University of Washington Publications in Anthropology 1(4): 113–70. Seattle.

1972 *Indian Life on the Northwest Coast of North America as Seen by the Early Explorers and Fur Traders during the Last Decades of the Eighteenth Century.* Chicago: University of Chicago Press.

Haeberlin, Hermann

1924 "Mythology of Puget Sound." *Journal of the American Folk-Lore Society* 37: 371–438.

Haines, Francis

1938 "The Northward Spread of Horses among the Plains Indians." *American Anthropologist* 40(3): 429–37.

Hajda, Yvonne

1984   "Regional Social Organization in the Greater Lower Columbia, 1792–1830." Ph.D. diss., University of Washington, Seattle.

Hale, Horatio

1846   *Ethnography and Philology.* Philadelphia: Lea and Blanchard.

Hall, Roberta, and Thomas German

1975   "Dental Pathology, Attrition, and Occlusal Surface Form in a Prehistoric Sample from British Columbia." *Syesis* 8: 275–89.

Hall, Roberta, Robert Morrow, and J. Henry Clarke

1986   "Dental Pathology of Prehistoric Residents of Oregon." *American Journal of Physical Anthropology* 69(3): 325–34.

Hancock, Samuel

1927   *The Narrative of Samuel Hancock, 1845–1860.* New York: R. M. McBride and Co.

Hare, Ronald

1967   "The Antiquity of Diseases Caused by Bacteria and Viruses: A Review of the Problem from a Bacteriologist's Point of View." In Don R. Brothwell and A. T. Sandison, eds., *Diseases in Antiquity,* pp. 115–31. Springfield: Charles C. Thomas.

Harkin, Michael

1997   *The Heiltsuks: Dialogues of Culture and History on the Northwest Coast.* Lincoln: University of Nebraska Press.

Harriott, John

1907   "Letter of February 25, 1831 to John McLeod." *Washington Historical Quarterly* 1(4): 260–61.

Harris, R. Cole

1994   "Voices of Disaster: Smallpox around the Strait of Georgia in 1782." *Ethnohistory* 41(4): 591–626.

Harrison, Gordon

1978   *Mosquitoes, Malaria, and Man: A History of the Hostilities since 1880.* New York: E. P. Dutton.

Harvey, Herbert

1967   "Population of the Cahuilla Indians: Decline and Its Causes." *Eugenics Quarterly* 14: 185–90.

Hastings, Loren

1847   Journal. MSS 660. Oregon Historical Society, Portland.

Heath, Joseph

1979   *Memoirs of Nisqually.* Edited by Lucille McDonald. Fairfield: Ye Galleon Press.

Heizer, Robert

1942   "Walla Walla Expeditions to the Sacramento Valley." *California Historical Quarterly* 21(1): 1–7.

Helmcken, John

1975   *The Reminiscences of Doctor John Sebastian Helmcken.* Edited by Dorothy Blakey Smith. Vancouver: University of British Columbia Press.

Henry, Alexander

1992   *The Journal of Alexander Henry the Younger.* Vol. 2, *The Saskatchewan and Columbia Rivers.* Edited by Barry Gough. Toronto: Champlain Society.

Henry, Anson

1856–58   Monthly medical reports, Grand Ronde reservation. Records of the Oregon Superintendency of Indian Affairs, 1848–73. National Archives, Washington.

Henry, Jules

1964   *Jungle People: A Kaingang Tribe of the Highlands of Brazil.* New York: Random House.

Hills, George

1863   "Extracts from the Journal of the Bishop of Columbia, 1862 and 1863." In *Fourth Annual Report of the Columbia Mission for the Year 1862,* vol. 4, pp. 56–64. London: Rivington's.

Hills, William

1853   "Journal on Board H.M.S. *Portland* and H.M.S. *Virago.*" Mf. AW1 R5028-2. University of British Columbia Library, Vancouver.

Hill-Tout, Charles

1978   *The Salish People: The Local Contribution of Charles Hill-Tout.* Vols. 2–4 edited by Ralph Maud. Vancouver: Torchbooks.

Hilton, Susanne

1971   "An Investigation of Bella Bella Tribes, Village Sites, and Population Movement to 1900." Typescript.

Hilton, Susanne, and Jennifer Gould

1973   *Bella Bella Stories.* Victoria: British Columbia Indian Advisory Committee.

Hinds, Richard

1836–40   Journal. MSS 1524. Microfilm. Oregon Historical Society, Portland. (Original in the British Museum, London.)

Hines, Gustavus

    1850   *A voyage round the world: with a history of the Oregon mission.* . . . Buffalo: G. H. Derby and Co.

    1868   *Oregon and its institutions.* . . . New York: Carlton and Porter.

Hirsch, August

    1883   *Handbook of Geographical and Historical Pathology.* London: New Sydenham Society.

Hodge, Frederick, ed.

    1907–10   *Handbook of American Indians North of Mexico.* 2 vols. Bureau of American Ethnology Bulletin 30. Washington.

Hodgson, Edward

    1957   "The Epidemic on the Lower Columbia." *Pacific Northwesterner* 1(4): 1–8.

Holman, James

    1853   "Three Shipwrecks—Four Bodies found, etc." Letter of 28–29 January in *Oregonian,* 19 February, p. 2.

Holmes, Silas

    1841   Journal kept by Assistant Surgeon Holmes on the U.S. Exploring Expedition, 1838–1842. . . . Mf. 426. Washington State Historical Society, Tacoma. (Original in Western Americana Collection, Beinecke Library, Yale University, New Haven.)

Howay, Frederic

    1931   "A List of Trading Vessels in the Maritime Fur Trade, 1795–1804." *Transactions of the Royal Society of Canada,* 3d ser., 25, sec. 2: 117–49.

    1934   "The Brig *Owyhee* on the Columbia, 1829–30." *Oregon Historical Quarterly* 35(1): 10–21.

———, ed.

    1941   *Voyages of the "Columbia" to the Northwest Coast, 1787–1790 and 1790–1793.* Collections of the Massachusetts Historical Society, vol. 79. Boston.

Howell, Nancy

    1973   "The Feasibility of Demographic Studies in 'Anthropological' Populations." In Michael Crawford and P. L. Workman, eds., *Methods and Theories of Anthropological Genetics,* pp. 249–62. Albuquerque: University of New Mexico Press.

    1979   *Demography of the Dobe !Kung.* San Francisco: Academic Press.

Hudson's Bay Company

    1838   "Census of Indian Population at Fort Vancouver: Klikitat Tribe,

Cathlacanasese Tribe, Cath-lal-thlalah Tribe." MS B. 223/z/1, fols. 26–28. Hudson's Bay Company Archives, Winnipeg.

Huggins, Edward

1833–39   "Journal of Occurrences." Fort Nisqually Records. Manuscripts and University Archives. University of Washington Libraries, Seattle. (Original in Huntington Library, San Marino, California.)

Hulbert, Archer, ed.

1938   *Marcus Whitman, Crusader.* Vol. 7 of *Overland to the Pacific.* Denver: Denver Public Library.

Hunn, Eugene

1990   *Nch'i-Wána, "The Big River": Mid-Columbia Indians and Their Land.* Seattle: University of Washington Press.

Hymes, Dell

1975   "Folklore's Nature and the Sun's Myth." *Journal of American Folklore* 88: 345–69.

1990   "Mythology." In Suttles 1990c: 593–601.

Irving, Washington

1964   *Astoria, or Anecdotes of an Enterprise beyond the Rocky Mountains.* Edited by Edgeley Todd. Norman: University of Oklahoma Press.

Isaac, Barry

1977   "The Siriono of Eastern Bolivia: A Reexamination." *Human Ecology* 5(2): 137–54.

Ivashintsov, Nikolai

1980   *Russian Round-the-world Voyages, 1803–1849.* Translated by Glynn Barratt. Kingston: Limestone Press.

Jackson, Donald, ed.

1978   *Letters of the Lewis and Clark Expedition with Related Documents, 1783–1854.* 2d ed. Urbana: University of Illinois Press.

Jackson, Robert

1983   "Epidemic Disease and Population Decline in the Baja California Missions, 1697–1834." *Southern California Quarterly* 63: 308–46.

1994   *Indian Population Decline: the Missions of Northwestern New Spain, 1687–1840.* Albuquerque: University of New Mexico Press.

Jacobs, Elizabeth

1959   *Nehalem Tillamook Tales.* University of Oregon Monographs, Studies in Anthropology 5. Eugene.

Jacobs, Melville

    1937   "Historic Perspectives in Indian Languages of Oregon and Washington." *Pacific Northwest Quarterly* 28(1): 55–74.

    1939   *Coos Narrative and Ethnologic Texts.* University of Washington Publications in Anthropology 8(1). Seattle.

    1945   *Kalapuya Texts.* University of Washington Publications in Anthropology 11. Seattle.

    1958–59   *Clackamas Chinook Texts.* 2 vols. University of Indiana Research Center in Anthropology, Folklore, and Linguistics Publication 8(11). Bloomington.

    1959   *The Content and Style of an Oral Literature.* Chicago: University of Chicago Press.

James, Maurice, and Robert Harwood

    1969   *Herms's Medical Entomology.* 6th ed. Toronto: Macmillan Co.

Jenness, Diamond

    1943   "The Carrier Indians of the Bulkley River: Their Social and Religious Life." In *Anthropological Papers 25,* pp. 469–586. Bureau of American Ethnology Bulletin 133. Washington.

    1955   *The Faith of a Coast Salish Indian.* Anthropology in British Columbia Memoir no. 3. Victoria: British Columbia Provincial Museum.

Jewitt, John

    1975   *Narrative of the Adventures and Sufferings of John R. Jewitt. . . .* Edited by Robert Heizer. Ramona, Calif.: Ballena Press.

Jilek, Wolfgang

    1982   *Indian Healing: Shamanic Ceremonialism in the Pacific Northwest Today.* Surrey, B.C.: Hancock House.

Jones, Roy

    1972   *Wappato Indians of the Lower Columbia River Valley.* Portland: privately printed.

Jones, William

    1909   *Malaria and Greek History.* Manchester: Manchester University Press.

Judson, Lewis

    1845   Letter of 16 March 1845. Canse Collection. Washington State Historical Society, Tacoma.

Kamakau, Samuel

    1961   *The Ruling Chiefs of Hawaii.* Honolulu: Kamehameha Schools Press.

Kan, Sergei

   1994   *Symbolic Immortality: The Tlingit Potlatch of the Nineteenth Century.* Washington, D.C.: Smithsonian Institution Press.

Kane, Paul

   1859   Appendix to *Wanderings of an Artist among the Indians of North America.* London: Longman, Brown, Green, Longmans, and Roberts.

   1971   *Paul Kane's Frontier.* Edited by J. Russell Harper. Austin: University of Texas Press.

Keddie, Grant

   1993   "The Victoria Small Pox Crisis of 1862." *Discovery: Friends of the R.B.C.M. Quarterly* 21(4): 6–7.

Kennedy, Alexander

   1824–25   "Report, Fort George District, Columbia Department." MS B. 76/e. Hudson's Bay Company Archives, Winnipeg.

Kew, Michael

   1990   "History of Coastal British Columbia since 1849." In Suttles 1990c: 159–68.

Khlebnikov, Kyrill

   1976   *Colonial Russian America: Kyrill T. Khlebnikov's Reports, 1817–1832.* Translated by B. Dmytryshyn and E. A. P. Crownhart-Vaughan. Portland: Oregon Historical Society Press.

Kiple, Kenneth, ed.

   1993   *The Cambridge World History of Human Disease.* New York: Cambridge University Press.

Knapp, Frances, and Rheta Childe

   1896   *The Thlinkets of Southeastern Alaska.* Chicago: Stone and Kimball.

Knight, Richard

   1982   *Parasitic Disease in Man.* New York: Churchill Livingstone.

Krause, Aurel

   1956   *The Tlingit Indians. . . .* Translated by Erna Gunther. Seattle: University of Washington Press.

Krauss, Michael

   1990   "Kwalhioqua and Clatskanie." In Suttles 1990c: 530–32.

Krech, Shepard

   1978   "Disease, Starvation, and Northern Athapascan Social Organization." *American Ethnologist* 5(4): 710–32.

1979   "The Nakotcho Kutchin: A Tenth Aboriginal Kutchin Band?" *Journal of Anthropological Research* 35(1): 109–21.

1981   "'Throwing Bad Medicine': Sorcery, Disease, and the Fur Trade among the Kutchin and Other Northern Athapascans." In Shepard Krech, ed., *Indians, Animals, and the Fur Trade: A Critique of Keepers of the Game*, pp. 73–108. Athens: University of Georgia Press.

Kroeber, Alfred

1923   "American Culture and the Northwest Coast." *American Anthropologist* 25(1): 1–20.

1939   *Cultural and Natural Areas of Native North America.* University of California Publications in American Archaeology and Ethnology 38. Berkeley.

Krupski, Edward, and Louis Fischer

1942   "A Phytochemical Study of the Root, Bark, and Fruit of *Cornus Nuttallii.*" *Journal of the American Pharmaceutical Association* (Scientific Edition) 31: 126–28.

Krzywicki, Ludwik

1934   *Primitive Society and Its Vital Statistics.* London: Macmillan and Co.

Kupreanov, Ivan

1836   Letters of 3 March (two), 26 March, 4 May, and 6 June. Microfilm. Records of the Russian-American Company, 1802–1867. National Archives, Washington.

Laderman, Carol

1975   "Malaria and Progress: Some Historical and Ecological Considerations." *Social Science and Medicine* 9: 587–94.

Landerholm, Carl

1956   *Notices and Voyages of the Famed Quebec Mission to the Pacific Northwest.* Portland: Oregon Historical Society.

Langdon, Steve

1979   "Comparative Tlingit and Haida Adaptation to the West Coast of the Prince of Wales Archipelago." *Ethnology* 18(2): 101–20.

Langer, William

1964   "The Black Death." *Scientific American* 210(2): 114–18.

Langsdorff, Georg von

1814   *Voyages and Travels in Various Parts of the World during the years 1803, 1804, 1805, 1806, and 1807.* 2 vols. London: Henry Colburn.

Larsell, Olof

1947 *The Doctor in Oregon.* Portland: Binfords and Mort.

Lauder, Colin [L. C.]

1789 *A Voyage Round the World in the years 1785, 1786, 1787, and 1788. . . .* London: R. Randal.

Laughlin, Charles, and Eugene d'Aquino

1979 "Ritual and Stress." In Eugene d'Aquino, Charles Laughlin, and John McManus, eds., *The Spectrum of Ritual: A Biogenetic Structural Analysis,* pp. 280–317. New York: Columbia University Press.

Lazenby, Richard, and Peter McCormack

1985 "Salmon and Malnutrition on the Northwest Coast." *Current Anthropology* 26(3): 379–83.

Lee, Anna Green

1847 "Account." MSS 283. Oregon Historical Society, Portland.

Lee, Daniel, and Joseph Frost

1844 *Ten Years in Oregon.* New York: J. Collard.

Lee, Jason

1841 Letter of 22 May 1840. *Christian Advocate,* 25 August.

1916 "Diary." *Oregon Historical Quarterly* 17: various pp.

Lee, Richard B.

1972 "Population Growth and the Beginnings of Sedentary Life among the !Kung Bushman." In Brian Spooner, ed., *Population Growth: Anthropological Implications,* pp. 329–42, Cambridge: MIT Press.

Lemert, Edwin

1954 "The Life and Death of an Indian State." *Human Organization* 13(3): 23–27.

Lévi-Strauss, Claude

1979 *The Way of the Masks.* Seattle: University of Washington Press.

Lewis, Meriwether, and William Clark

1990 *The Journals of the Lewis and Clark Expedition.* Vol. 6, *November 2, 1805–March 22, 1806.* Edited by Gary Moulton. Lincoln: University of Nebraska Press.

1991 *The Journals of the Lewis and Clark Expedition.* Vol. 7, *March 23, 1806–June 9, 1806.* Edited by Gary Moulton. Lincoln: University of Nebraska Press.

Lindenbaum, Shirley

1979 *Kuru Sorcery: Disease and Danger in the New Guinea Highlands.* Palo Alto: Mayfield Publishing Co.

Linton, Ralph

1943   "Nativistic Movements." *American Anthropologist* 45: 230–40.

Lisiansky, Urey

1814   *A Voyage Round the World in the Years 1803, 4, 5, & 6.* . . . London: John Booth.

Litke, Fedor [Feodor Lütke]

1835   *Voyage Autour du Monde.* Paris: Diderot Frères.

Livi, Livio

1949   "Considérations théoriques et pratiques sur le concept de 'minimum population.'" *Population* 4: 754–56.

Livingstone, Frank

1958   "Anthropological Implications of Sickle Cell Gene Distribution in West Africa." *American Anthropologist* 60(3): 533–62.

Lockley, Fred

1916   "Reminiscences of Mrs. Frank Collins nee Martha Elizabeth Gilliam." *Oregon Historical Quarterly* 17(4): 358–72.

Lowe, Thomas

1843–48   "Private Journal Kept at Fort Vancouver." MSS E/A/1.95A. Royal British Columbia Archives, Victoria.

Ludington, E. H.

1871   *Report, 12/30/70.* 42d Cong., 1st sess. House Executive Doc. 5 (Serial no. 1470), pp. 26–32. Washington.

Lundy, John

1981   "Spondylolysis of the Lumbar Vertebrae in a Group of Prehistoric Upper Puget Sound Indians at Birch Bay, Washington." In Jerome Cybulski, ed., *Contributions to Physical Anthropology, 1978–1980,* pp. 107–14. Archaeological Survey of Canada Mercury Series, paper no. 106. Ottawa: National Museum of Canada.

Lyman, Horace

1902   "Reminiscences of James Jory." *Oregon Historical Quarterly* 3(3): 271–86.

MacCluer, Jean, and Bennett Dyke

1976   "On the Minimum Size of Endogamous Populations." *Social Biology* 23(1): 1–12.

MacDonald, George

1983   *Haida Monumental Art: Villages of the Queen Charlotte Islands.* Vancouver: University of British Columbia Press.

1989   *Kitwanda Fort Report.* Mercury Series Directorate Paper no. 4. Hull: Canadian Museum of Civilization.

Malaspina, Alejandro

1934   "Appendix: Physical Description of the Coast of NorthWest America Visited by the Corvette." In *Politico-Scientific Voyage around the World . . . 1789–1794,* pp. 198–235. Translated by Carl Robinson. Typescript. University of British Columbia Library, Vancouver.

Manby, Thomas

1790–93   "Manuscript Journal of the Voyage of H.M.S. *Discovery* and *Chatham:* 12/20/90–6/22/93." Mf. A6610. Microforms. University of Washington Libraries, Seattle. (Original at Yale University, New Haven.)

Marino, Cesare

1990   "History of Western Washington since 1846." In Suttles 1990c: 169–79.

Martin, W. Kay

1969   "South American Foragers: Case Study in Cultural Devolution." *American Anthropologist* 71(2): 243–60.

Martinez, Esteban

1915   "Diary of the Voyage. . . . " 1789. Translated by Herbert Priestly. Mf. A409. Microforms. University of Washington Libraries, Seattle. (Original at the Bancroft Library, University of California, Berkeley.)

Marwick, Max

1965   *Sorcery in Its Social Setting.* Manchester: Manchester University Press.

May, Jacques, ed.

1961   *Studies in Disease Ecology.* New York: Hafner.

McArthur, Norma

1961   *Introducing Population Statistics.* Melbourne: Oxford University Press.

1967   *Island Populations of the Pacific.* Canberra: Australian National University Press.

McClellan, Catherine

1950   "Culture Change and Native Trade in Southern Yukon Territory." Ph.D. diss., University of California, Berkeley.

McClellan, George

1853   Journal, 20 May–11 December 1853. Mf. A228. Microforms, University of Washington Libraries, Seattle.

McDonald, Archibald

1830   Letter of 25 February. MS D. 4/123, fol. 120. Hudson's Bay Company Archives, Winnipeg.

McGillivray, Simon
  1831–32   "Fort Nez Perces Journal." MS B. 146/a. Hudson's Bay Company
            Archives, Winnipeg.

McGrath, Janet
  1991   "Biological Impact of Social Disruption from Epidemic Disease."
            American Journal of Physical Anthropology 84(4): 407–19.

McIlwraith, Thomas
  1948   *The Bella Coola Indians.* 2 vols. Toronto: University of Toronto Press.

McKay, William
  1878   Address of J. Henry Brown, pp. 3–8. *Transactions of the Annual Reunion
            of the Oregon Pioneer Association for 1877.* Salem: E. M. Waite.

McKechnie, Robert
  1972   *Strong Medicine: History of Healing on the Northwest Coast.* Vancouver:
            J. J. Douglas.

McKenzie, Alexander
  1825   "Journal of Mr. Alex. McKenzie on Board Brig *William & Ann.*" MS B.
            223/a/1. Hudson's Bay Company Archives, Winnipeg.

McKerrow, James, Judy Sakanari, and Thomas Deardorff
  1988   "Anisakiasis: Revenge of the Sushi Parasite." *New England Journal of
            Medicine* 319: 1228–29.

McLoughlin, John
  1832   Letters of 12 September, 3 October, and 10 October. MS B. 223/b/8.
            Hudson's Bay Company Archives, Winnipeg.

  1833a   Letter of 3 March. MS D. 5/4. Hudson's Bay Company Archives,
            Winnipeg.

  1833b   Letter of 23 October. MS B. 223/b/9. Hudson's Bay Company Archives,
            Winnipeg.

  1837   Letter of 29 August. MS B. 223/b/17, fol. 31. Hudson's Bay Company
            Archives, Winnipeg.

  1908   Letter of 1 March 1832. *Washington Historical Quarterly* 2(1): 40–41.

McNeil, William
  1859–62   "Fort Simpson Journal, 9/15/59–12/31/62." Manuscript. Royal British
            Columbia Archives, Victoria.

  1862   Letter of 25 October 1862. MS B. 226/c/2, fol. 320. Hudson's Bay
            Company Archives, Winnipeg.

McNeill, William H.
  1976   *Plagues and Peoples.* Garden City: Anchor Books.

1979   "Historical Patterns of Migration." *Current Anthropology* 20(1): 95–102.

McWhorter, Lucullus

1910   "The First White Man among the Klickitats." Collected from William Charley, 10 March. MS 1528. McWhorter Collection. Holland Library. Washington State University, Pullman.

1918   "Vision of Wa-til-ki." Collected from Ie-keep-swah, July. MS 1514. McWhorter Collection. Holland Library. Washington State University, Pullman.

Meares, John

1790   *Voyages Made in the Years 1788 and 1789 from China to the North West Coast of America.* London: Logographic Press.

Mengarini, Gregory

1977   *Recollections of the Flathead Mission.* Translated by Gloria Lothrop. Glendale: Arthur H. Clark.

Menzies, Archibald

1793   Journal. Mf. 27, Microforms. University of Washington Libraries, Seattle.

1923   *Menzies' Journal of Vancouver's Voyage, April to October, 1792.* Edited by C. F. Newcombe. Archives of British Columbia Memoir 5. Victoria: W. H. Cullin.

Merbs, Charles

1992   "A New World of Infectious Disease." *Yearbook of Physical Anthropology* 35: 3–42.

Millemann, Raymond, and Stuart Knapp

1970   "Biology of *Nanophyetus salmincola* and 'Salmon Poisoning' Disease." In B. Dawes, ed., *Advances in Parasitology,* vol. 8, pp. 1–41. New York: Academic Press.

Minor, Rick

1983   "Settlement and Subsistence at the Mouth of the Columbia River." In Robert Greengo, ed., *Prehistoric Places on the Southern Northwest Coast,* pp. 195–210. Thomas Burke Memorial–Washington State Museum Research Report no. 4. Seattle.

Minto, John

1895   "The Indians of Oregon fifty years ago." *Oregonian,* 7 November, p. 8.

Mitchell, Donald

1984   "Predatory Warfare, Social Status, and the North Pacific Slave Trade." *Ethnology* 23(1): 39–47.

1985 "A Demographic Profile of Northwest Coast Slavery." In Marc Thompson et al., eds., *Status, Structure, and Stratification: Current Archaeological Reconstructions*, pp. 227–36. Calgary: University of Calgary.

Moffat, Hamilton

1862 Letter of 9 August. Hamilton Moffat Letter Book, 1857–1867. Royal British Columbia Archives, Victoria.

Møller-Christensen, Vilhelm, and R. G. Inkster

1965 "Cases of Leprosy and Syphilis in the Osteological Collection of the Department of Anatomy, University of Edinburgh." *Danish Medical Bulletin* 12(1): 11–18.

Mooney, James

1928 *The Aboriginal Population of America North of Mexico*. Smithsonian Miscellaneous Publications 80(7). Washington.

Morison, Samuel

1927 "New England and the Opening of the Columbia River Salmon Trade, 1830." *Oregon Historical Quarterly* 28(2): 111–32.

Morse, Jedediah

1822 *A Report to the Secretary of War of the United States, on Indian Affairs, Comprising a Narrative of a Tour Performed in the Summer of 1820. . . .* New Haven: S. Converse.

Moser, Charles, ed.

1926 *Reminiscences of the West Coast of Vancouver Island*. Victoria: Acme Press.

Moses, Israel

1855 "On the Medical Topography of Astoria, Oregon Territory. . . . " *American Journal of Medical Science*, n.s., 29: 32–46.

Moss, Madonna

1992 "Shellfish, Gender, and Status on the Northwest Coast: Reconciling Archaeological, Ethnographic, and Ethnohistorical Records of the Tlingit." *American Anthropologist* 95(3): 631–52.

Moulton, Gary

1983 *Atlas of the Lewis & Clark Expedition*. Lincoln: University of Nebraska Press.

Mozino, José

1970 *Noticias de Nutka*. Translated by Iris Wilson. Seattle: University of Washington Press.

Mudge, Zachariah

    1848   *The Missionary Teacher: A Memoir of Cyrus Shepard.* New York: Lane and Tippett.

Munnick, Harriet, ed.

    1972   *Catholic Church Records of the Pacific Northwest: Vancouver,* vols. 1–2, and *Stellamaris Mission.* St. Paul: French Prairie Press.

    1979   *Catholic Church Records of the Pacific Northwest: St. Paul, Oregon, 1839–1898,* vol. 1. Portland: Binfords and Mort.

Murdock, George

    1938   "Notes on the Tenino, Molala, and Paiute of Oregon." Pp. 395–402 in Verne Ray et. al., "Tribal Distribution in Eastern Oregon and Adjacent Regions." *American Anthropologist* 40(3): 384–415.

Murphy, Robert

    1960   *Headhunter's Heritage: Social and Economic Change among the Mundurucu.* Berkeley: University of California Press.

Nakano, James, and M. Colin Jordan

    1994   "Smallpox and Other Poxvirus Infections." In Paul Hoeprich, M. Colin Jordan, and Allan Ronald, eds., *Infectious Diseases: A Treatise of Infectious Processes,* pp. 943–51. Philadelphia: J. B. Lippincott Co.

Neel, James, et al.

    1970   "Notes on the Effect of Measles and Measles Vaccine in a Virgin Soil Population of South American Indians." *American Journal of Epidemiology* 91(4): 418–29.

Newell, Robert

    1959   *Robert Newell's Memoranda.* Edited by Dorothy Johansen. Portland: Champoeg Press.

Newman, Marshall

    1976   "Aboriginal New World Epidemiology and Medical Care, and the Impact of Old World Disease Imports." *American Journal of Physical Anthropology* 45(3): 667–72.

Nichols, Lucius

    1921   "Malaria and the Lost Cities of Ceylon." *Indian Medical Gazette* 56: 121–30.

Noli, Dieter, and Graham Avery

    1988   "Protein Poisoning and Coastal Subsistence." *Journal of Archaeological Science* 15(4): 395–401.

Norton, Helen H.

1981   "Plant Use in Kaigani Haida Culture: Correction of an Ethnohistorical Oversight." *Economic Botany* 35(4): 434–49.

Norton, Helen H., Robert Boyd, and Eugene Hunn

1983   "The Klickitat Trail of South-Central Washington: A Reconstruction of Seasonally Used Resource Sites." In Robert Greengo, ed., *Prehistoric Places on the Southern Northwest Coast,* pp. 121–52. Thomas Burke Memorial–Washington State Museum Research Report no. 4. Seattle.

Nunis, Doyce

1968   "Michel LaFramboise." In LeRoy Hafen, ed., *The Mountain Men of the Fur Trade of the Far West,* vol. 5, pp. 145–70. Glendale: Arthur H. Clark.

Ogden, Adele

1941   *The California Sea Otter Trade, 1784–1848.* University of California Publications in History 26. Berkeley.

Ogden, Peter Skene

1848   Letter of 10 March. Donald Ross Collection. A 833. Add. MSS 635. Royal British Columbia Archives, Victoria.

1853   Letters of 15 May, 15 June, 12 July, and 2 August. MS B. 223/b/41. Hudson's Bay Company Archives, Winnipeg.

———— ["Fur Trader"]

1933   *Traits of American Indian Life and Character.* 1853. San Francisco: Grabhorn Press.

Olson, Ronald

1936   *The Quinault Indians.* University of Washington Publications in Anthropology 6. Seattle.

1940   *The Social Organization of the Haisla of British Columbia.* Anthropological Records 2(5): 169–200. Berkeley and Los Angeles: University of California Press.

1955   *Notes on the Bella Bella Kwakiutl.* Anthropological Records 14(5): 319–48. Berkeley and Los Angeles: University of California Press.

Omran, Abdel

1971   "The Epidemiological Transition." *Milbanke Memorial Fund Quarterly* 49(4): 509–38.

Ordway, John

1916   "Sergeant Ordway's Journal." In Milo Quaife, ed., *The Journals of*

Captain Meriwether Lewis and Sergeant John Ordway, pp. 77–402. Madison: State Historical Society of Wisconsin.

Oregonian (Portland)

1900   Obituary of James Taylor. 6 April, p. 8.

Oregon Spectator (Oregon City)

1848   Article. 13 July, p. 2.

O'Reilly, Peter

1883   Letter of 27 October 1882 to the Indian Reserve Commission, Victoria. In Canada, *Sessional Papers,* no. 5, pp. 106–9. Ottawa.

Ortner, Donald, Noreen Tuross, and Agnes Stix

1992   "New Approaches to the Study of Disease in Archaeological New World Populations." *Human Biology* 64(3): 337–60.

Ortner, Donald, and Charles Utermohle

1981   "Polyarticular Inflammatory Arthritis in a Pre-Columbian Skeleton from Kodiak Island, Alaska." *American Journal of Physical Anthropology* 56(1): 23–31.

Ostler, H. Bruce

1994   "Conjunctivitis and Scleritis." In Paul Hoeprich, M. Colin Jordan, and Allan Ronald, eds., *Infectious Diseases: A Treatise of Infectious Processes,* pp. 1447–50. Philadelphia: J.B. Lippincott Co.

"Our Indian Population"

1859   *Victoria Weekly Gazette,* 28 April, p. 2.

Palmer, H. Spencer

1863   *Report of a Journey of Survey from Victoria to Fort Alexandria, via North Bentinck Arm.* New Westminster: Royal Engineer Press.

Palmer, Joel

1853   Letter of 27 May. Records of the Oregon Superintendency of Indian Affairs, 1848–73. National Archives, Washington.

Panum, Peter

1940   *Observations Made during an Epidemic of Measles on the Faroe Islands in the Year 1846.* New York: Delta Omega Society.

Parker, Samuel

1837   "Indians on the Northwest Coast." *Missionary Herald* 33(8): 348–49.

1838   *Journal of an Exploring Tour Beyond the Rocky Mountains, Under the Direction of the A.B.C.F.M., Performed in the Years 1835, '36, and '37.* Ithaca.

1936 "The Report of Rev. Saml. Parker: Tour West of the Rocky Mountains in 1835–7." In Archer Hulbert and Dorothy Hulbert, eds., *Marcus Whitman, Crusader*, pt. 1, *1802–1839*, pp. 90–135. Denver: Denver Public Library.

Parrish, Josiah

1855 "Annual Report, Port Orford, 10 July 1854." In *Annual Report of the Commissioner of Indian Affairs*, 33d Cong., 2d sess. Senate Executive Doc. 1 (Serial no. 747), pp. 494–500 Washington.

Passmore, Reginald, and Martin Eastwood

1986 *Davidson and Passmore Human Nutrition and Dietetics*. 8th. ed. New York: Churchill Livingstone.

Perkins, Henry

1843 "History of the Oregon Mission." *Christian Advocate and Journal*, 20 September. (Reprinted in Boyd 1996b: 263–70.)

Pethick, Darrel

1978 *British Columbia Disasters*. Langley: Stagecoach.

Petrov, Ivan

1884 *Report on the Population, Industries, and Resources of Alaska*. Department of the Interior, Census Office. 10th Census, 1880. Washington: Government Printing Office.

Pirie, Peter

1972 "The Effects of Treponematosis and Gonorrhoea on the Populations of the Pacific Islands." *Human Biology in Oceania* 1: 187–206.

Plattzgraff, Roy, and Anthony Bryceson

1985 "Clinical Leprosy." In Robert Hastings, ed., *Leprosy*, pp. 134–76. New York: Churchill Livingstone.

Polgar, Steven

1964 "Evolution and the Ills of Mankind." In Sol Tax, ed., *Horizons of Anthropology*, pp. 200–11. Chicago: Aldine.

Polk, James

1848 *Message of the President of the United States on the Number of Indians in Oregon, California, and New Mexico*. 30th Cong., 1st sess. House Executive Doc. 76 (Serial no. 521), pp. 1–12. Washington.

Polunin, Ivan

1967 "Health and Disease in Contemporary Primitive Societies." In Don R. Brothwell and A. T. Sandison, eds., *Diseases in Antiquity*, pp. 69–97. Springfield: Charles C. Thomas.

1977 "Some Characteristics of Tribal Peoples." In *Health and Disease in Tribal Societies,* pp. 5–23. CIBA Foundation Symposium 49. Amsterdam: Mouton.

Poole, Francis

1872 *Queen Charlotte Islands: a narrative of discovery and adventure in the North Pacific.* London: Hurst and Blackett.

Portlock, Nathaniel

1789 *Voyage Around the World but more particularly to the North-West Coast of America: performed in 1785, 1786, 1787 and 1788 in the King George and Queen Charlotte. . . .* London: John Stockdale.

Puget, Peter

1792 Log of the *Discovery,* 12 June–19 August 1792. Microfilm 274. Microforms. University of Washington Libraries, Seattle. (Original in Public Record Office, Adm. 55/27.)

1793 Log of the *Discovery* and other papers. Microfilm 635. Microforms. University of Washington Libraries, Seattle.

1939 "Log of the *Discovery,* May 7–June 11, 1792." *Pacific Northwest Quarterly* 30(2): 177–217.

Quimby, George

1985 "Japanese Wrecks, Iron Tools, and Prehistoric Indians of the Northwest Coast." *Arctic Anthropology* 22(2): 7–15.

Rae, William [probable author]

1845 "Census of Stikine Population." MS B. 209/z/1. Hudson's Bay Company Archives, Winnipeg.

Ramenofsky, Ann

1987 *Vectors of Death: The Archaeology of European Contact.* Albuquerque: University of New Mexico Press.

1993 "Diseases of the Americas, 1492–1700." In Kiple 1993: 317–28.

Ramsay, Marina

1976 *Documents on the History of the Russian-American Company.* Kingston, Ont.: Limestone Press.

Ray, Arthur

1974 *Indians in the Fur Trade: Their Role as Trappers, Hunters, and Middlemen in the Lands Southwest of Hudson Bay, 1660–1870.* Toronto: University of Toronto Press.

1976 "Diffusion of Diseases in the Western Interior of Canada, 1830–1850." *Geographical Review* 66(2): 139–57.

Ray, Dorothy

   1975   *The Eskimos of Bering Strait, 1650–1898.* Seattle: University of Washington Press.

Ray, Verne

   1938   "Tribal Distribution in Northeastern Oregon." Pp. 384–95 in Verne Ray et al., "Tribal Distribution in Eastern Oregon and Adjacent Regions." *American Anthropologist* 40(3): 384–415.

Raymond, W.

   1854   Letter of 27 March. Records of the Oregon Superintendency of Indian Affairs, 1848–73. National Archives, Washington.

Reagan, Albert

   1935   "Some Myths of the Hoh and Quillayute Indians." *Transactions of the Kansas Academy of Science* 38: 43–85.

Reagan, Albert, and L. Walters

   1933   "Tales from the Hoh and Quileute." *Journal of American Folk-Lore* 46: 297–346.

Rees, Williard

   1880   "Donald Manson. Born April 6, 1800; Died January 7, 1880." In *Transactions of the Seventh Annual Reunion of the Oregon Pioneer Association; for 1879 . . .* , pp. 56–63. Salem: E. M. Waite.

Reff, Daniel

   1991   *Disease, Depopulation and Culture Change in Northwestern New Spain, 1518–1764.* Salt Lake City: University of Utah Press.

Reinhard, Karl

   1990   "Archaeoparasitology in North America." *American Journal of Physical Anthropology* 82(2): 145–63.

   1992   "Parasitology as an Interpretive Tool in Archaeology." *American Antiquity* 57(2): 231–45.

Rich, Edwin E., ed.

   1941   *The Letters of John McLoughlin from Fort Vancouver to the Governor and Committee: First Series, 1825–38.* Toronto: Champlain Society.

   1947   *Part of Dispatch from George Simpson . . . 1829.* Hudson's Bay Record Society, vol. 10. London.

Richardson, H. D.

   1874   History of the Foundation of the City of Vallejo, dictated 30 June 1874. In "Pioneer Sketches." MS C-E 65: 3. Bancroft Library. University of California, Berkeley.

Riddle, George

1920   *History of Early Days in Oregon.* Riddle, Oreg.: Riddle Enterprise.

Rivers, William H., ed.

1922   *Essays on the Depopulation of Melanesia.* Cambridge: Cambridge University Press.

Roberts, George B.

1878   Letter of 28 November to Frances Fuller Victor. Microfilm. Regional Research Library. Oregon Historical Society, Portland. (Original in Bancroft Library, University of California, Berkeley. Published in George B. Roberts, "Letters to Mrs. F. F. Victor, 1878–83," *Oregon Historical Quarterly* 63[2] [1962]: 175–244.)

1880   "Sauvie's Island." *Oregonian,* 9 July, p. 1.

1962   "The Round Hand of George B. Roberts: The Cowlitz Farm Journal, 1847–51." *Oregon Historical Quarterly* 63(2): 101–74.

Romanov, Vladimir

1825   "O Kolyuzhakh ili Koloshakh voobsche." *Severny archiv* 17: 3–28.

Romanowsky and Frankenhauser [*sic*]

1962   "Five Years of Medical Observations in the Colonies of the Russian-American Company, Parts I and II." Translated and edited by Levi Browning. *Alaska Medicine* 4(2–3): 33–37, 62–64.

Roquefeuil, Camille de

1823   *Journal d'un Voyage autour du Monde.* 2 vols. Paris: Lebel.

Rosebury, Theodor

1962   *Microorganisms Indigenous to Man.* New York: McGraw-Hill.

Rosen, George

1958   *A History of Public Health.* New York: MD Publications.

Ross, Alexander

1849   *Adventures of the First Settlers on the Oregon or Columbia River.* London: Smith, Elder and Co.

1956   *The Fur Hunters of the Far West.* Norman: University of Oklahoma Press.

Ross, Charles

1842   Letter of 1 October, Fort McLoughlin, to Sir George Simpson. MS D. 5/7, fol. 292. Hudson's Bay Company Archives, Winnipeg.

Rosse, Irving

1883   "Medical and Anthropological Notes on Alaska." In *Cruise of the Revenue-Steamer "Corwin" in Alaska and the N.W. Arctic Ocean 1881,* pp. 9–43. Washington: Government Printing Office.

Rothschild, Bruce, and Christine Rothschild

1996   "Treponemal Disease in the New World." *Current Anthropology* 37(3): 555–61.

Rothschild, Bruce, Christine Rothschild, Kristi Turner, and M. A. DeLuca

1988   "Symmetrical Erosive Peripheral Polyarthritis in the Late Archaic Period of Alabama." *Science* 241: 1498–1501.

Ruby, Robert, and John Brown

1976   *The Chinook Indians: Traders of the Lower Columbia River.* Norman: University of Oklahoma Press.

Russell, Julia

1902   "Testimony." In "The Lower Band of Chinook Indians of the State of Washington vs. the United States Court of Claims," pp. 204–14. MS 5. Oregon Historical Society, Portland.

Rutman, Darrett, and Anita Rutman

1976   "Of Agues and Fevers: Malaria in Early Chesapeake." *William and Mary Quarterly* 33(1): 31–60.

Saavedra, Ramon

1794   "Informe de lo ocurrido en Noutka del 7 de Junio de 93 al 15 de Julio de 94." In "Official Documents Relating to Spanish and Mexican Voyages of Navigation, Exploration, and Discovery Made in North America in the Eighteenth Century." Translated by Mary Daylton, WPA project no. 2749. Seattle, 1939–40. Special Collections. University of Washington Libraries, Seattle.

Sackett, Russell

1979   *The Chilkat Tlingit: A General Overview.* Anthropology and Historic Preservation Cooperative Park Studies Unit. University of Alaska Occasional Paper no. 23. Fairbanks.

Sahagun, Bernardino

1975   *Florentine Codex,* Vol. 12, *Conquest of Mexico.* Translated by Arthur Anderson and Charles Dibble. Santa Fe: School of American Research.

Saint-Amant, Pierre

1854   *Voyages en Californie et dans l'Oregon.* Paris: L. Maison.

Saleeby, Becky, and Richard Pettigrew

1983   "Seasonality of Occupation of Ethnohistorically-Documented Villages on the Lower Columbia River." In Robert Greengo, ed., *Prehistoric Places on the Southern Northwest Coast,* pp. 169–94. Thomas Burke Memorial–Washington State Museum Research Report no. 4. Seattle.

Salo, Wilmar, et al.

1994   "Identification of Mycobacterium Tuberculosis DNA in a Pre-Columbian Peruvian Mummy." *Proceedings of the National Academy of Sciences* 91(6): 2091–94.

Sampson, Martin

1972   *The Indians of Skagit County.* Mount Vernon: Skagit County Historical Society.

Samwell, David

1957   "Observations respecting the Introduction of the Venereal Disease into the Sandwich Islands." 1786. In *Captain Cook and Hawaii,* pp. 35–41. San Francisco: David Magee.

Sapir, Edward, and Morris Swadesh

1939   *Nootka Texts: Tales and Ethnological Narratives.* Philadelphia: Linguistic Society of America.

Sarafian, Winston

1977   "Smallpox Strikes the Aleuts." *Alaska Journal* 7(1): 46–49.

Schaeffer, Claude

1965   "The Kutenai Female Berdache: Courier, Guide, Prophetess, and Warrior." *Ethnohistory* 12(3): 193–236.

Schmidt, Gerald, and Larry Roberts

1989   *Foundations of Parasitology.* St. Louis: Times Mirror/Mosby.

Schmitt, Robert

1968   *Demographic Statistics of Hawaii: 1778–1965.* Honolulu: University of Hawaii Press.

1970   "The Oku'u—Hawaii's Greatest Epidemic." *Hawaii Medical Journal* 29: 359–64.

Schoolcraft, Henry

1851   *Historical and Statistical Information Respecting the History, Condition and Prospects of the Indian Tribes of the United States. . . .* 6 vols. Philadelphia: Lippincott, Grambo.

Schurz, William

1939   *The Manila Galleon.* New York: E. P. Dutton.

Scouler, John

1905   "Journal of a Voyage to N.W. America." *Oregon Historical Quarterly* 6: various pp.

Service, Elman

1971   *Primitive Social Organization.* 2d ed. New York: Random House.

1979   *The Hunters.* Englewood Cliffs, N.J.: Prentice-Hall.

Sheepshanks, John

1864   "A Lecture . . . The 'Red Indians of the West.'" In *Sixth Annual Report of the Columbia Mission for the Year 1864,* pp. 39–50. London: Rivington's.

Shepard, Cyrus

1834–35   Diary. Beinecke Library. Yale University, New Haven. Xerox copy in the Archives of the Oregon-Idaho Conference of the United Methodist Church. Willamette University, Salem.

1933   Letter of 10 January 1835. *Washington Historical Quarterly* 24(1): 53–57.

Shortess, Robert

1851   Letter of 5 February to Anson Dart. Records of the Oregon Superintendency of Indian Affairs, 1848–73. National Archives, Washington.

Sierra, Benito de la

1930   "Fray Benito de la Sierra's account of the Hezeta expedition to the Northwest Coast in 1775." Edited by H. R. Wagner and A. J. Baker. *California Historical Society Quarterly* 9(3): 209–42.

Sievers, Maurice, and Jeffrey Fisher

1981   "Diseases of North American Indians." In Henry Rothschild, ed., *Biocultural Aspects of Disease,* pp. 191–251. New York: Academic Press.

Silverstein, Michael

1990   "Chinookans of the Lower Columbia." In Suttles 1990c: 533–46.

Simpson, George

1832   Report, 8 August. MS A. 12/1, fol. 435. Hudson's Bay Company Archives, Winnipeg.

1834   Report, 21 July. MS D. 4/100. Hudson's Bay Company Archives, Winnipeg.

1841   Letter of 25 November. MS D. 4/110. Hudson's Bay Company Archives, Winnipeg.

1847   *An Overland Journey Round the World.* 2 vols. Philadelphia: Lea and Blanchard.

1968   *Fur Trade and Empire: George Simpson's Journal . . . 1824–1825.* Edited by Frederick Merk. Cambridge: Harvard University Press.

Slacum, William

1972   *Memorial to the Senate Committee on Foreign Relations, December 18, 1837.* Fairfield: Ye Galleon Press.

"Small Pox"

    1862   *San Francisco Bulletin,* 11 March, p. 3.

Smith, C. J.

    1928   "Malaria." Typescript. Oregon Health Sciences University Library, Portland.

Smith, Eric

    1981   "The Application of Optimal Foraging Theory to the Analysis of Hunter/ Gatherer Group Size." In Eric Smith and Bruce Winterhalder, eds., *Hunter/Gatherer Foraging Strategies: Ethnographic and Archaeological Analyses,* pp. 36–65. Chicago: University of Chicago Press.

Smith, Harlan

    1929   "Materia Medica of the Bella Coola and Neighbouring Tribes." In *National Museum of Canada Annual Report for 1927,* bulletin 56, pp. 47–68. Ottawa.

Smith, Howard

    1975   "The Introduction of Venereal Disease into Tahiti: A Re-examination." *Journal of Pacific History* 10(1–2): 38–45.

Smith, Marvin

    1987   *Archaeology of Aboriginal Culture Change in the Interior Southeast: Depopulation during the Early Historic Period.* Gainesville: University Presses of Florida.

Snow, Dean, and Kim Lanphear

    1988   "European Contact and Indian Depopulation in the Northeast: The Timing of the First Epidemics." *Ethnohistory* 35(1): 15–33.

Snow, John

    1936   *Snow on Cholera, Being a Reprint of Two Papers by John Snow, M.D. . . .* New York: Oxford University Press.

Sokoloff, Vassili

    1878   "The Voyage of Alexander Markoff." Dictated to Ivan Petrov, Sitka. MS P-K24. Bancroft Library. University of California, Berkeley.

Spalding, Henry

    1851   Letters of 22 March and 27 August. Records of the Oregon Superintendency of Indian Affairs, 1848–73. National Archives, Washington.

Speth, John

    1991   "Protein Selection and Avoidance Strategies of Contemporary and Ancestral Foragers: Unresolved Issues." *Philosophical Transactions of the Royal Society of London* B 334(1270): 265–70.

Speth, John, and Katherine Spielmann

    1983   "Energy Source, Protein Metabolism, and Hunter-Gatherer Subsistence Strategies." *Journal of Anthropological Archaeology* 2(1): 1–31.

Spier, Leslie

    1935   *The Prophet Dance of the Northwest and Its Derivatives: The Source of the Ghost Dance.* General Series in Anthropology 1. Menasha, Wis.

Splawn, Andrew J.

    1944   *Ka-Mi-Akin: Last Hero of the Yakimas.* Portland: Metropolitan Press.

Sproat, Gilbert

    1868   *Scenes and Studies of Savage Life.* London: Smith, Elder.

Starling, E. A.

    1853   Letters of 15 June, 4 December, and 10 December. Records of the Washington Superintendency of Indian Affairs, 1853–74. National Archives, Washington.

Stearn, Esther Wagner, and Allen Stearn

    1945   *The Effect of Smallpox on the Destiny of the Amerindian.* Boston: Bruce Humphries.

Stern, Bernhard

    1934   *The Lummi Indians of Northwest Washington.* Columbia University Contributions to Anthropology 17. New York: Columbia University Press.

Stevens, Isaac I.

    1854   Report. 33d Cong., 2d sess. Senate Executive Doc. 1 (Serial no. 747), pp. 392–462. Washington.

Steward, Julian

    1960   "Carrier Acculturation: The Direct Historical Approach." In Stanley Diamond, ed., *Culture in History: Essays in Honor of Paul Radin,* pp. 732–44. New York: Columbia University Press.

Storie, Susanne. See Hilton, Susanne.

Strange, James

    1929   *James Strange's Journal and Narrative of the Commercial Expedition from Bombay to the North-West Coast of America.* Madras, India: Government Press.

Strong, Emory

    1959   *Stone Age on the Columbia River.* Portland: Binfords and Mort.

Stuart, Robert

    1935   *The Discovery of the Oregon Trail: Robert Stuart's Narratives of His*

    Overland Trip Eastward from Astoria, 1812–13. Edited by Philip Rollins. New York: Charles Scribner's Sons.

Stuart-Macadam, Patty

 1992 "Porotic Hyperostosis: A New Perspective." *American Journal of Physical Anthropology* 87(1): 39–47.

Sturgis, William

 1978 *The Journal of William Sturgis.* Edited by S. W. Jackman. Victoria: John Booth.

Suckley, George

 1857 "Report on the Fauna and Medical Topography of Washington Territory." *Transactions of the American Medical Association* 10: 183–217.

Sutter, John

 1939 *New Helvetia Diary.* San Francisco: Grabhorn Press.

Suttles, Wayne

 1947–48 Field notes. In Suttles's possession.

 1951 "The Early Diffusion of the Potato among the Coast Salish." *Southwestern Journal of Anthropology* 7(3): 272–88. Reprinted in Suttles 1987a.

 1954 "Post-contact Culture Change among the Lummi Indians." *British Columbia Historical Quarterly* 18(1–2): 29–102.

 1955 *Katzie Ethnographic Notes.* Anthropology in British Columbia Memoir no. 2. Victoria: British Columbia Provincial Museum.

 1957 "The Plateau Prophet Dance among the Coast Salish." *Southwestern Journal of Anthropology* 13(4): 352–96. Reprinted in Suttles 1987a.

 1982 "The Halkomelem Sxwayxwey." *American Indian Art Magazine* 8(1): 56–65.

 1987a *Coast Salish Essays.* Vancouver: Talonbooks.

 1987b "Cultural Diversity within the Coast Salish Continuum." In Reginald Auger et al., eds., *Ethnicity and Culture,* pp. 243–49. Calgary: Archaeological Association, University of Calgary.

 1990a "Introduction." In Suttles 1990c: 1–15.

 1990b "Central Coast Salish." In Suttles 1990c: 453–75.

————, ed.

 1990c. *Northwest Coast.* Vol. 7 of William Sturtevant, ed., *Handbook of North American Indians.* Washington: Smithsonian Institution Press.

Swan, James

 1870 "The Indians of Cape Flattery. . . . " *Smithsonian Contributions to Knowledge* 16(8): 1–106.

1883   Diary extract, 1883: "Cruise to Queen Charlotte Islands, B.C." Manuscripts and University Archives. University of Washington Libraries, Seattle.

1972   *The Northwest Coast; or, Three Years Residence in Washington Territory.* 1857. Seattle: University of Washington Press.

Swanton, John

1905a   *Contributions to the Ethnology of the Haida.* Publications of the Jesup North Pacific Expedition 5. New York: G. E. Stechert.

1905b   *Haida Texts and Myths, Skidegate Dialect.* Bureau of American Ethnology Bulletin 29. Washington.

1908   *Haida Texts, Masset Dialect.* Publications of the Jesup North Pacific Expedition 10(2). New York: G. E. Stechert.

1909   *Tlingit Myths and Texts.* Bureau of American Ethnology Bulletin 39. Washington.

Talbot, Horace

1862   Letter of 13 July. MS 1557. Oregon Historical Society, Portland.

Tappan, William

1854   "Annual Report, Southern Indian District, Washington Territory." Records of the Washington Superintendency of Indian Affairs, 1853–74. National Archives, Washington.

Taylor, Herbert

1961   "The Utilization of Archaeological and Ethnohistorical Data in Estimating Aboriginal Population." *Bulletin of the Texas Archaeological Society* 32: 121–40.

1963   "Aboriginal Populations of the Lower Northwest Coast." *Pacific Northwest Quarterly* 54(4): 158–65.

Taylor, Herbert, and Wilson Duff

1956   "A Post-contact Southward Movement of the Kwakiutl." *Washington State College Research Studies* 24(1): 55–66.

Taylor, Herbert, and Lester Hoaglin

1962   "The Intermittent Fever Epidemic of the 1830s on the Lower Columbia River." *Ethnohistory* 9(2): 160–78.

Taylor, John

1977   "Sociocultural Effects of Epidemics on the Northern Plains: 1734–1850." *Western Canadian Journal of Anthropology* 7(4): 55–81.

Teichmann, Emil

1963   *A Journey to Alaska in 1868.* Edited by Oskar Teichmann. New York: Argosy-Antiquarian.

Teit, James

1900 "The Thompson Indians of British Columbia." *American Museum of Natural History Memoir* 2(4): 163–392.

1912a "Mythology of the Thompson Indians." *American Museum of Natural History Memoir* 12: 199–416.

1912b "Traditions of the Lillooet Indians of British Columbia." *Journal of American Folk-Lore* 25: 287–358.

1917 "Tales from the Lower Fraser River." *Memoirs of the American Folk-Lore Society* 11: 129–34.

1928 *The Middle Columbia Salish.* University of Washington Publications in Anthropology 2(4): 83–128. Seattle.

1930 "The Salishan Tribes of the Western Plateaus." In *Forty-fifth Annual Report of the Bureau of American Ethnology for the Years 1927–1928*, pp. 23–396. Washington.

Tennant, Paul

1990 *Aboriginal Peoples and Politics: The Indian Land Question in British Columbia, 1849–1989.* Vancouver: University of British Columbia Press.

Thompson, David

1962 *David Thompson's Narrative, 1784–1812.* Edited by Richard Glover. Toronto: Champlain Society.

Thorne, J.

1847–48 Log of S.S. *Beaver*. MS C. 1/207. Hudson's Bay Company Archives, Winnipeg.

Thornton, Jesse

1849 *Oregon and California in 1848.* New York: Harper and Bros.

Thornton, Russell

1986 *We Shall Live Again: The 1870 and 1890 Ghost Dance Movements as Demographic Revitalization.* New York: Cambridge University Press.

Thornton, Russell, Tim Miller, and Jonathan Warren

1991 "American Indian Population Recovery Following Smallpox Epidemics." *American Anthropologist* 93(1): 28–45.

Tikhmenev, Petr

1978 *A History of the Russian-American Company.* 1861. Translated and edited by Richard Pierce and Alton Donnelly. Seattle: University of Washington Press.

Tolbert, Carter

    1907   "Pioneer Days." In *Transactions of the Thirty-Fourth Annual Reunion of the Oregon Pioneer Association, June 14, 1906*, pp. 65–103. Portland: Peaslee Bros. and Chausse.

Tolmie, William

    1847–48   Letterbook. Fort Nisqually Papers. Manuscripts and University Archives. University of Washington Libraries, Seattle.

    1856   "Indian Population of the Northwest Coast of America, 10 December 1856." W. F. Tolmie Collection. Add. MSS 557, vol. 1, fol. 10. Royal British Columbia Archives, Victoria.

    1878   "History of Puget Sound and the Northwest Coast." Manuscript. Bancroft Library. University of California, Berkeley.

    1885   Letter of 3 June, 1884. In *Transactions of the Twelfth Annual Reunion of the Oregon Pioneer Association for 1884 . . .*, pp. 25–37. Salem: E. M. Waite.

    1963   *The Journals of William Fraser Tolmie: Physician and Fur Trader.* Vancouver: Mitchell Press.

Top, Franklin, and Paul Wehrle

    1981   "Measles." In Paul F. Wehrle and Franklin H. Top, eds., *Communicable and Infectious Diseases*, pp. 407–14. 9th ed. St. Louis: C. V. Mosby.

Townsend, John

    1978   *Narrative of a Journey across the Rocky Mountains to the Columbia River.* 1839. Lincoln: University of Nebraska Press.

Trigger, Bruce

    1976   *The Children of Aataentsic.* Montreal: McGill University Press.

    1981   "Ontario Native Peoples and the Epidemics of 1634–1640." In Shepard Krech, ed., *Indians, Animals, and the Fur Trade: A Critique of Keepers of the Game*, pp. 19–38. Athens: University of Georgia Press.

Trimble, Michael

    1988   "Chronology of Epidemics among Plains Village Horticulturalists: 1738–1838." *Southwestern Lore* 54(4): 4–31.

Turner, Nancy

    1979   *Plants in British Columbia Indian Technology.* British Columbia Provincial Museum Handbook no. 38. Victoria.

UBC Museum of Anthropology

    1994   First Nations of British Columbia (map: 5 March 1996 revision). Vancouver.

Ubelaker, Douglas

1976   "The Sources and Methodology for Mooney's Estimates of North American Indian Populations." In Denevan 1976: 243–88.

1988   "North American Indian Population Size, A.D. 1500 to 1985." *American Journal of Physical Anthropology* 77(3): 289–94.

U.S. Bureau of the Census

1893   *Report on Population and Resources of Alaska at the Eleventh Census: 1890*. Washington.

1922   *Fourteenth Census of the United States*. Vol. 3, *Population*. Washington.

U.S. Congress

1868   *Message on Russian America*. 40th Cong., 2d sess. House Executive Doc. 177, vol. 13 (Serial no. 1339). Washington.

Valle, Rosemary

1973a   "James Ohio Pattie and the 1827–1828 Alta California Measles Epidemic." *California Historical Quarterly* 52(1): 28–36.

1973b   "Prevention of Smallpox in Alta California during the Franciscan Mission Period (1769–1833)." *California Medicine* 119: 73–77.

Vallejo, Mariano

n.d.   "Historia de California." Translated by Earl Hewitt. MS C-D 19. Bancroft Library. University of California, Berkeley.

Van Blerkom, Linda

1991   "Zoonoses and the Origins of Old and New World Viral Diseases." In Lola Romanucci-Ross, Daniel Moerman, and Laurence Tancredi, eds., *The Anthropology of Medicine: From Culture to Method*, pp. 196–218. 2d ed. New York: Bergin and Garvey.

Vancouver, George

1798   *A Voyage of Discovery to the North Pacific and Round the World. . . .* 3 vols. London: G. G. and J. Robinson.

Vansina, Jan

1985   *Oral Tradition as History*. Madison: University of Wisconsin Press.

VanStone, James

1967   *Eskimos of the Nushagak River: An Ethnographic History*. Seattle: University of Washington Press.

1979   *Ingalik Contact Ecology: An Ethnohistory of the Lower Middle Yukon*. Fieldiana: Anthropology, vol. 71. Chicago.

Vaughan, J. Daniel

1984   "Toward a New and Better Life: Two Hundred Years of Alaskan

Haida Culture Change." Ph.D. diss., University of Washington, Seattle.

Vaughan, Warren

n.d.   "Early History of Tillamook." Typescript. Multnomah County Library, Portland.

Veniaminov, Ivan

1836   Letter of 24 April to Fedor Litke. In Ivan Barsukov, ed., *Pis'ma Innokentiia, Mitropolita Moskovskago i Kolomenskago,* vol. 1, pp. 29–30. St. Petersburg, 1897.

1972   "The Condition of the Orthodox Church in Russian America." 1840. Translated by Robert Nichols and Robert Croskey. *Pacific Northwest Quarterly* 63(2): 41–54.

1981   "Notes on the Atka Aleuts and Koloshi." Part 3 of "Notes on the Islands of the Unalaskan District." Saint Petersburg, 1840. Translated by Edward Vajda, Dept. of Slavic Languages, University of Washington, Seattle.

Verano, John, and Douglas Ubelaker, eds.

1992   *Disease and Demography in the Americas.* Washington: Smithsonian Institution Press.

Vibert, Elizabeth

1995   "'The Natives Were Strong to Live': Reinterpreting Early Nineteenth-Century Prophetic Movements in the Columbia Plateau." *Ethnohistory* 42(4): 197–229.

Victor, Frances

1901   "Flotsom and Jetsom of the Pacific—The Owyhee, The Sultana, and the May Dacre." *Oregon Historical Quarterly* 2(1): 36–54.

Vogel, Virgil

1970   *American Indian Medicine.* New York: Ballantine Books.

Wagley, Charles

1940   "The Effects of Depopulation upon Social Organization as Illustrated by the Tapirape Indians." *Transactions of the New York Academy of Sciences,* ser. 2, 3(1): 12–16.

1951   "Cultural Influences on Population: A Comparison of Two Tupi Tribes." *Revista do Museu Paulista* (São Paulo) 5: 95–104.

Walker, Alexander

1982   *An Account of a Voyage to the North West Coast of America in 1785 and 1786.* Edited by Robin Fisher and J. Bumsted. Seattle: University of Washington Press.

Walker, Deward

1966   "The Nez Perce Sweat Bath Complex: An Acculturational Analysis."
        Southwestern Journal of Anthropology 22(2): 133–71.

Wallace, Anthony

1956   "Revitalization Movements." *American Anthropologist* 58(2): 264–81.
1970   *Culture and Personality.* New York: Random House.

Waller, Alvan

1844   Diary, 25 July to 12 September. Alvan Waller Papers. MSS 1210. Regional
        Research Library. Oregon Historical Society, Portland.

Warre, Henry, and Mervyn Vavasour

1909   "Documents Relative to Warre and Vavasour's Military Reconnoisance
        in Oregon, 1845–6." Edited by Joseph Schafer. *Oregon Historical Quar-
        terly* 10(1): 1–99.

Watt, James

1979   "Medical Aspects and Consequences of Cook's Voyages." In Robin
        Fisher and Hugh Johnson, eds., *Captain James Cook and His Times,* pp.
        129–57. Seattle: University of Washington Press.

Weiss, Kenneth

1975   "Demographic Disturbance and the Use of Life Tables in Anthro-
        pology," In Alan Swedlund, ed., *Population Studies in Archaeology and
        Biological Anthropology: A Symposium,* pp. 46–56. Memoirs of the
        Society for American Archaeology 30. Washington.

Wells, Oliver

1987   *The Chilliwacks and Their Neighbors.* Vancouver: Talonbooks.

White, Fred

1940   "Bones of Ancient Indians Exposed by Dike Builders." *Oregon Journal,*
        20 December, p. 6.

White, J. W.

1869   *A Cruise in Alaska.* 40th Cong. 3d sess. Senate Executive Doc. 8 (Serial
        no. 1360). Washington.

White, Richard

1991   *"It's Your Misfortune and None of My Own": A New History of the
        American West.* Norman: University of Oklahoma Press.

Wilkes, Charles

1845   *Narrative of the United States Exploring Expedition During the Years 1838,
        1839, 1841, 1842.* Vols. 4–5. Philadelphia: Lea and Blanchard.

1925–26.   "Diary of Wilkes in the Northwest." *Washington Historical Quarterly* 16–17: various pp.

Williams, Joseph

1921   *Narrative of a Tour from the State of Indiana to the Oregon Territory in the Years 1841–42.* New York: Cadmus Book Shop.

Winthrop, Theodore

1913   *The Canoe and the Saddle: or Klalam and Klickatat. . . . To Which Are Now first Added His Western Letters and Journals.* Edited by John Williams. Tacoma.

Wolfe, Robert

1982   "Alaska's Great Sickness, 1900: An Epidemic of Measles and Influenza in a Virgin Soil Population." *Proceedings of the American Philosophical Society* 126(2): 90–121.

Wood, Corinne

1979   *Human Sickness and Health: A Biocultural View.* Palo Alto: Mayfield.

Work, John

1838   Letter of 20 October to James Douglas. MS B. 223/c/1 no. 25, fol. 113. Hudson's Bay Company Archives, Winnipeg.

1848a   Letter of 10 February. MS A. 11/67, fols. 5–6. Hudson's Bay Company Archives, Winnipeg.

1848b   Letter of 9 November. MSS 319. Oregon Historical Society, Portland.

1907   "Letter of 6 September 1831." *Washington Historical Quarterly* 1(4): 263–64.

1908   "Letter of 24 February 1834." *Washington Historical Quarterly* 2(2): 163–641.

1912   "Journal of John Work, November and December 1824." Edited by T. C. Elliott. *Washington Historical Quarterly* 3(3): 198–228.

1923   *The Journal of John Work.* Edited by William Lewis and Paul Phillips. Cleveland: Arthur Clark.

1945a   *Fur Brigade to the Bonaventura: John Work's California Expedition, 1832–1833. . . .* Edited by Alice Maloney. San Francisco: California Historical Society.

1945b   *The Journal of John Work, January to October 1835.* Archives of British Columbia, Memoir 10. Victoria.

Wright, Edgar, ed.

1895   *Lewis & Dryden's Marine History of the Pacific Northwest.* New York: Lewis and Dryden Printing Co.

Wyeth, Nathaniel

    1899   "Correspondence and Journals." In Frederick Young, ed., *Sources of Oregon History,* vol. 1 (3–6). Eugene: University of Oregon.

Yarmie, Andrew

    1968   "Smallpox and the British Columbia Indians: Epidemic of 1862." *British Columbia Library Quarterly* 31(3): 13–21.

Yesner, David

    1980   "Maritime Hunter-Gatherers: Ecology and Prehistory." *Current Anthropology* 21(6): 727–50.

    1987   "Life in the 'Garden of Eden': Causes and Consequences of the Adoption of Marine Diets by Human Societies." In Marvin Harris and Eric Roth, eds., *Food and Evolution: Toward a Theory of Human Food Habits,* pp. 285–310. Philadelphia: Temple University Press.

Zagoskin, Lavrentiy

    1967   *Lieutenant Zagoskin's Travels in Russian America, 1842–1844.* Translated and edited by Henry Michael. Toronto: University of Toronto Press.

Zenk, Henry

    1976   "Contributions to Tualatin Ethnography: Subsistence and Ethnobiology." M.A. thesis, Portland State University.

    1990   "Kalapuyans." In Suttles 1990c: 547–53.

Index

aboriginal (precontact) populations, 262–65, table 3

Alaska, southwest, 122 n. 6, 136. *See also* Kodiak Island

Aleutian Islands, 33, 122 n. 6, 157; Aleuts, 27 n. 4, 34, 118, 144, 157, 159

Alseans, 60 n. 34, 164–65, 267, 268, tables 16–17

Amazon River, 17–20 passim, 275, 276

Andean region, 16, 62; tropical Ecuador, 232

anemia, 269, 290, table 5

Anglicans, 128, 173, 177–83 passim, 278; Green, Jonathan, 26–27, 32 n. 10, 205, tables 7, 9, and 11. *See also* Duncan, Rev. William

archeology, 16, 21, 29–30 n. 7, 103, 207, 274, fig. 3

arthritis, 12, table 5, fig. 20; rheumatoid, 14, tables 2 and 6

Athapascans (lower Columbia), 95, 232, 236–39, 268, tables 15–17; Clatskanie, 235 n. 6, 240, 298; Kwalhioqua (Willapa), 256

Ball, John, 85 n. 1, 104, 108

Barclay, Dr. Forbes, 50, 100–101 n. 14, 138–39, 141, 146 n. 2, 149, 150 n. 8, 297, fig. 10

Beaver. See seagoing vessels

Belcher, Edward, 131, 246

Blackfoot, 32, 37, 38, 99

Boas, Franz, 28, 55, 58, 94, 125

Bolduc, Jean-Baptiste, 106, 141

Brabant, Augustin, 303–4

Brown, Robert, 77, 184 n. 9, 188, 190

burial. *See* canoe burial; cemeteries

California, 32, 35, 36, 50, 74, 75 n. 15, 97–99, 103, 119, 128–34, 145–47, 158, 159, 256, 272, 294, map 5

Campbell, Sarah, 16, 21, 207, 274

Library of Congress Cataloging-in-Publication Data

Boyd, Robert T. (Robert Thomas), 1945–
The coming of the spirit of pestilence : introduced infectious diseases and
population decline among Northwest Coast Indians, 1774–1874 / Robert Boyd.
p.   cm.
Includes bibliographical references and index.
ISBN 0-295-97837-6 (alk. paper)
1. Epidemiology—Northwest, Pacific—History—18th century.
2. Epidemiology—Northwest, Pacific—History—19th century.
3. Indians of North America—Diseases—Northwest, Pacific—
History—18th century.
4. Indians of North America—Diseases—Northwest, Pacific—
History—19th century.
I. Title.
RA650.55.N67B69   1999   99-28736
614.4'9795—dc21   CIP

Canadian Cataloging in Publication Data

Boyd, Robert, 1945–
The coming of the spirit of pestilence
Includes bibliographical references and index.
ISBN 0-7748-0755-5
1. Indians of North America—Diseases—Northwest Coast
of North America—History.
2. Indians of North America—Northwest Coast
of North America—Population—History.
I. Title.
RA650.55.N67B69   1999   614.4'2'089970795   C99-910856-5